Adenoid Cystic Cancer of the Head and Neck

Adenoid Cystic Cancer of the Head and Neck

John Conley and John D. Casler

with a contribution on pathology by Karl Perzin

164 illustrations

1991

Georg Thieme Verlag
Stuttgart · New York

Thieme Medical Publishers, Inc.
New York

John Conley, M.D.
211 Central Park West, New York, NY 10024
Clinical Professor of Otolaryngology (Emeritus),
Columbia University, College of Physicians and Surgeons;
Attending Otolaryngologist,
Columbia Presbyterian Medical Center;
Attending Otolaryngologist, Head and Neck Service,
St. Vincent's Hospital and Medical Center of New York,
NY, USA

Major John D. Casler, MC, USA, M.D.
Assistant Chief, Otolaryngology Service
Letterman Army Medical Center
Presidio of San Francisco
San Francisco, CA 94129-6700 USA

Karl H. Perzin, M.D.
Professor of Clinical Pathology,
Columbia Presbyterian Medical Center
College of Physicians and Surgeons
Columbia University
630 West 168th Street, New York, NY 10032 USA

Library of Congress Cataloging-in-Publication Data

Conley, John J. (John Joseph), 1912–
    Adenoid cystic cancer of the head and neck / John Conley and John Casler, with a contribution on pathology by Karl Perzin.
      p. cm.
    Includes bibliographical references and index.
    1. Adenoid cystic carcinoma. 2. Head--Cancer.
3. Neck--Cancer.
    I. Casler, John. II. Perzin, Karl. III. Title.
    [DNLM: 1. Cylindroma. 2. Head and Neck Neoplasms.
WE 707 C752a]
RC280.H4C68   1991
616.99'491--dc20
DNLM/DLC
for Library of Congress   91-729

Some of the product names, patents and registered designs referred to in this book are in fact registered trademarks or proprietary names even though specific reference to this fact is not always made in the text. Therefore, the appearance of a name without designation as proprietary is not to be construed as a representation by the publisher that it is in the public domain.

This book, including all parts thereof, is legally protected by copyright. Any use, exploitation or commercialization outside the narrow limits set by copyright legislation, without the publisher's consent, is illegal and liable to prosecution. This applies in particular to photostat reproduction, copying, mimeographing or duplication of any kind, translating, preparation of microfilms, and electronic data processing and storage.

Important Note: Medicine is an ever-changing science undergoing continual development. Research and clinical experience are continually expanding our knowledge, in particular our knowledge of proper treatment and drug therapy. Insofar as this book mentions any dosage or application, readers may rest assured that the authors, editors and publishers have made every effort to ensure that such references are in accordance with the state of knowledge at the time of production of the book.

Nevertheless this does not involve, imply, or express any guarantee or responsibility on the part of the publishers in respect of any dosage instructions and forms of application stated in the book. Every user is requested to examine carefully the manufacturers' leaflets accompanying each drug and to check, if necessary in consultation with a physician or specialist, whether the dosage schedules mentioned therein or the contraindications stated by the manufacturers differ from the statements made in the present book. Such examination is particularly important with drugs that are either rarely used or have been newly released on the market. Every dosage schedule or every form of application used is entirely at the user's own risk and responsibility. The authors and publishers request every user to report to the publishers any discrepancies or inaccuracies noticed.

Cover drawing by Renate Stockinger

© 1991 Georg Thieme Verlag, Rüdigerstraße 14,
D-7000 Stuttgart 30, Germany
Thieme Medical Publishers, Inc., 381 Park Avenue South, New York, NY 10016

Typesetting by Druckhaus Götz KG, D-7140 Ludwigsburg
(Linotype System 5 – [Linotron 202])
Printed in Germany by K. Grammlich, D-7401 Pliezhausen

ISBN 3-13-766001-7 (GTV, Stuttgart)
ISBN 0-86577-396-3 (TMP, New York)   1 2 3 4 5 6

Dedication

This book is dedicated to those who knowingly and unwittingly contributed to the advancement of the knowledge of this disease and to those patients who gave us their lives with trust and hope for help.

Preface

The purpose of writing this book was to consolidate the germane knowledge of adenoid cystic carcinoma as it has developed over the past one hundred years and to attempt to present this view so that it would measure the "state of the art" in the management of this neoplasm today. This consisted of a review of 406 cases of this tumor occurring in the aerodigestive system with an attempt, as far as was possible, to correlate this information to illustrate some of its enigmatic features, its lethality, the attempts at different modalities of treatment and their outcomes, and to emphasize the axiom that the patient has the best chance for cure when all of the cancer cells are removed from his or her body at the earliest possible date. This idealistic hope was severely diminished by the anatomy and biology of this cancer, which automatically delayed an early diagnosis and set the stage for the development of advanced disease with its demands for aggressive treatment and its result of a very poor prognosis. These facts have led to consternation and disappointment with the management of the majority of these cases and have created a climate of therapeutic uncertainty. This book does not dispel that uncertainty but creates a knowledge about it that will hopefully assist in planning management.

New York, Spring, 1991

John Conley
John D. Casler

Acknowledgments and Thanks

Acknowledgment and thanks are given to Dr. John Casler and Dr. James Mihalcik, who accomplished the computer print-outs, and Dr. Karl Perzin, who produced a chapter on the histopathology of this disease. Margaret Hadler and the staff at Georg Thieme organized this semi-raw material, gave it their hallmark of distinction, and shaped it into this text. Gertrud Thiel organized and typed the manuscript. Acknowledgments and thanks also go to Winifred Weber and Jack Guz for their generous support.

Contents

1 **Introduction** *1*
General Considerations *1*
Some Unsettling Aspects of Adenoid
Cystic Carcinoma *2*
Differences of Opinion *3*

2 **Pathology** *5*
Karl H. Perzin
General Features *5*
Gross Features *5*
Histologic Features *6*
Histogenesis *13*
Clinicopathologic correlations *13*

3 **Adenoid Cystic Carcinoma at Aberrant Sites** *15*
Lacrimal Gland *15*
Skin *16*
Tracheobronchial Tree *17*
Esophagus *17*
Breast *18*
Uterine Cervix *19*
Bartholin's Gland *20*
Prostate *20*
Summary *20*

4 **Data and Statistics** *21*

5 **Diagnosis** *27*
Signs and Symptoms *27*
Age, Sex, Incidence, and Sites *28*
Biopsy *28*
Pain and Nerve Involvement *29*
Prognosis *30*

Staging *30*
Imaging *31*

6 **Tumor Behavior** *41*
Predictables *41*
Unexplained Clinical Behavior and Unusual
Cases *42*
Reflections *46*

7 **Management** *49*
Philosophy of Management *49*
Therapeutic Planning *49*
Radiotherapy *50*
Chemotherapy *51*

8 **Surgical Treatment** *53*
Minor Salivary Glands *53*
Nasal Cavity and Sinuses *53*
Oral Cavity *60*
Pharynx *70*
Upper Trachea and Paralaryngeal Regions *71*
Major Salivary Glands *73*
Parotid Gland *73*
The Facial Nerve in Adenoid Cystic Cancer of
the Parotid Gland *84*
Submandibular Gland *90*
Sublingual Gland *97*
Ear Canal *98*

9 **Management of Persistent Tumor** *109*
Local Recurrence *109*
Regional Metastasis *112*
Systemic Metastasis *112*

10 Risk Factors *113*
  Morbidity and Mutilation *113*
  Rehabilitation *114*

11 References *117*
  General *117*
  Adenoid Cystic Carcinoma at Aberrant Sites *118*
  Chemotherapy *119*
  Imaging *119*
  Pathology *120*

12 Index *121*

1
Introduction

General Considerations

Everyone who has ever treated adenoid cystic cancer has been impressed with its threatening unpredictability. The difficulty experienced in trying to control this tumor by all therapeutic means has resulted in very emotional attitudes toward it and very subjective decision-making concerning the type of treatment program necessary, which reflects the professional analysis of the responsible doctor, his or her scientific and human background, the medical mores as to "what should be done," and the frustrations associated with the perniciousness of this disease in spite of what is done. There is a marked uncertainty today as to what denotes optimal treatment of patients suffering from this disease. A certain amount of scientific data has been accumulated regarding the histopathology, natural history, classification, risk factors, and response of this tumor to a variety of therapies and protocols. All of this is extremely helpful in establishing a rational program, but it is far from complete. It would appear that the best way to cure this disease would be to remove all of it from the human body at the first operation. However, there are so many factors that work against this ideal that other concepts must be included in treatment in an attempt to minimize the deficiencies of incomplete or inadequate surgical excision.

Fast frozen-section techniques have added significant security to the definition of adequate surgical margins, but these techniques are often defeated by occult extensions, extensions into vital structures, unacceptable mutilations, patient resistance, and the ultimate decision of the surgeon.

Irradiation has established itself as an effective palliative treatment in many of the advanced cases, and also as an effective adjunct in the postoperative program, but has not yet proved itself to be curative. We must also appreciate that there has not yet been a controlled trial on the treatment of early adenoid cystic cancer with irradiation, as the majority of these cases are treated surgically. It is recognized that control rates, when irradiation is used for definitive treatment after biopsy only, are significantly less than after surgical excision, and this may be an indication of what to expect with irradiation for curing small lesions, but not necessarily so. It must also be understood that the correct radiobiological factors in terms of the dose, the size of the field, and the precise type of ionization and equipment have not been determined and are still undergoing study and revision.

A great number of chemotherapeutic agents have been tried in treating this disease, and no agent or planned protocol has been accepted as routine treatment to date. This is naturally under intensive investigation, with combinations of drugs and new drugs coming into the picture, along with the possible improvement that might come from advances in the genetic and immunological fields.

The professional attitude of the responsible doctor, and his or her background, have an influence on therapy. Doctors specialize in surgery or radiotherapy or medical oncology, and advise sick patients with malignant tumors regarding treatment from their particular perspective. They justifiably have a certain power and prestige because of their training and skills and use that in the process of deciding how each patient will be managed. Surgeons usually prefer surgical treatment, radiotherapists prefer irradiation, and medical oncologists are eager to find a niche for their proposals. In many respects, this is a quite simple and efficient approach, but in certain cases it can be biased and inefficient. The process of selection for treatment has become more democratic and more composite through discussion and cooperative decision-making by a group of surgeons, radiotherapists, medical oncologists and other support personnel. It is assumed at this time that this democratic trend is worthwhile, but this policy has not been universally applied. The tendency is to take the cases you think you can treat successfully and best, and refer the others for a different type of therapy. There is, of course, not always agreement about these matters for reasons of scientific prestige and administration. Also, there is gradual but constant change in treatments, depending on what is available and what its chances of success are.

In adenoid cystic cancer, most types of curative and palliative therapy will be ultimately defeated because of the behavior of the tumor itself. Its nature calls for all of the therapist's professional and humanistic resources at the beginning, when making a therapeutic decision, and then challenges his or her decision as the life of the patient extends into decades.

Some Unsettling Aspects of Adenoid Cystic Carcinoma

1. It took one hundred years to classify this tumor microscopically so that pathologists and clinicians could coordinate the diagnosis with the treatment and with the results. There is obviously room for considerable improvement in the the accepted classification, which will ultimately go far beyond measurement of the size and volume of the cancer and determination of its histologic type.

2. It took at least 80 years to fully appreciate the malignant nature of this tumor. At first it was considered to be benign in its behavior pattern and was originally classified as a mixed tumor, a type which had been considered malignant by certain pathologists at one time until this view was corrected. It was also confused with neoplasms of the skin that were identified as cylindromas, as were other ductal cancers found throughout the body. When first recognized as malignant, it was identified as a low-grade cancer. This classification established a philosophy about treatment that emphasized conservative local resection and thus prevented adequate resection. The tumor is now appreciated by both the pathologist and the clinician as a pernicious tumor with a protracted morbidity in many instances and ultimately an unacceptably low cure rate.

3. At one time, irradiation was used as the sole method of treatment for these neoplasms. It lost this "most-favored" status to radical surgery, but over the past three decades, irradiation has been rehabilitated as an effective palliative modality and also as an adjunct to surgical excision. The criteria for its application today are still being tested in spite of this general acceptance.

4. Since the beginning there have been significant discrepancies in the surgical management of these tumors. The general opinion moved from conservative local resection at first toward a crescendo of radical ablation. Reassessment of this radicalism was followed by an attempt to reintroduce some of the form and style of conservative management. It is fair to say at this moment that there is no universally accepted standard treatment.

5. Conservative surgery proved ineffective. Radical surgery evolved as a consequence and, although it was more effective as far as cure rate was concerned, it also created an extended morbidity and, in some instances, serious disfigurement. Radical surgery has endured these necessary but unwanted sequelae and remains the dominant type of treatment today. Some doctors, however, still favor minimum surgery and palliative techniques and are willing to accept the consequences. This is a direct result of the frustration experienced by the surgeons in dealing with the low cure rate of this pernicious disease.

6. There may be no universally accepted standard of treatment, but there are certain criteria that are basic. One is the possibility of removing all of the cancer cells from the patient at initial surgery. The important consideration here is the chance of success weighed against the morbidity associated with this effort. It is not to be expected that all surgeons would assess these factors in precisely the same way. Consequently, there is still a dichotomy, a confusion, and a fatalistic attitude in the management of many of these problems.

7. Everyone agrees that local recurrence is a strong clinical characteristic of this disease; it is inevitable in gross subtotal resection and in cases with positive margins. This troublesome feature can be eliminated in certain instances where it is possible to attain completely safe margins. Most clinicians and patients would accept this as desirable. This optimal therapeutic situation is often negated by the duration of the life of the tumor, the massivity of the tumor, the technical inaccessibility of the tumor, the necessity to sacrifice vital structures in order to gain clearance, and the unexpected and occult extensions beyond the surgical field. Any of these conditions can nullify a well-planned and well-executed therapeutic program.

8. Everyone agrees that inaccessibility, advanced tumor, large size, and manifest systemic spread are incurable conditions. The treatment ultimately ends in a chronic repetition of local recurrence and, finally, in systemic spread. There are, however, options and variables that must be assessed in the therapeutic program in spite of these hopeless factors. The surgeon must be prepared for the fact that there is no single therapeutic technique that solves this problem. In most instances, the treatment depends on the condition itself. Ultimately, persistent and massive local recurrence overwhelms the attempt at ablative treatment and becomes not only an anatomical part of the disease process, but an accepted part of the morbidity as the quality of life diminishes toward its end.

Some metastases are inadvertently discovered and some cause symptoms. There is certainly no rigid rule as to what should be done. Some are observed, some are treated by conservative surgical excision, some by irradiation, and some by chemotherapy and general oncological management. This program is depressing for all concerned, not because it does not cause a temporary respite, but because it is condemned to ultimate defeat. Partial temporary relief for the patient in the dying process is hardly ever adequately satisfying for the therapist.

9. Everyone agrees that irradiation can affect this tumor and in some instances cause its disappearance. No one, however, has presented a series of cases with cure rates of ten or twenty years with radiotherapy. There is no question about the temporary advantages of this type of management; in many instances, it must be incorporated into the therapeutic program. These remissions in neoplastic growth and presentation may last for one to eight years, and when planned and pursued in its most effective manner, may prove invaluable in attaining adequate palliation. The delicate balance between regional tissue necrosis and tumor control, however, is not always predictable when large doses are used and when the treatment is repetitive. Unwanted necrosis about the bones of the skull, vertebrae, and mandible, as well as serious effects on the brain, orbit, and spinal cord understandably nullify the hoped-for palliation. This must be weighed against the fact that, in some instances, the cancer can be retarded significantly in its growth and destructive pattern. The radiotherapist who uses minimal doses will, of course, never encounter any of these sequelae and, most likely, will also never experience significantly favorable results or prolongation of life.

10. Everyone agrees that the cancer itself is the greatest crippling and mutilating factor in this type of illness. The surgeon's response to this is to try to prevent the overwhelming effects of the cancer, or to slow it down, or to make it more bearable. It is within this milieu of risk and uncertainty that certain decisions must be made regarding the possibilities of living and dying and the consequences of these decisions on the quality of the patient's life and dying process. None of these decisions come easily and there is no guarantee that they are right.

Differences of Opinion

One should not be overwhelmed by the differences of opinion on the management of adenoid cystic carcinoma in the area of the head and neck. There is hopefully a difference of opinion—to one degree or another—on almost everything in life. This is the result of time, change, personalities, leadership, and experience.

Changes in the treatment of adenoid cystic carcinoma are inevitable. All therapists are trying to improve their meager successes by way of different operations and modalities of therapy. Very few of these efforts and innovations have been successful with adenoid cystic carcinoma. Consequenctly, some therapists are convinced at this time that radicality has very few rewards to offer the patient. These doctors may prefer no treatment at all, or conservative surgical treatment combined with radiotherapy, or irradiation alone, or chemotherapy combined with other modalities. These opinions come from serious and active clinicians who have experience with this tumor and who are in a position to make these judgments on the basis of their knowledge of this tumor's behavior. The strict criteria they use in this decision-making process are unquestionably rational in certain instances. Other surgeons consider these judgments to be nihilistic. These differences are best explained on the basis of their philosophical reaction to the relative value of extensive surgical excisions in advanced cases with a poor prognosis. On the whole, however, surgeons with a strong tendency toward surgery are inclined to operate even when the chance for cure is minimal and the chance for palliation debatable. The vast majority of patients with this disease status are willing to take the smallest chance to try do help themselves. Neither group of doctors or the patients are to be criticized at this stage, as it is in compliance with our mores and with human nature.

This position will undoubtedly change with the passage of time as these therapeutic attitudes are limited to a historical framework that is ultimately influenced by scientific and technological advances which are brought about by certain leaders who introduce change, practice it, and teach it. This change is gradually tested by other surgeons and it either proves itself worthy or is relegated to oblivion. Understandably, there is argumentation and rivalry during this period of trial. There will be mistakes made on both sides, but in the end, a position close to the truth will evolve. This is part of empiricism and the learning process. When one realizes that it has taken over one hundred years to classify this family of tumors, and that neither its classification not its treatment is by any means perfect or complete, then there should be no anxiety about differences of opinion.

A large portion of this opinion is generated by the clinical course of adenoid cystic carcinoma. It is not possible to state how this tumor will behave in every instance, so the clinical course is, except in general terms, quite unpredictable. Nevertheless, some distinct hallmarks have emerged. In most cases there is a relentless growth characteristic that is usually slow in the first five years without the production of significant symptoms. Occasionally, these tumors are more aggressive within this period of time, but very few fulminate at this stage. It is precisely this characteristic that first brought the malignant potential of this neoplasm into question and added confusion to its management. Another general characteristic is its high tendency to recur after local resection and, after a period of five, ten or fifteen years, to manifest systemic metastases. This is the natural course of events in the vast majority of cases, with the lethal nature of the disease in some instances not becoming apparent for twenty to thirty years.

These tumors have been divided histologically into the tubular, cribriform, and basaloid types, and a correlation between these patterns and the clinical course of the disease has been made. The tubular and cribriform types behave in a less aggressive manner than the basaloid. In many instances, however, there is a mixture of these types in one neoplasm, but even here, usually one pattern prevails and determines the clinical course. This simplistic classification has been augmented by a variety of other staining techniques in addition to electron-microscopic analysis. There are findings in the aerodigestive system consistent with adenoid cystic carcinoma that are distinct from similar tumors in other areas of the body. These identifications are indeed impressive, but none of them state or measure the biological behavior of the tumor in the human subject. The research that needs to be done to understand these tumors properly will provide the ideal climate for the development of different opinions in management.

2
Pathology

Karl H. Perzin

General Features

Adenoid cystic carcinoma (ACC) arises most often in salivary glands, but tumors with the histologic features of ACC can occasionally be found originating in various other sites, including the breast, skin, ear canal, lacrimal gland, lung, prostate and uterine cervix.

Adenoid cystic carcinoma arises in both major and minor salivary glands. The latter are the serous and mucous glands found in the oral cavity, nasal cavity, paranasal sinuses, nasopharynx, pharynx, esophagus, larynx, trachea, and bronchi. When arising in minor salivary glands, ACC occurs most often in the oral cavity, especially the palate. The distribution of ACC arising in major and minor salivary glands varies considerably from report to report, depending upon the type of patient seen in individual institutions, the selection of cases for reports, and the criteria used by pathologists to diagnose ACC. Table 2.1 illustrates the distribution of ACC reported in one series (Perzin et al., 1978).

In most reported series, adenoid cystic carcinoma is the second most common type of carcinoma arising in major and minor salivary glands, following mucoepidermoid carcinoma. However, ACC is the most common malignant tumor arising in the submandibular gland, the sublingual gland, the lacrimal gland and in the minor salivary glands. ACCs are more common than acinic cell carcinomas and malignant mixed tumors (carcinomas arising in benign mixed tumors). Overall, fewer than 5% of all salivary gland neoplasms are adenoid cystic carcinomas.

Gross Features

At gross pathologic examination, ACC tends to have a uniformly firm, grey, cut surface. These lesions are not encapsulated. In some cases, the lesion obviously invades, sending tentacles of firm, grey tumor tissue into adjacent tan, lobulated salivary gland tissue. In many cases, the tumor appears fairly well circumscribed at gross examination and the invasive nature of the lesion can be determined only when the tumor is studied histologically. These neoplasms usually do not exhibit areas of hemorrhage and necrosis, as may be seen in some other malignant salivary gland tumors.

Table 2.1 **Distribution of adenoid cystic carcinoma** reported by Perzin, Gullane, and Clairmont, 1978

Site of tumor	Number of cases
Parotid gland	12
Submandibular gland	10
Sublingual gland	2
Palate	7
Oral Cavity, Other	9
Nasal Cavity and Sinuses	14
Nasopharynx	4
Trachea	2
Total	60

Histologic Features

The histologic diagnosis of adenoid cystic carcinoma is based on certain distinctive features seen only in this tumor. These neoplasms, however, also frequently produce growth patterns that can be found in other types of salivary gland tumors, especially in mixed tumors, both benign and malignant. Therefore, the pathologist may not be able to make the correct diagnosis in small biopsy specimens, because some of the histologic features of ACC overlap with those of other salivary gland neoplasms.

Differentiating adenoid cystic carcinomas from benign mixed tumors (pleomorphic adenomas) and from monomorphic adenomas may be difficult. Table 2.2 contains a list of pathologic features that are useful in differentiating between these lesions.

The most distinctive histologic finding observed in ACC is the cribriform pattern. Nests of tumor cells contain randomly distributed, punched-out holes, producing a "swiss-cheese" pattern (Figs. 2.1–7).

Table 2.2 Pathologic features differentiating benign mixed tumors, monomorphic adenomas, and adenoid cystic carcinomas

Benign mixed tumor	Monomorphic adenoma	Adenoid cystic carcinoma
Well circumscribed borders	Well circumscribed borders	Invasive
Usually solitary nodule	Usually solitary nodule	Multiple separate nests
May have "satellite" nodules	May have "satellite" nodules	No "satellite" nodules
Epithelial structures: usually show various patterns	Epithelial structures: usually show one dominant pattern	Epithelial structures: usually show various patterns
Cribriform structures unusual, only focal	Cribriform structures unusual, only focal	Cribriform structure prominent, should be present
Myxoid or chondroid tissue usually present	Large stroma not prominent; usually fibrous	Fibrous stroma, rarely myxoid, not chondroid
Hyalinized fibrous tissue variable	Hyalinized fibrous tissue variable	Hyalinization often prominent, producing cylindromatous pattern
Ductular structures have double layer of cells, outer myoepithelial cell layer flat	If ductules present, double layer of cells present, outer layer flat	Ductules with a double layer may be seen; outer layer usually similar to inner layer
Cells of epithelial structures often merge into surrounding spindle-shaped myoepithelial cells	Epithelial cells usually well demarcated from adjacent stroma	Epithelial structures clearly demarcated from adjacent stroma
Myoepithelial cells should be present, may be prominent	Myoepithelial cells may be prominent, or predominate	Myoepithelial cells rarely seen

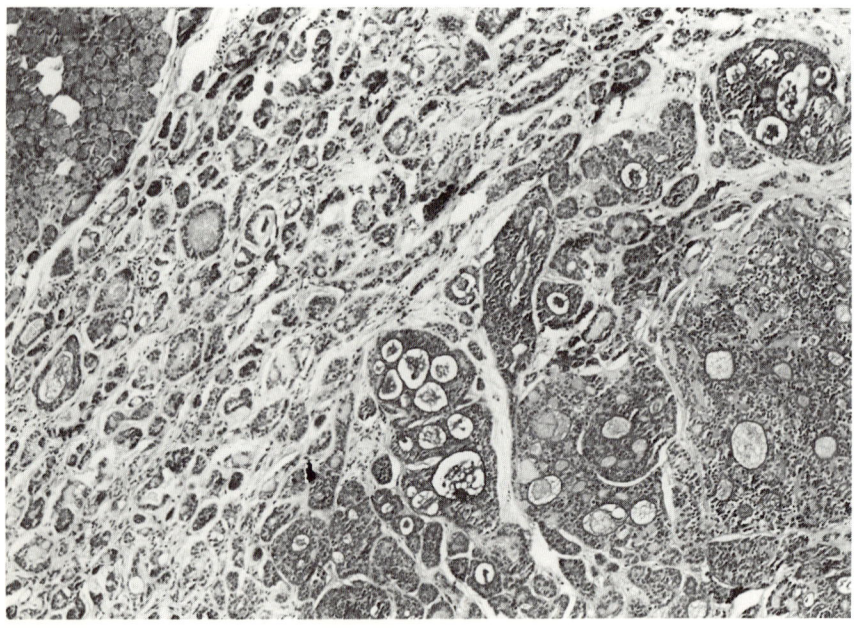

Fig. 2.1 **Low-power view of an adenoid cystic carcinoma.** Normal salivary gland tissue can be seen at the upper left. At the middle left, the tumor is composed mainly of small tubular structures. At the middle right, several nests of tumor have a cribriform pattern; here the neoplasm has a "swiss-cheese" pattern in which holes contain mucinous secretions (63×)

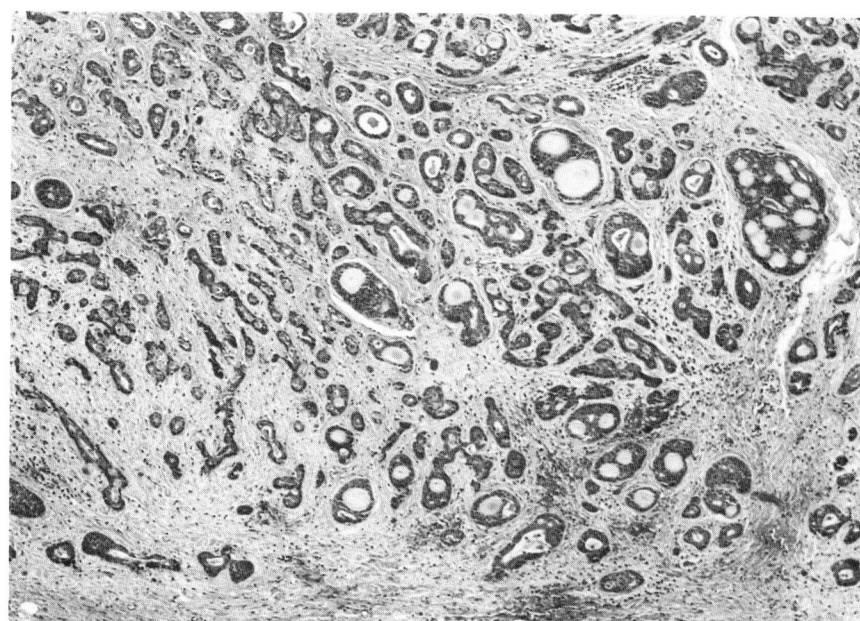

Fig. 2.**2 Adenoid cystic carcinoma with a predominantly tubular pattern,** with a few scattered nests showing a cribriform pattern (63×)

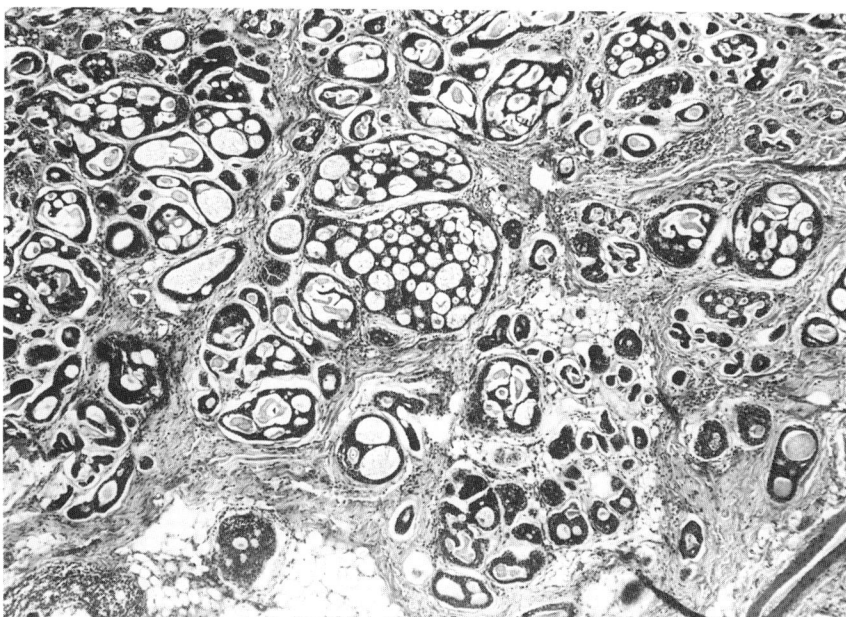

Fig. 2.**3 Adenoid cystic carcinoma with a predominantly cribriform pattern.** The holes in the nests of tumor cells contain predominantly mucinous secretions. The tumor invades fat (40×)

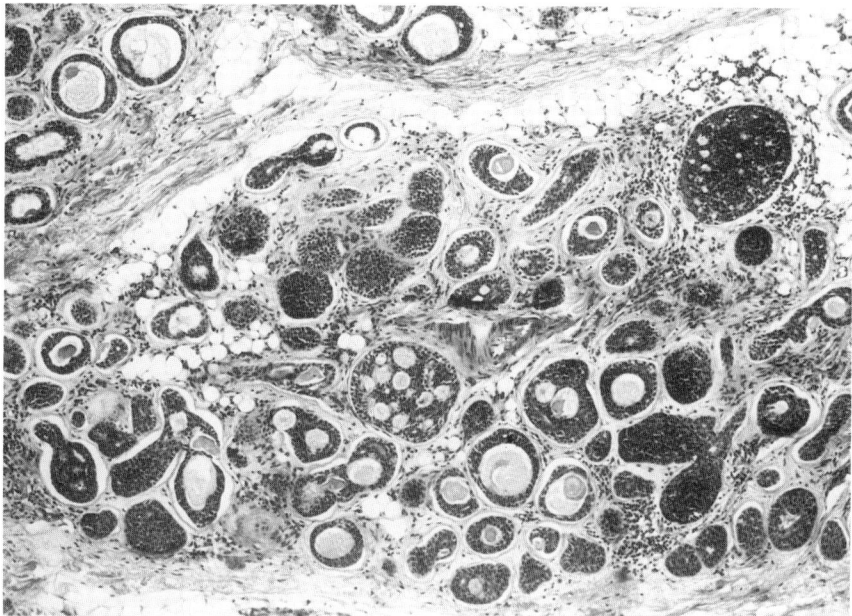

Fig. 2.**4 Adenoid cystic carcinoma with an admixture of tubules, cribriform structures and a few solid nests.** The tumor invades adipose tissue (63×)

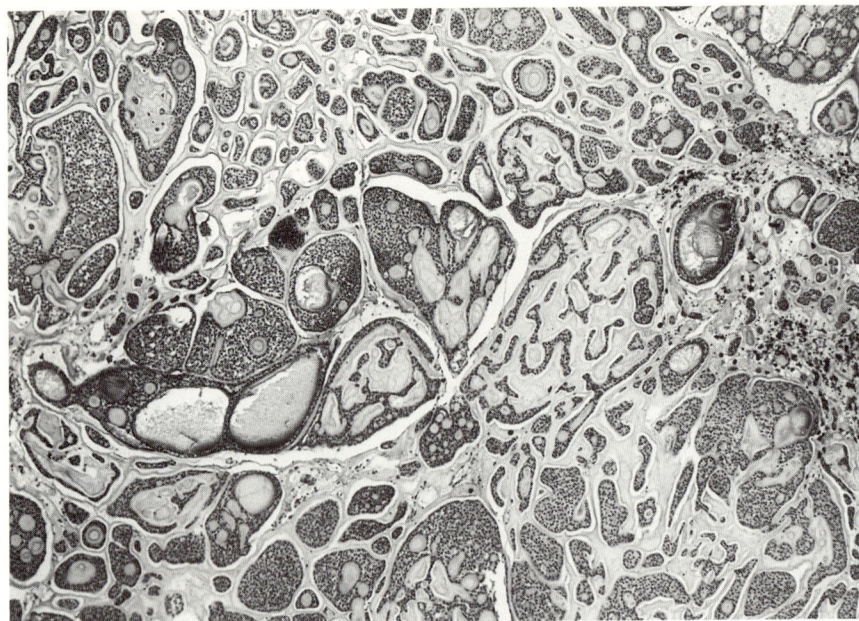

Fig. 2.**5 Adenoid cystic carcinoma with tubules, cribriform nests and solid nests.** Dense hyalinized fibrous tissue found within some cribriform nests, and surrounds small tubules and trabecular structures (40×)

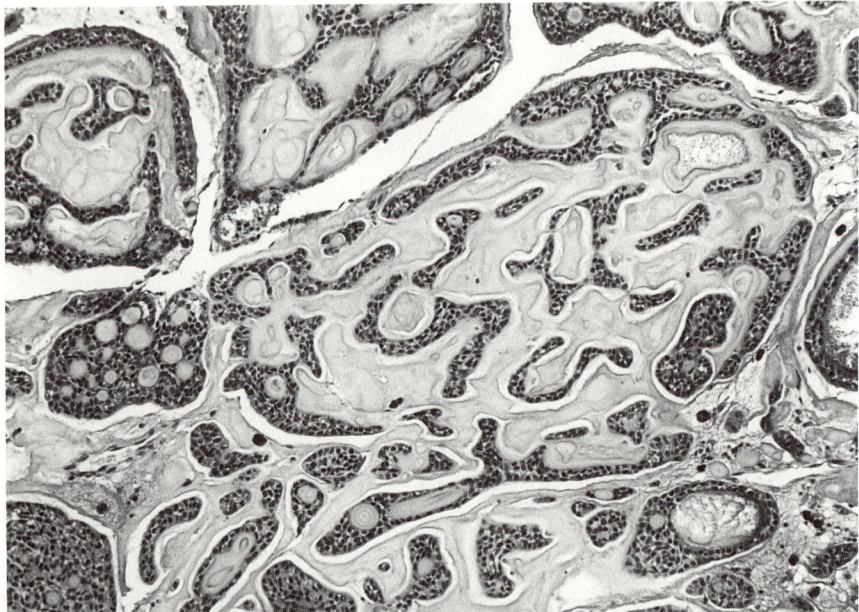

Fig. 2.**6 Hyalinized fibrous tissue found within cribriform nests.** In some areas, this fibrous tissue is continuous with dense fibrous tissue outside of these nests (Higher-power view of Fig. 2.**5**, 100×)

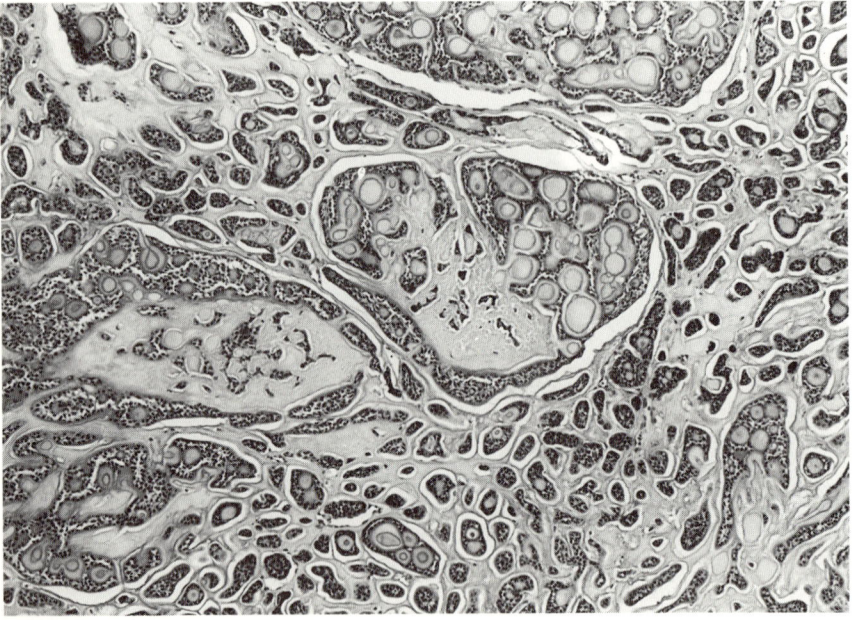

Fig. 2.**7 Densely hyalinized fibrous tissue** surrounding small tubules, continuous with the hyalinized fibrous tissue found within cribriform nests (63×)

The pathologist should not make a definite diagnosis of ACC unless this pattern is identified. In some ACC, many nests of tumor cells show a cribriform pattern; in other lesions, only a few nests may exhibit this feature. Thus, in a small biopsy specimen, cribriform nests may not be present, and the pathologist may not be able to make the correct diagnosis.

However, a cribriform pattern may occasionally be found in benign salivary gland lesions also, especially in benign mixed tumors (pleomorphic adenomas), and in a type of monomorphic adenoma which has been termed a "membranous" adenoma by Batsakis (1979). Thus, a diagnosis of ACC cannot be based only on the presence of cribriform nests.

In attempting to differentiate between these lesions, the pathologist should always examine the edge of a salivary gland tumor; ACC usually invades adjacent structures (Figs. 2.3, 2.4, 2.8–10), while monomorphic and pleomorphic adenomas (mixed tumors) generally have smoothly circumscribed borders.

The cribriform pattern can be found in nests of cells in which the punched-out holes appear empty. In other nests, these holes can contain mucinous secretions (Figs. 2.3, 2.4), as demonstrated in mucin stains such as the mucicarmine stain, or the PAS stain. In other nests, these holes contain a hyalinized fibrous tissue stroma (Figs. 2.5–7). Because of extensive hyalinization (fibrosis), the underlying cribriform pattern may be obscured in these nests, but may be more readily recognized during low-power examination (Figs. 2.5–7).

At ultrastructural examination, the spaces in these nests lined or filled by hyaline material show an accumulation of fine microfibrils of the type associated with collagen or elastic fibers (Chaudry et al., 1986). In both light-microscopic and electron-microscopic examination, these spaces show a continuity with surrounding connective tissue, where hyalinization may also be seen (Figs. 2.5–7).

Another common pattern found in ACC is the tubular pattern, in which multiple, small, elongated tubular structures are identified; these are frequently accompanied by elongated solid cords of cells, producing a trabecular pattern (Figs. 2.1, 2.2, 2.7–12). Whether or not all of these trabecular structures actually have central lumens is not clear. The presence of trabeculae without lumens may merely reflect the level at which these structures have been sectioned histologically; deeper levels in the block of tissue often show that these structures contain lumens. In some instances, both tubules and solid cords may be identified in the same nest of tumor cells. While most of these tubular and trabecular structures appear to be discrete, they occasionally interconnect, producing an interlacing branching pattern (Fig. 2.12). When such a pattern is seen in a salivary gland neoplasm, the tumor is most often benign, but ACC is an exception to this rule. If histologic examination shows that the tubular and trabecular structures predominate, the lesion may be classified as a tubular-predominant form of adenoid cystic carcinoma. This type of ACC has the best prognosis. As is discussed below, the predominant pattern found at histologic examination appears to influence prognosis.

Tubular structures, similar to those found in ACC can be seen in various benign tumors, especially benign mixed tumors (pleomorphic adenomas) and various monomorphic adenomas. In general, the tubular structures found in the benign tumors are lined by a double layer of cells, an inner cuboidal cell, and an outer, flattened myoepithelial cell. A double layer of cells may be found lining the tubules in ACC, but in general, the cells in the two layers appear similar or identical histologically (Fig. 2.12). An outer, flattened myoepithelial cell layer is usually not seen. In many areas, the tubular structures may not be sufficiently distinctive (Figs. 2.9, 2.11); thus, again, the pathologist may not be able to correctly differentiate between an ACC and a benign tumor in a small biopsy specimen composed predominantly of tubular structures.

A solid pattern can also be found in ACC. Solid nests of tumor cells can be seen in almost all ACC, but in most cases, they are not numerous (Fig. 2.4). In some cases, however, the solid nests predominate; in these cases, the tumor cells are generally more anaplastic, having nuclei showing greater hyperchromasia, pleomorphism and mitotic activity than the cells found in most ACC. These tumors are more aggressive and have a worse prognosis than the other types of ACC.

The solid-predominant form of ACC may be difficult to differentiate from a type of monomorphic adenoma called "basal cell adenoma". In the latter lesion, solid nests of tumor cells are present, but these nests usually show prominent palisading of cells at the edge of the tumor cell nests. In addition, the tumor cells are cytologically benign in contrast to the cytologically malignant cells seen in the solid-predominant type of ACC.

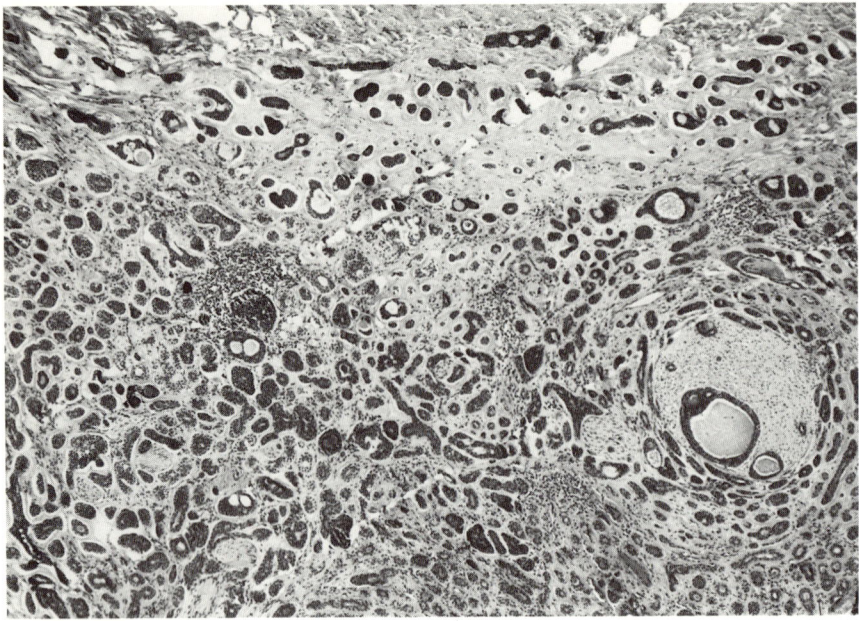

Fig. 2.**8 Adenoid cystic carcinoma composed mainly of small tubular structures;** only a few cribriform nests are seen. On the far right, tumor invades a nerve (40×)

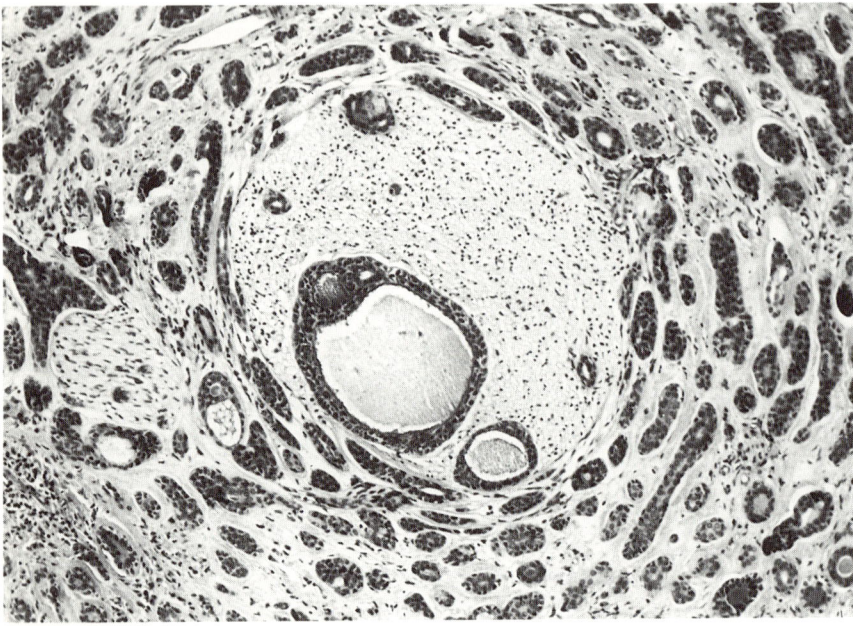

Fig. 2.**9 Tumor found within a nerve.** Small tubular structures surround the nerve (Higher-power view of Fig. 2.**8**, 100×)

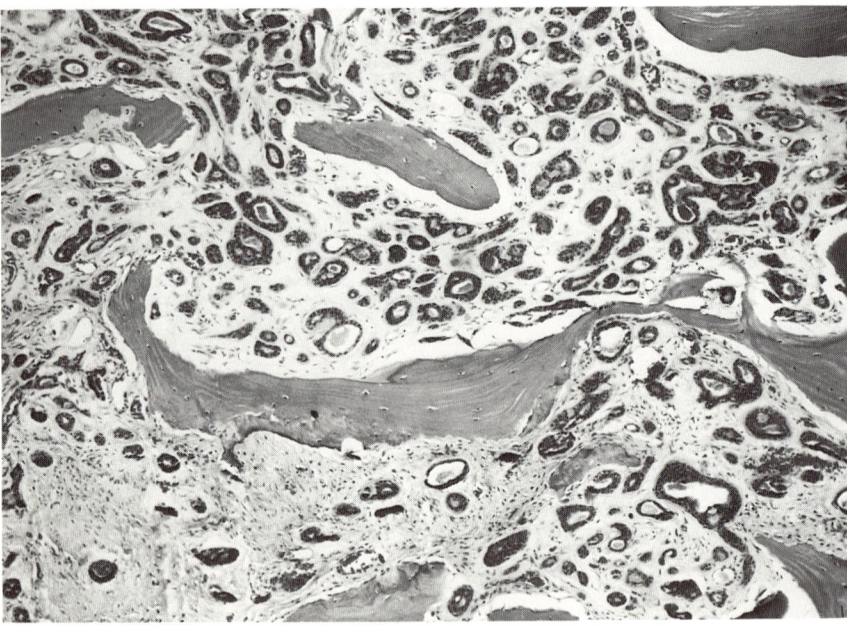

Fig. 2.**10 A predominantly tubular adenoid cystic carcinoma invading bone** (63×)

Histologic Features

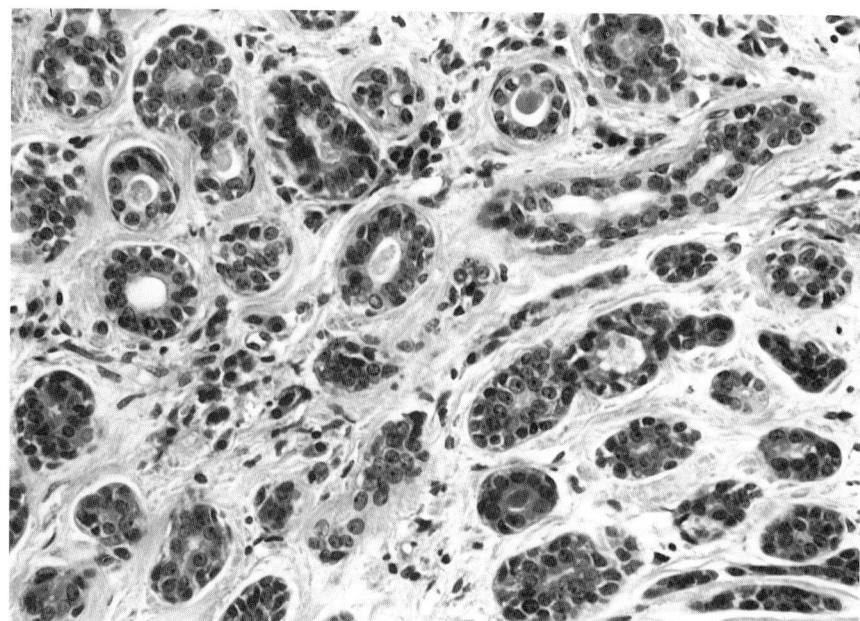

Fig. 2.11 **Tumor composed of small tubular structures.** In some foci, tubules are lined by a double layer of cells, an inner epithelial cell layer, and a flattened outer myoepithelial cell layer. These structures are identical to those that can be seen in benign mixed tumors (pleomorphic adenomas, monomorphic adenomas). However, other tubules are surrounded by a double row of cells in which the outer cell layer also has large and somewhat hyperchromatic nuclei. the tumor cells demonstrate mild nuclear pleomorphism and hyperchromasia. Occasional nuclei contain prominent nucleoli. In most cases, adenoid cystic carcinoma shows only minimal nuclear atypia (Higher-power view of Fig. 2.**8**, 250×)

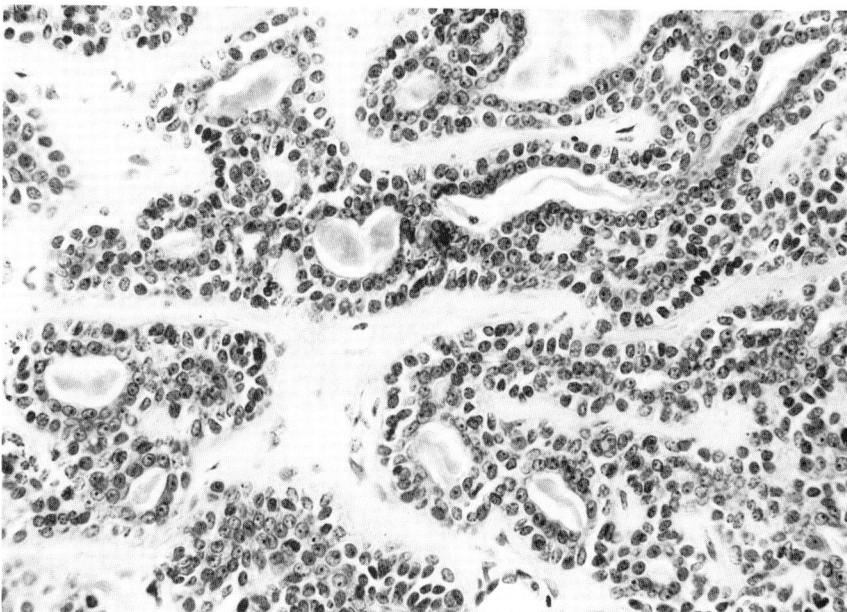

Fig. 2.**12** **Adenoid cystic carcinoma consisting of branching tubules lined by a double layer of cells;** the outer cell layer is similar to the inner cell layer. The tumor cells have medium-sized nuclei which show minimal nuclear atypia. The nuclei are uniform, show a good polarity, and have occasional prominent nucleoli (250×)

As reported in one series (Perzin et al., 1978), the distribution of subtypes of ACC is illustrated in Table 2.3.

Table 2.3 **Predominant growth pattern of ACC** from Perzin, Gullane, and Clairmont, 1978

Type	Number	%
Tubular	22	35
Cribriform	27	44
Solid	13	21
Total	62	100

In ACC composed predominantly of tubular or cribriform structures, the tumor cells have relatively little cytoplasm. The nuclei are usually round to ovoid and exhibit minimal pleomorphism (Figs. 2.**11**, 2.**12**). Minimal hyperchromasia may be present. In the tubular-predominant form of ACC, relatively few mitotic figures are seen. More mitotic figures, but not many, are usually found in the cribriform-predominant form. As more and more solid nests are produced, the tumor cells generally tend to show greater nuclear pleomorphism and hyperchromasia, and they exhibit more mitotic figures. Prominent nucleoli may be found in the tumor cells as these lesions become less differentiated.

Adenoid cystic carcinomas are invasive tumors; the pathologist should probably not diagnose ACC in the case of a non-invasive, well-circumscribed neoplasm. As mentioned above, benign mixed tumors (pleomorphic adenomas) and monomorphic adenomas may contain nests of tumor cells with cribriform and other patterns similar to those found in ACC. The presence of these structures may lead to an incorrect diagnosis of ACC, especially in small biopsy specimens. In biopsy and large resection specimens in which the edge of the tumor can be seen, ACC should demonstrate invasion.

Adenoid cystic carcinomas may invade adjacent salivary gland tissue directly. These tumors frequently demonstrate perineural and intraneural invasion (Figs. 2.**8**, 2.**9**). These are treacherous neoplasms, since the neural invasion may be found at a great distance from the primary lesion. The nerve leading from the primary site may be thickened at palpation, but in other cases, the neural invasion may be demonstrated only microscopically. When performing a large resection for ACC, the surgeon should ask the pathologist to perform frozen sections on the nerves near the line of resection, even if the nerves are not grossly involved. ACC also frequently sends long tentacles of tumor between lobules of otherwise normal salivary gland tissue, so that tumor is often found far beyond the area where the lesion is palpable.

Thus, when the pathologist studies surgical resection specimens, tumor is frequently found on the lines of resection, even though the surgeon felt that the margin of resection was adequate during the operative procedure. ACC also frequently penetrates into bone in an unusual manner. These lesions often send long tentacles of tumor tissue through the canal system of the involved osseous tissue; this may be associated with minimal or no bone resorption, so that extensive bone involvement may be present in the absence of radiologic abnormalities in the bone. ACC may extend directly into adjacent lymph nodes, such as intraparotid and periparotid nodes, but it metastasizes via lymphatics to regional nodes in only 10% of cases. Lymph node metastasis usually occurs only in ACC in which solid nests of cells predominate. As mentioned above, in these cases, the tumor cells usually exhibit greater pleomorphism and mitotic activity as compared to the usual ACC. The tumor may occasionally invade veins, leading to pulmonary metastases.

Can adenoid cystic carcinomas arise in preexisting benign mixed tumors? In general, the carcinomas that arise in benign mixed tumors (malignant mixed tumors) are poorly differentiated carcinomas or poorly differentiated adenocarcinomas. Occasionally, the poorly differentiated adenocarcinoma may have features suggesting a poorly differentiated mucoepidermoid carcinoma. Only occasionally does the malignant lesion have features diagnosable as an adenoid cystic carcinoma. In general, the diagnosis of ACC arising in a benign mixed tumor should be made only when the ACC invades tissue outside of the main mass of the benign mixed tumor. Can ACC be found within the confines of a benign mixed tumor without invading adjacent tissues? This is difficult to diagnose, because, as mentioned above, ACC and benign mixed tumors have overlapping histologic features. In general, as long as a malignant change is found within the confines of a preexisting benign mixed tumor or monomorphic adenoma, without evidence of invasion of adjacent tissues, the lesion will behave clinically as a benign tumor. Thus, for practical clinical purposes, any malignant histologic change found within the confines of a benign mixed tumor is generally not associated with a malignant clinical course. Thus, when pathologists disagree as to whether areas within a benign mixed tumor do or do not exhibit the features of an ACC, there is little clinical significance, unless the lesion is invasive, or is identified on the lines of surgical excision. In such a case, the lesion may recur locally; the recurrence may contain benign areas, malignant tumor, or both.

For a more extensive discussion of the pathologic features of ACC, the reader is referred to the studies of Evans and Cruikshank (1970), and of Thackray and Lucus (1974).

Does fine-needle biopsy aid in diagnosing ACC? This is a subject of debate. Because ACC and mixed tumors have overlapping histologic features, unless the specimen contains tissue from an absolutely diagnostic area, the tissue may not differentiate reliably between these two lesions. In some cases, the needle-biopsy tissue may contain tumor cells with dense hyperchromatic nuclei; cells such as these are usually not found in typical benign mixed tumors or in monomorphic adenomas. Thus, cells such as these would suggest the presence of an adenoid cystic carcinoma.

Histogenesis

Recently, immunhistologic studies have been performed in order to further identify the cell types present in ACC (Azumi and Battifora, 1987 and Caselitz et al., 1986). These studies have demonstrated that some tumor cells show epithelial ductal differentiation, while others show evidence of myoepithelial differentiation. Myoepithelial differentiation is found most commonly in areas of pseudocyst formation and stromal hyalinization. These studies also support the interpretation that adenoid cystic carcinomas are derived from intercalated ducts, where epithelial duct cells and myoepithelial cells are normally present. Substantial evidence supports the concept that benign mixed tumors (pleomorphic adenomas) and various monomorphic adenomas are also composed of varying combinations of epithelial and myoepithelial cells. Thus, the fact that adenoid cystic carcinomas and these various benign tumors have overlapping histologic features should not be surprising, since all these neoplasms appear to be composed of various combinations of ductal and myoepithelial cells.

Clinico-Pathologic-Correlations

The following results come predominantly from the clinicopathologic study of adenoid cystic carcinomas reported by Perzin, Gullane, and Clairmont (1978). Subsequent studies have supported these findings (Matsuba et al., 1986 and Nascimento et al., 1986).

When examining surgical resection specimens of ACC, the pathologist should carefully study the lines of surgical excision. The presence or absence of tumor on the lines of resection is the most important factor influencing prognosis. The pathologist should take multiple sections showing the relationship between the tumor and the margin. As described above, ACC frequently sends tentacles of tumor far beyond the area where the lesion can be palpated, so that neoplastic tissue is often found beyond where the surgeon believes the tumor is present; as a result, the neoplasm is frequently found on the lines of surgical resection. In one series of surgical resection cases in which the lines of excision were carefully studied and could be evaluated in the sections, no tumor was found on the lines of excision in only 12 of 58 cases (20%). Of these 12 patients, 10 were alive without recurrence (84%), one was living with disease (8%) and one had died of disease (8%). In contrast, of the 46 cases with tumor found on the lines of surgical excision, 2 patients (4%) had no recurrence, 6 (13%) developed recurrent tumor, but following further treatment, had no evidence of disease at follow-up; 12 (26%) were living with persistent disease; and 26 (57%) had died of their disease. These data demonstrate that the presence or absence of tumor on the lines of surgical resection strongly influences prognosis.

Another important feature influencing prognosis is the histologic pattern exhibited by the tumor, as illustrated in Table 2.4. Only 12 of 62 patients had no evidence of recurrence; of these, 9 (75%) had a tubular-predominant form of ACC, even though this type of ACC constituted only 35% of all the forms of ACC. Overall, 50% of patients with the tubular-predominant form of ACC had a good outcome, either never having a recurrence or having no evidence of disease following treatment of a recurrence. In contrast, only 26% of patients with a cribriform-predominant tumor had a favorable outcome. None of the patients with a solid-predominant form of ACC had a good outcome, all either living with persistent disease or having died of their tumor.

Table 2.4 **Histologic pattern and clinical course in ACC** from Perzin, Gullane, and Clairmont, 1978

Pattern	Total	NER	NED–RC	LWD	DOD
Tubular	22	9 (41%)	2 (9%)	2 (9%)	9 (41%)
Cribriform	27	3 (11%)	4 (15%)	5 (19%)	15 (55%)
Solid	13	0	0	6 (46%)	7 (54%)
Total	62	12 (19%)	6 (10%)	13 (21%)	31 (50%)

NER: no evidence of recurrence
NED–RC: no evidence of disease, recurrence controlled
LWD: living with persistent disease
DOD: dead of disease

The histologic pattern of the tumor also influences whether or not neoplastic tissue is found on the lines of excision. Of cases in which the margins of resection could be studied, 9 of 21 (43%) tubular-predominant ACC had negative margins, while only 3 of 24 (13%) cribriform-predominant tumors and none of 13 (0%) solid-predominant tumors had negative margins.

The site of the origin of the tumor also appears to influence prognosis, but the numbers of cases at each site are so small that the findings may not be significant. The most favorable site appears to be the sublingual gland; two tumors at this site did not recur. Of 10 submandibular gland tumors, 4 had no evidence of recurrence, while only 2 of 12 parotid gland tumors, 2 of 7 palatal lesions, and 1 of 9 oral-cavity lesions did not recur. All 4 nasopharyngeal lesions and all 14 nasal-sinus and paranasal-sinus lesions recurred. The site of origin probably influences prognosis based on the ability of the surgeon to perform an adequately wide resection of the involved site.

The size of the primary tumor also affects prognosis. Of 8 lesions measuring 2 cm or less, 7 did not recur; in another case, a recurrence was apparently successfully treated. In contrast, of 28 tumors measuring more than 2 cm, only 5 did not recur; in another 3 cases, recurrences were successfully treated. Thus, the larger the lesion, the worse the prognosis.

Of 8 tumors measuring 2 cm or less, 6 were tubular-predominant lesions. Thus, tubular-predominant forms of ACC appear to be relatively slowly growing tumors, so that when they are discovered clinically, they tend to be relatively small and are less likely to be found on the lines of excison. Thus, they have a better prognosis than other forms of ACC.

Lymph node involvement also appears to affect prognosis. Of 18 patients with nodes negative for tumor, 8 had no evidence of recurrence, 2 had recurrences controlled, 2 were living with disease, and 6 had died of disease. In contrast, of 7 patients with nodes positives for tumor, 5 had died of disease, 1 was living with a presistent tumor, and 1 had recurrent tumor apparently controlled.

Adenoid cystic carcinoma involving the external auditory canal represents an unusual problem (Perzin et al., 1982). In some cases, ACC arising in the parotid gland may extend directly into the ear canal and initially present clinically with ear canal obstruction. However, ACC may arise primarily within the ear canal, presumably from apocrine ceruminous glands, or eccrine sweat glands. These lesions are histologically identical to ACCs arising primarily in salivary glands. That such lesions may arise primarily in the ear canal is proved by large resection specimens in which careful histologic examination shows the lesion confined to the ear canal wall, with no evidence of involvement of the adjacent parotid salivary gland tissue. The prognosis in these cases mainly depends on the presence or absence of tumor on the lines of surgical excision.

3
Adenoid Cystic Carcinoma at Aberrant Sites

Adenoid cystic carcinoma may be found in any location in the head and neck where salivary or mucoserous glands have been identified. However, this tumor does not confine itself to these areas; its characteristic histologic features have been recognized in neoplasms arising at numerous sites throughout the body. These include the lacrimal gland, the skin, the tracheobronchial tree, the esophagus, the breast, the uterine cervix, Bartholin's gland, and the prostate.

Some researchers have questioned whether tumors which appear at these sites bearing the morphologic characteristics of cylindromas of the head and neck are indeed true adenoid cystic carcinomas or whether they are adenocarcinomas exhibiting a histologic variation which mimics the cribriform pattern found in true adenoid cystic tumors. Several elegant studies have addressed this issue. One particular work by Lawrence and Mazur (1982) compares the histologic, histochemical, and ultrastructural characteristics of adenoid cystic carcinomas found in salivary gland, breast, lung, and uterine cervical tissue. These authors analyzed material from these areas using a combination of selective staining of specimens for light microscopy as well as for electron microscopy. Results of histochemical staining with alcian blue and PAS stain were variable. Though each tumor contained hyaluronidase-digestible stromal mucins, only five of eight showed the expected differential staining of stromal and epithelial mucins. This latter finding is thought to be characteristic of true ACC of salivary-gland origin. Electron microscopy was more elucidating, since it revealed ultrastructural features of adenoid cystic carcinomas in all specimens. Specific findings included the presence of intercellular spaces, pseudocysts (rounded extracellular spaces, lined by tumor cells, containing basal lamina and a variable amount of collagen and other forms of fibrils and particles), true glandular lumens lined by microvilli, myofilaments, and a ubiquitous basal lamina. Though the presence of intercellular spaces and the propensity for forming large quantities of basal lamina are not conditions specific to adenoid cystic carcinoma, the presence of pseudocysts is thought to be quite characteristic of it.

The consistent finding of myofilaments, verified by immunofluorescent staining for actomyosin, gives further support to the theory of a myoepithelial origin of these tumors. Myoepithelium has not been identified in the uterine cervix, but the similarity of the fine ultrastructural patterns gives credence to the belief that true adenoid cystic carcinomas may arise at varying sites, though the histogenesis may not be identical.

Lacrimal Gland

Tumors of the lacrimal gland are relatively infrequent. Adenoid cystic carcinoma, however, ranks as the most common epithelial malignancy found in this gland. Estimates of its incidence range from 30% to 40% of all primary epithelial neoplasms in the lacrimal gland. This is proportionally higher than in the parotid or submandibular glands.

Patients with this tumor most commonly present with proptosis. Henderson describes a "forward and downward displacement of the eye, a palpable orbital mass in the superior temporal quadrant, and swelling, drooping, or fullness of the adjacent upper eyelid." Whether a mass can be palpated depends on how far forward the tumor originates in the orbit and its size upon presentation. Pain is not usually observed except in lesions that have been present for a year or more. Pain is much more common in recurrent disease and is usually referred to the eyebrow, forehead, or temple. Of interest is a report by Lee et al. (1985) in which pain was associated with 58% of the primary cases. The average time span from onset of symptoms to diagnosis was 10 months in their series.

Vision may be interfered with in both primary and recurrent settings. Initially, there is a mechanical obstruction to the upward and outward gaze, causing diplopia in that direction. In advanced primary disease or with a recurrence, invasion of the extraocular muscles causes additional limitation of movement.

Treatment of these tumors is primarily surgical. The initial procedure (which is done prior to making the diagnosis of ACC) should remove as much of the mass as possible to avoid spillage. Lesions located anteriorly in the orbit may be reached by an anterior approach. Those tumors located more posteriorly are best accessed by way of an anterotemporal approach. Once the diagnosis is made, further surgery, usually in the form of an orbital exenteration, is required to insure adequacy of margins.

The role of radiotherapy has not been concretely established. Some authors suggest treating postoperatively with 60 Gy if there has been any involvement of bone. Others routinely prescribe postoperative irradiation.

The clinical course of this neoplasm is such that many authors consider it to be the most malignant primary tumor in the orbit. Recurrences are frequent; many occur a year or so after even the most aggressive surgical therapy. It is significant that Billroth's (1856) description of cylindroma includes a case of an orbital tumor in a 22-year-old male that recurred on multiple occasions and led to the slow, painful death of the patient in spite of seven attempts at resection over the course of two and a half years.

Recurrent tumors have three main patterns of spread. The most common pathway leads out laterally into the temporal region. An intracranial spread via the skull base foramina of the region is also common. Spread into adjacent sinus cavities is less likely to occur, but can involve the maxillary, ethmoidal, or sphenoidal sinuses.

Adenoid cystic carcinoma of the orbit has traditionally been associated with a grave prognosis. Many series cite mortality rates of over 90%. Gamel and Font (1982) review 74 cases of lacrimal ACC. They found a significantly greater survival rate for patients whose tumors did not contain any areas of the basaloid or solid cellular pattern. Results were obtained using a blind retrospective analysis. The 5-year survival rate for the entire group was 47%. Patients showing no basaloid component had a 71% 5-year survival rate. If any basaloid pattern was found, the 5-year survival rate dropped to 21%. The 10-year and 15-year survival rates for the entire group were 20% and 12%, respectively. Lee et al. (1985) report a 2.5-year survival rate of 50%. Fifty percent of the patients in their series experienced distant metastases.

The poor prognosis associated with this lesion has led clinicians to question the validity of radical surgery for this tumor. In a series from the Mayo Clinic, eight of nine patients died of their diseases, regardless of whether an exenteration alone was used or whether exenteration was combined with bone removal and postoperative radiotherapy. The ninth patient had recurrent disease at four years and was lost to follow-up after an exenteration.

Henderson alludes to the frustration experienced by many clinicians in caring for patients with lacrimal gland ACC. He expresses doubt as to whether any of these tumors are curable, attributing this to early bony invasion in spite of negative radiographic evidence. Histologic examination of bony specimens has led him to believe that the tumor spreads more rapidly in bone than in the orbital soft tissues. In his opinion, initially definitive surgery should include a monobloc resection of tumor and adjacent bone.

Skin

Our knowledge of the existence of a cutaneous variety of adenoid cystic carcinoma predates much of our understanding of its salivary gland counterpart, however, a clear definition of its biology is still lacking. The tumor is usually considered to be benign, though metastases and malignant degeneration have been reported on rare occasions. ACC of the skin may exist as a single lesion or may occur as a multiplicity of tumors, often concentrated on the scalp (the so-called "turban tumor"). In the latter instance, there appears to be a genetic component to the disease; many cases are transmitted in an autosomal dominant pattern.

Adenoid cystic carcinoma has been referred to as "dermal cylindroma," although some authors use this term to refer to a separate eccrine gland tumor that has histologic characteristics which are slightly different from adenoid cystic carcinoma of salivary-gland origin. ACC of the skin has been thought to arise from apocrine or eccrine glands in the skin, or from hair follicles. Most authors now favor the theory of eccrine-gland origin. This disease may occur more frequently in women than in men. The tumor is most commonly found in the ear canal. One must differentiate ACC of the skin from adenoid basal-cell carcinoma, mucinous carcinoma of the skin, and ordinary basal-cell carcinoma, which undergo a cystic degeneration. One must also exclude the possibility that what appears to be ACC originating in the skin may actually represent an underlying salivary gland lesion with extension into the skin or a cutaneous metastasis from another primary source.

ACC in the skin is less aggressive than lesions in salivary-gland tissue. Recurrence after local resection is common and may develop after 20 years. Local recurrence is found more frequently when perineural invasion is noted. Treatment has been primarily surgical excision, though the extent of the surgical margins required has been debated in the literature. Adequate treatment of the turban-tumor variety has resulted in total scalp replacement in several patients. Lang et al. (1986) report on the use of the Mohs' technique to achieve surgical surgical removal. The patient in their report had no recurrence in the 18 months of follow-up, but this may not be an adequate amount of time to demonstrate the validity of this technique, since recurrences often take much longer to develop. Radiotherapy has been relatively useless in controlling these tumors and is regarded as palliative.

Tracheobronchial Tree

In many series, adenoid cystic carcinoma ranks second behind squamous-cell carcinoma as the most common malignant neoplasm of the trachea. The lesion was thought to represent a benign adenoma in many early reports. Though now accepted as a malignancy, the tumor may be slow in its growth. It has often been mistaken for asthma or chronic bronchitis. ACC in this area is usually confined to the trachea and main-stem bronchi, though involvement at more peripheral sites has been reported (Gallagher et al. 1986).

Prognosis of ACC in the tracheobronchial tree depends on the size of the primary tumor, the degree of submucosal spread, and the histologic grade of the tumor. Nomori (1988) review 12 cases of ACC in the trachea and main-stem bronchi. Infiltration into the submucosa and into perineural lymphatics was common in this series. The lesions were graded 1 to 3 based on the proportion of cribriform to solid pattern in the specimen. Lesions with more of the solid pattern were considered to represent a more undifferentiated form of the disease. Though patients with higher-grade tumors tended to have a worse prognosis, follow-up in the patients with lower-grade lesions was less than sufficient to show a significant difference between groups. Metastatic spread was more common in patients with higher-grade lesions.

Surgery has been the main form of treatment for ACC of the tracheobronchial tree. Resections are usually performed through a cervical collar incision combined with a median sternotomy. Most lesions are removed by segmental sleeve resection with primary anastomoses. Prosthetic replacement of segments of trachea or bronchi has been very hazardous. Earlier attempts were associated with a high perioperative mortality from erosion of the innominate artery.

Pearson et al. (1984) report on 28 cases. Twelve patients were thought to have received a potentially curative operation with safe margins. Mean survival in this group was 8.3 years. Eight of nine patients with surgical margins involved by tumor died of their diseases two to nine years after surgery. Adjuvant radiotherapy was used routinely in this series, with some patients receiving a partial dose preoperatively. Metastatic spread occurred in ten patients. Pulmonary metastases were found in nine, spread to the brain was seen in two patients, and osseus involvement was found in one patient.

Unfortunately, not all lesions are amenable to surgical resection. There are several options available for palliation including radiotherapy, chemotherapy, and partial endoscopic resection with or without the use of the endoscopic laser (Huber et al., 1986). Occasionally, intraluminal stenting may be required to prevent obstruction from progressive tumor growth or from swelling resulting from radiotherapy (Munsch et al., 1987).

Esophagus

Adenoid cystic carcinoma of the esophagus is quite rare. Large series of carcinomas of the esophagus may not contain a single case. Pourzand et al. (1975) present a single case and review the cases in the literature of the time for a total of 15 cases. Patients ranged from 51 to 72 years of age (an average of 64.9 years). The lesion was noted to occur in the middle third of the esophagus in most of the cases. Dysphagia was the most common symptom. One patient presented with massive gastrointestinal bleeding. Similar descriptions are found in reports by Petursson in 1986 (44 cases from the literature) and Akamatsu et al., also in 1986 (23 cases from the literature).

The tumor is thought to arise in the submucosal glands of the esophagus. Some authors have suggested that the neoplasms arise from embryonal nests of the tracheobronchial tree located in the esophagus. Others argue that the tumor is a form of adenocarcinoma originating in the resident submucosal glands of the esophagus.

ACC in this location tends to be less differentiated than in the salivary-gland tissue of the head and neck, however, Akamatsu et al. were able to show three different areas of differentiation within a single tumor using immunohistochemical staining techniques. Esophageal ACC is thought to have a poorer prognosis than similar lesions in the head and neck. Metastatic spread to the mediastinum, lungs, liver, cerebellum, bones, and soft tissues has been documented at autopsy. One reason for this is that most of these tumors present quite late. Only two cases have been reported where the lesions were confined to the submucosa.

Treatment is similar to squamous-cell cancers in the same location. Most patients undergo a surgical resection, some receive primary radiotherapy, others undergo a combination of surgery and irradiation. Some receive no therapy at all. Chemotherapy has been used on several occasions. Petursson (1986) reports the case of a 55-year-old man who obtained a transient complete response of his metastatis disease with a combination of cisplatin, cyclophosphamide, vincristine, and doxorubicin. The patient died 21 months after diagnosis. Other authors have described only a partial response to chemotherapy, and Wobbes et al. (1984) report progression of the disease on cisplatin, doxorubicin, and bleomycin. The majority of patients die within two years. There have been only three cases in which the reported survival rates were greater than 3.5 years.

Breast

The first reports of adenoid cystic carcinoma originating in breast tissue were from Gerschickter in 1945 and from Foote and Stewart in 1946. Since that time there have been over 50 cases documented in various reports. Within large series of carcinoma of the breast, ACC comprises between 1 in 525 and 1 in 640 cases.

Patients are typically postmenopausal women, although in at least two reported instances, this lesion has occurred in males. The neoplasm is usually found near the nipple or areolar tissue. The most common presenting symptom is a breast mass. Pain or tenderness is not an infrequent finding.

Therapy has been primarily surgery. Most authors have advocated wide excision of the tumor, usually in the form of a simple mastectomy. Others have advocated therapy ranging from lumpectomy with subsequent radiotherapy to radical mastectomy with axillary dissection. The more radical approach has been tempered somewhat by the fact that there has been only one reported case of metastatic spread of breast ACC to axillary lymph nodes. Metastatic spread to the lungs has been reported on several occasions. Koller et al. (1986) report one case in which metastasis to the brain occurred. Radiotherapy is generally viewed as unnecessary for most lesions, provided that the size is less than 3–4 cm and that an adequately wide excision has been performed.

Similar to salivary gland lesions, ACC of the breast has been noted to display some diversity in its histologic appearance. In addition to the characteristic pattern of epithelial and myoepithelial cells, tubular, cribriform, and solid patterns have been identified. Ro et al. (1987) recommend classifying the lesions into three grades based on the proportion of the solid histologic component in the tumor. They propose local resection for grade 1 lesions (no solid component) and simple mastectomy for higher grades. No recurrences were noted for grade 1 lesions, while two of six patients with grade 2 tumors had recurrences.

Adenoid cystic carcinoma of the breast may occasionally be confused with other primary breast lesions. This most commonly occurs with certain forms of intraductal carcinoma. Both tumors may exhibit a cribriform pattern. The differentiation is important, however, because the treatment and prognosis is different, since the intraductal carcinoma is a more aggressive lesion. Harris (1977) analyzes both neoplasms using electron microscopy. He describes a case of breast cancer initially diagnosed as adenoid cystic carcinoma based on its light microscopy appearance with hemotoxin and exosin staining. Electron microscopy failed to demonstrate the "pseudocyst" characteristic of adenoid cystic carcinoma. Subsequently, a diagnosis of intraductal carcinoma with cribriform features was made. Harris recommends electron microscopy to differentiate between the two lesions on the basis of the presence or absence of pseudocysts in equivocal cases. Several authors have commented on the lack of hormonal receptors in adenoid cystic carcinoma of the breast. Only one case of an ACC with estrogen receptors has been documented in the literature.

It is difficult to ascertain precise information regarding survival statistics for adenoid cystic carcinoma of the breast, since few reports contain more than a five-year follow-up. Weitzner et al. (1970) reviewed the then-current literature and found 46 cases to analyze. They found that in 41 of the 46 cases, the patients still were alive at the time of their report. Of these, 22 had had less than five years of follow-up. Nineteen were followed for over five years, but only 11 had had more than a ten-year follow-up. By 1987, at least 110 cases had been recorded in the literature. Metastatic spread was documented in 7 and local recurrence was known to have occurred in 10.

It is well-known that patients with ACC in the head and neck may die of their diseases twenty or more years after diagnosis. It is not clear whether this holds true for ACC of the breast. In contrast to its counterpart in the salivary tissue of the head and neck, breast ACC does not tend to recur locally after adequate excision. Indeed, this tumor has a relatively favorable prognosis when compared to ACC of salivary origin and to other forms of breast cancer.

Several explanations have been offered to account for the more favorable prognosis associated with ACC of the breast. Tavassoli and Norris (1986) examined the ultrastructure of several cases of breast ACC with sebaceous differentiation. Myoepithelial differentiation was not observed. They attribute the limited aggressiveness of mammary ACC to a tendency of the tumor to differentiate along dermal appendage cell lines, rather than along mesenchymal lines. Sumpio et al. (1987) comment on the lack of perineural invasion in 37 tumors examined. They feel that this feature could explain the paucity of recurrences and the generally more favorable outlook associated with the lesion in this location.

Uterine Cervix

Adenoid cystic carcinoma in the uterine cervix occurs in postmenopausal women, usually in their sixties. It comprises 0.4% to 3% of cervical cancers. Interestingly, a significant number of patients (up to 30%) are found to have another coexisting malignancy of the cervix. Postmenopausal vaginal bleeding is the most common presenting complaint. Occasional cases present with abdominal pain. Most tumors are diagnosed in stage I or stage II (Table 3.**1**). While some tumors may be exophytic, others can be deeply infiltrating. Musa et al. (1985) report that 6 of 17 cases they studied were asymptomatic and were picked up on Papanicolaou cytopathologic smears.

The histologic features are typical of adenoid cystic carcinoma located elsewhere: "clusters of small, uniform, basaloid cells with regular, darkly staining nuclei and scanty cytoplasm ... arranged in irregular anastomosing cords, pseudoglands, and varying sized cribriform nests". Perineural or intraneural invasion is observed here less often than in other locations, but lymphatic invasion is frequent. One author noted the scant amount of associated inflammatory response and minimal stromal reaction. This neoplasm has been associated with concurrent squamous-cell carcinomas and adenocarcinomas.

The lesion is thought to arise from endocervical glands in a manner similar to that in which primary adenocarcinomas of the cervix arise. As mentioned above, myoepithelial cells have not been identified in the cervix, which suggests the possible existence of a histogenesis different from adenoid cystic carcinomas elsewhere in the body. Ferry and Scully (1988) suggest that ACC of the cervix is a fundamentally different lesion than ACC found in salivary glands. Some authors have suggested that the lesions may arise following metaplasia in the cervical epithelium.

Treatment of cylindromas in the cervix varies from institution to institution. Some centers treat primarily with radiotherapy while others advocate surgical excision. The statistics in the literature have an average five-year survival rate of approximately 50%. Fowler et al. (1978) broke the survival rate down according to stage (Table 3.**2**). They combined 9 new cases with 38 cases reported in the literature. Eight of 18 patients in this series treated with primary irradiation died of their diseases. Fowler et al. thus advocate radical pelvic surgery with lymph node dissection in qualified surgical candidates. He felt that "adjuvant chemotherapy should be considered in view of the high incidence of lung metastases". Prempree et al. (1980) treated five of six patients with primary radiotherapy. One patient (stage 0) received a modified hysterectomy. They felt that radiotherapy was more effective than surgery for stage I disease. Survival rates for stages I, II, and III in his series were 56.2%, 27.3%, and 0%, respectively. Follow-up in this series was limited, however, and ranged from one to eight years in length. Musa et al. (1985) advocate the use of external radiotherapy for early lesions, pointing out that two patients treated with this modality survived for 9 and 11 years.

Table 3.1 **Staging system for carcinoma of the cervix** (adapted from the International Federation of Gynecology and Obstetrics)

Stage 0	Carcinoma in situ, intraepithelial carcinoma
Stage I	Carcinoma confined to the cervix
Stage II	Carcinoma extending beyond the cervix, but not to the pelvic wall
Stage III	Carcinoma involving the pelvic wall
Stage IV	Carcinoma extending beyond the limits of the true pelvis or involving the bladder or rectum

Table 3.2 **Survival rates by stage** (from Fowler et al., 1978)

Stage	%	Surviving patients	Total cases
I	42	7	17
II	22	2	9
III	0	0	3
IV	One patient living with disease		

Metastatic spread from adenoid cystic carcinoma of the cervix ranges from 0% to 47%. Pulmonary metastases are the most common. The incidence appears to be related to the length of follow-up. Metastatic spread appears to occur once the lesion has extended beyond the confines of the cervix.

Bartholin's Gland

Carcinoma arising in Bartholin's glands of the vulva is relatively rare. Adenoid cystic carcinoma is thought to account for about 10% of all cases. 41 cases were collected by Amichetti and Aldovini (1988). ACC at this location usually presents with a painful palpable mass. The disease has a poor prognosis. Recurrences are frequent, as is metastatic spread. Lung and bone metastases are the most common, although several cases of lymph node spread have been documented. Perineural and intravascular spread, characteristic of ACC in salivary glands, has been observed in many cases (Abrao et al., 1985 and Copeland et al., 1986).

Proposed treatment has varied from author to author. Amichetti and Aldovini recommend wide excision of the lesion, followed by radiotherapy, bilateral lymphadenectomy in all cases. They state that radiotherapy is not very effective, especially when surgery fails to obtain clear margins. Chemotherapy has shown little or no effect in controlling the disease at this location.

Early local recurrence has been associated with a poorer survival. In the review by Copeland et al. (1986), patients who developed a recurrence within two years did not survive longer than three years after surgery, whereas all patients who developed a recurrence after three years were alive five years after surgery. In spite of some long term survivors, Amichetti and Aldovini express the view that ACC located in Bartholin's glands appears to be incurable.

Prostate

Adenoid cystic carcinoma is extremely rare in the prostate, with less than ten cases reported in the world's literature. This paucity of clinical material has made it difficult to characterize the biologic behavior of the tumor at this location. Shong-San and Walters (1984) report no perineural invasion in the one case they describe.

The tumor is believed to arise either from ectopic salivary-gland tissue, or from glands contained in the prostatic epithelium. The differential diagnosis for adenoid cystic carcinoma at this location includes a cribriform variant of adenocarcinoma of the prostate, carcinoma of the anus (including cloacogenic carcinoma), carcinoma of the rectum, and Cowper's gland cancers. Treatment has been primarily transurethral resection. Antiandrogenic therapy has been unsuccessful. Lack of long-term follow-up data makes comments on survival rates impossible.

Summary

This chapter has reviewed the various manifestations of adenoid cystic carcinoma at non-salivary gland sites throughout the body. Though many features remain relatively constant, others show considerable variation from site to site. The prognosis for tumors in the skin and breast is much better than at salivary gland locations, while the survival rates of patients with lacrimal or esophageal ACC appear to be much worse. The reasons for these discrepancies have not been completely elucidated. While the tumors seem to exhibit a commonality in their predilection for secretory tissues, there appears to be some hormonal influence which may impact on the degree of malignancy exhibited by these neoplasms. At this point, we may state that adenoid cystic carcinomas found throughout the body appear to be at least somewhat related, though subtle ultrastructural variations may occur. They appear to represent a family of glandular malignancies and, as a family, display certain similarities. For example, a tendency toward perineural invasion, a propensity for local recurrence, and a predisposition for hematogenous spread to lung and bone have been consistently demonstrated. That we do not completely understand the reason why the biologic manifestation of the tumor differs from site to site indicates that much research is still required.

4 Data and Statistics

A significant amount of valuable information can be gathered from a computer analysis of 406 cases of adenoid cystic carcinoma in the head and neck. There are many ways to analyze this material, but none are completely satisfactory. Definitive actuarial tables and computer print-outs can be used to bring out certain points, but no method alone can present the entire clinical picture. A large volume of cases which has been followed for three or four decades has the best chance of presenting germane clinical features and outcomes. These data cannot predict how individual cases will behave, but they can provide general impressions, highlight weaknesses and strengths in the prognosis, and create a framework for the philosophy of management, the concepts of treatment, the consequences of the treatment and the disease, and the results. The data are not considered "hard data" because of the variabilities in their acquisition the unpredictables in tumor behavior, and the decisional and technical factors of tumor management.

In the 406 cases studied, this disease was more common in women (56% of the cases), and it occurred in all age groups (Figs. 4.1, 4.2). There were very few cases with patients below the age of 20 and a small number with patients over 80 years of age. The vast majority—over 90%—occurred between 30 and 70, with the highest peak between 50 and 60 years of age.

This tumor was most prevalent in the aerodigestive system; 39% occurred in the major salivary glands and 59% in the minor salivary glands (Fig. 4.3). The major salivary gland tumors occurred in the parotid gland (26%), in the submandibular gland (9%) and in the sublingual gland (4%). The preponderance of this tumor in the minor salivary glands had a significant influence on prognosis. Of these, 54% occurred in the oral cavity, 33% in the nasal and sinus cavities, and 13% in the pharyngotracheal areas (Table 4.1, Fig. 4.4). There was no correlation between the concentration of minor salivary gland parenchyma and the increase of adenoid cystic carcinoma.

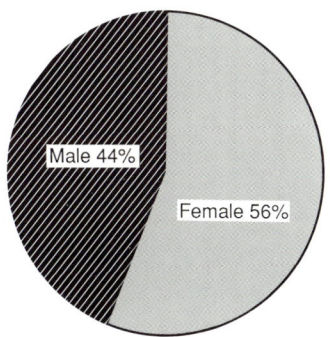

Fig. 4.1 **Sex ratio.** There was a modest preponderance of women

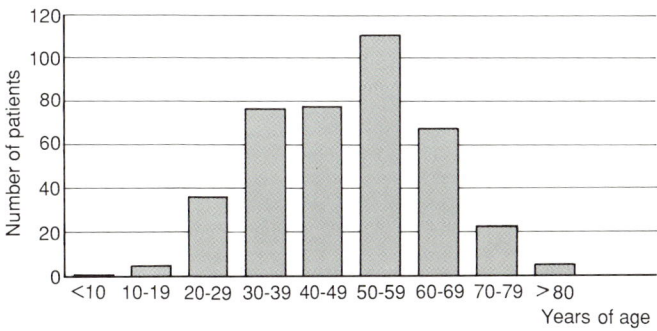

Fig. 4.2 **Age distribution.** The majority of adenoid cystic carcinomas occurred in middle age. There were very few before the age of 10 and few after the age of 80

Tumor histology proved to be significant in treatment and prognosis. Tumors of the cribriform type made up 62% of the group and 16% of the tumors were of the tubular type. In many cases, these histologic types were mixed together. Both of these types were classified as having a more favorable prognosis than the basaloid (compact small-cell) type, which composed 22% of the group (Fig. 4.5).

The primary tumor dominated the classification by staging because of the very low incidence of regional and systemic metastases discovered at the initial examination. Only 5% had enlarged cervical lymph nodes at the initial examination, the majority of which were associated with the submandibular gland, tongue, and pharynx, and with a more undifferentiated histologic pattern. Only 1% had pulmonary metastases at the initial examination. The T classification applied primarily to the major salivary glands and these linear measurements underestimated the size of the tumor in the majority of these cases. The T classification was also applied to minor salivary glands, when realistic, with the understanding that there was a gross underestimation of the pernicious effects of the extensions of these tumors, because their size in relation to their surroundings was much more advanced than their measurements indicated when classified together with the tumors of the major salivary glands. Many of the tumors classified as T2 and T3 would likely have been T4B grossly and microscopically, if their location in a minor salivary gland had been taken into consideration. The category T1 comprised 27% of the tumors; 66% were classified as T2 and T3 (Fig. 4.6).

Perineural invasion was observed in 46% of the cases (Fig. 4.7). This figure is most likely too low, as these tumors tend toward perineural involvement and grow in an environment that is rich in motor and sensory nerve filaments. Nerve involvement had a significant effect on prognosis. In one group of 43 studied to assess facial nerve involvement in relation to prognosis, 7% had preoperative facial paresis. There is little question that, in this group, the incidence of involvement of other nerves would also be significant. In addition, in adenoid cystic carcinomas in other locations, particularly in advanced lesions, the incidence of perineural involvement is likely to be much higher than reported from the laboratory.

Local recurrence and the number of operations form a strategic part of the data in that these figures establish the chronicity of this disease and document the frustrated, repetitive attempts to control it. There was local recurrence in 74% of the cases; most of these occurred within five years after surgery at all tumor sites and continued to occur for more than 20 years after surgery in minor salivary glands and parotid glands (Fig. 4.8). This powerful example of surgical inadequacy is also shown in the number of operations performed in an attempt to control the failed primary tumor. Approximately 5% underwent at least four operations, and some had five or six operations without success at local control (Fig. 4.9).

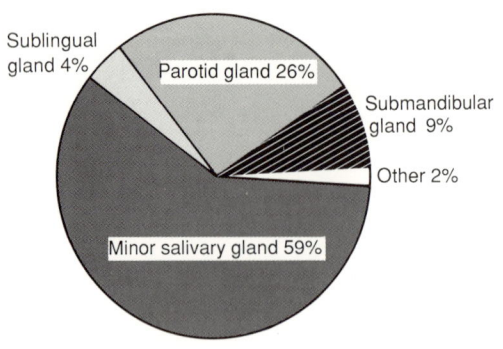

Fig. 4.3 **Tumor location.** The majority of the tumors were located in the minor salivary glands. The parotid gland was the dominant location for tumors of the major salivary glands

Table 4.1 **Minor salivary gland tumor distribution**

Site	%
Oral cavity	**54**
Palate	26
Tongue	14
Lip	7
Retromolar	4
Buccal	3
Nasal cavity	**33**
Maxillary sinus	17
Turbinates and septum	14
Ethmoidal sinus	2
Pharynx	**13**
Supraglottic / Subglottic	13
Total	**100**

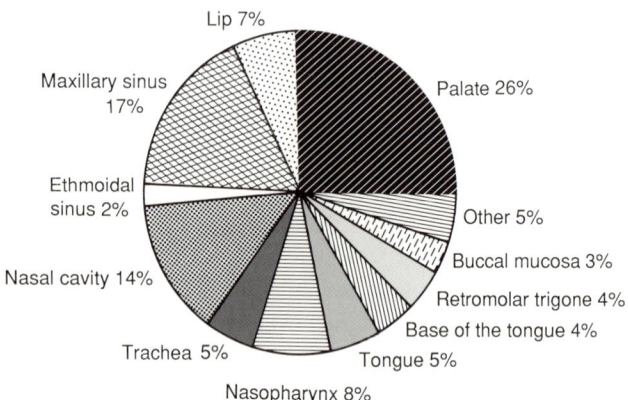

Fig. 4.4 **Breakdown of minor salivary gland tumors.** There is a very wide distribution of minor salivary gland adenoid cystic carcinomas in the aerodigestive system. The palate contains the largest number

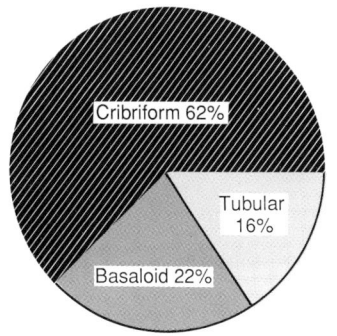

Fig. 4.5 **Tumor histology.** The cribriform pattern dominated

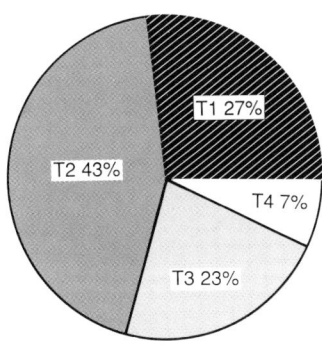

Fig. 4.6 **Staging.** The majority of tumors were classified T2

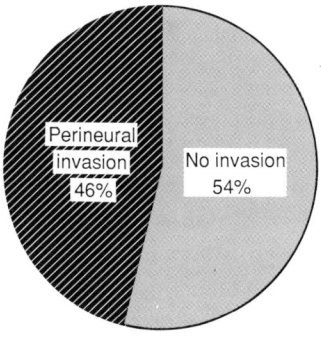

Fig. 4.7 **Perineural invasion** was documented in 46% of the cases, but the incidence is unquestionably higher than this

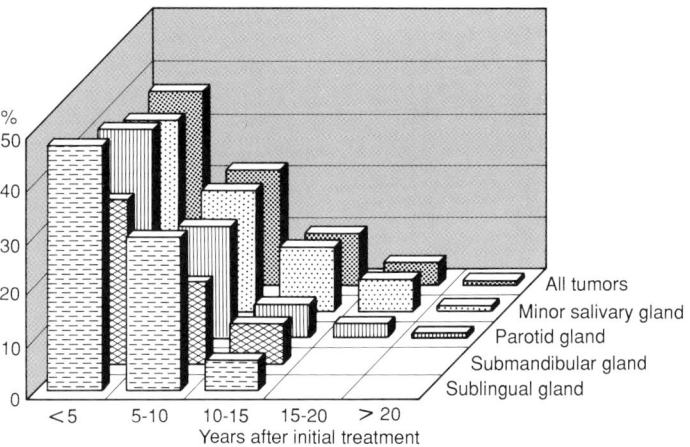

Fig. 4.8 **Local recurrence** was most common in the periods of less than five years after surgery and up to ten years; however, local recurrences can be expected on rare occasions up to 20 years after initial surgery

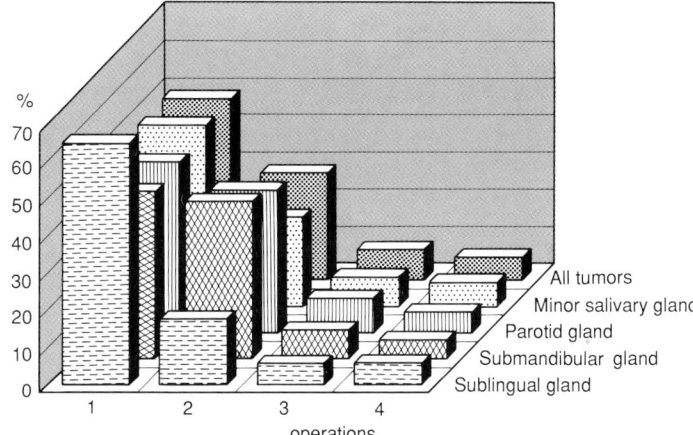

Fig. 4.9 **Number of operations.** There was a crescendo of operations in the first two years, but by the third and fourth year this diminished; however, it persisted for 10–20 years

The reasons for these failures are the surgeon's underestimation of the extent of the primary tumor, the patient's resistance to undergoing a mutilating procedure, the doctor's misconception regarding the potential lethality of this disease, and the tumor's pernicious occult extensions, which create a false sense of security by deceiving both the patient and the doctors. The diagrams in Figures 4.**8** and 4.**9** demonstrate these weaknesses and frustrations graphically.

At the initial examination, the tumor had metastasized regionally in 5% of the cases and systemically in 3%. Within five years, however, there was a dramatic increase in systemic spread and a decrease in regional spread. From 5 to 10 years after initial examination to over 20 years, there is a diminuendo, but persistence, of these metastases. Lungs, bone, and brain are the primary sites of systemic spread (Fig. 4.**10**).

A general review of the outcome at ten years after initial surgery establishes the clinical nature of this disease and its potential lethality. Thirty percent of patients were free of disease at the time, 36% were dead of disease, 17% living with disease, 13% free of

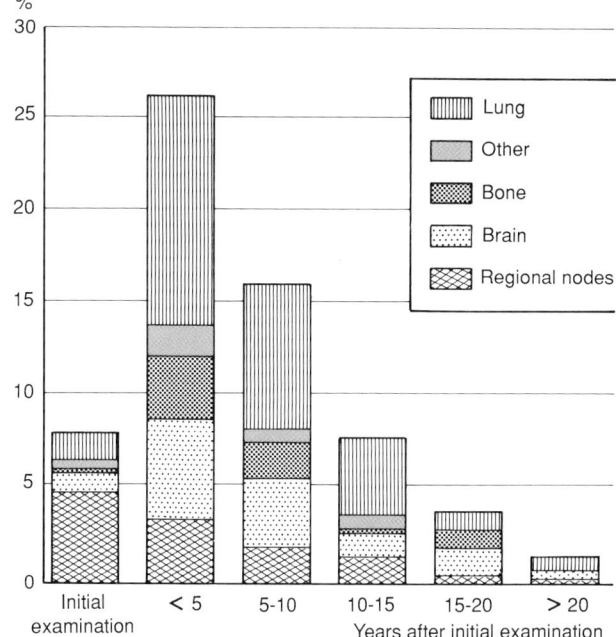

Fig. 4.**10** **Metastasis** was most common in the period of less than five years after initial examination, but persisted for more than ten years. Metastases were also discovered after 20 years

disease after recurrence, and 4% dead of other causes (Fig. 4.11). Those listed as free of disease will understandably be reduced in number by local recurrence. Those living with disease will eventually join those dead of disease, and those free of disease after recurrence will shift to living with diesease, and then shift again to dead of disease. The only stable figures at ten years are those indicating the patients dead of disease and dead of other causes. It is realistic to project that those who have had recurrent tumor (30%) and some of those who are free of disease (10 to 15%) may develop a recurrence, to add these potentially fatal cases to those dead of disease (36%), and thus, to figure a mortality rate of 75 to 80% over a 30-year period.

These grim figures are, however, ameliorated by the fact that 176 patients out of 406 were alive 15 years after initial surgery (Fig. 4.12). This 43% survival rate at this point in time proves that somewhat less than half the patients gained this period of life, in part, as a result of their treatments. There is some consolation in this, but it is certainly possible to improve these statistics.

There is little question that adenoid cystic carcinoma in the minor salivary glands is more lethal than in the major salivary glands. The reasons for this are discussed in chapter 4, under "staging." A 24% survival rate for minor salivary glands 15 years after surgery (Fig. 4.13) would realistically decrease to approximately 12% by 30 years after surgery.

Fifteen years after surgery, submandibular gland tumors had a survival rate of 59%, parotid gland tumors 54%, and sublingual gland 44% (Figs. 4.14–16). A physical factor that perhaps influences this data is that the submandibular gland is technically the most accessible. The parotid gland is the largest major salivary gland, but is technically more difficult to manage because of the presence of the facial nerve. The sublingual gland is smaller and located in the anterior portion of the oral cavity, making adequate resection an awkward and often mutilating procedure. One can realistically subtract 20–25% from these 15-year figures to estimate their final disposition.

Sixty-three percent of tumors in the minor salivary glands received postoperative irradiation, 37% did not. There is an almost 20% difference in the survival rates appearing 3 years after surgery and persisting through 10 and 15 years after surgery (Fig. 4.17). The improvement in the survival rates of patients with tumors in the major salivary glands is less impressive.

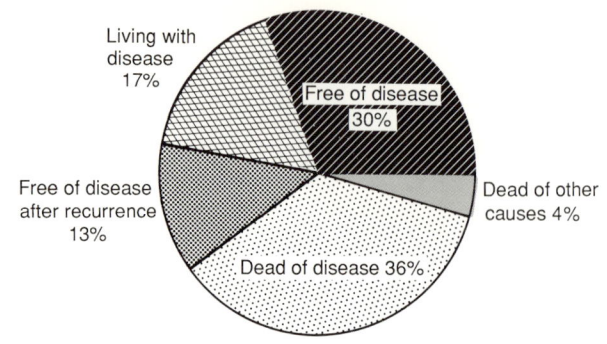

Fig. 4.11 **The outcome at ten years** indicated that 36% were dead of their disease, 13% were free of disease after at least one local recurrence, 17% were living with disease, and 30% were free of disease. This general figure indicates the lethality of this neoplasm. Five percent died of other causes

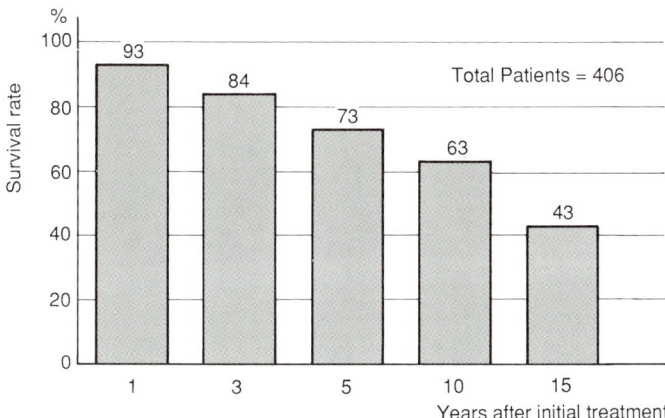

Fig. 4.12 **The overall survival rates** indicated that 93% were living one year after surgery and 43% were living 15 years later. This latter figure is expected to decrease as the years go on

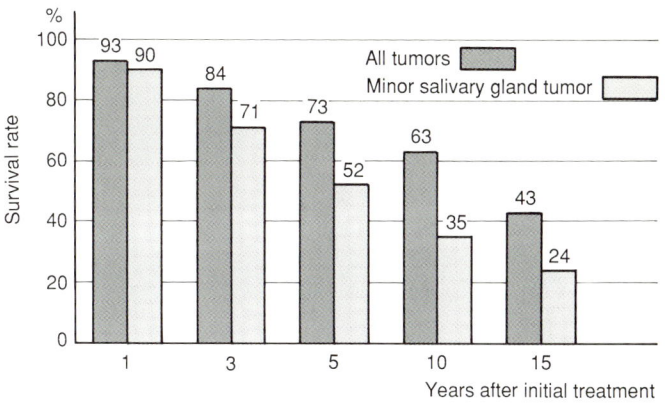

Fig. 4.13 **The survival rates for minor salivary gland tumors** are lower than for major salivary gland tumors. This becomes apparent at three years after initial surgery and persists beyond 15 years. At 15 years the cure rate for minor salivary gland tumors was only 24% and this is expected to decrease as the years go by

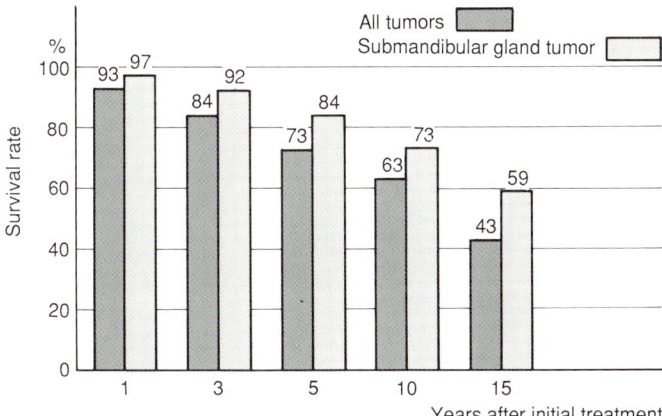

Fig. 4.14 **The survival rates for submandibular gland adenoid cystic carcinomas** were better than all tumors combined. At 15 years after surgery it was 59%

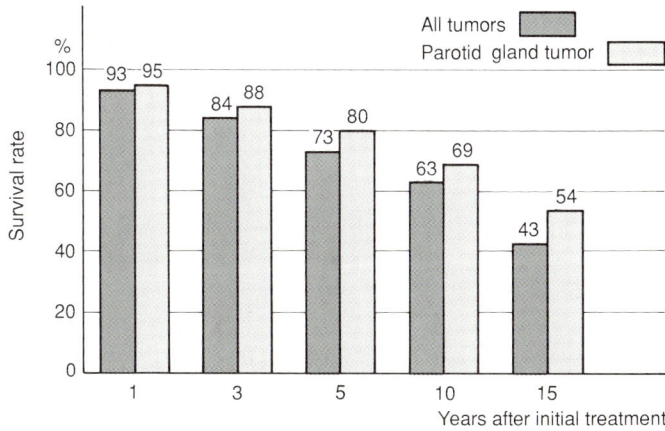

Fig. 4.15 **The survival rates for parotid gland adenoid cystic carcinomas** were somewhat better than all tumors combined. It was 54% at 15 years after surgery

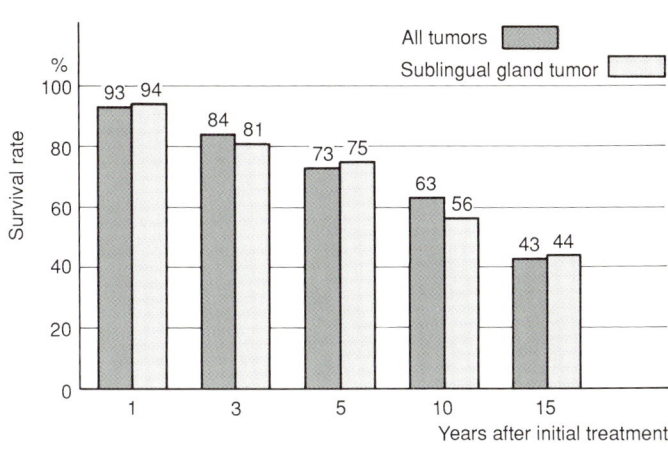

Fig. 4.16 **The survival rates for sublingual gland adenoid cystic carcinomas** were quite similar to those for all tumors. At 15 years after surgery it was 44%

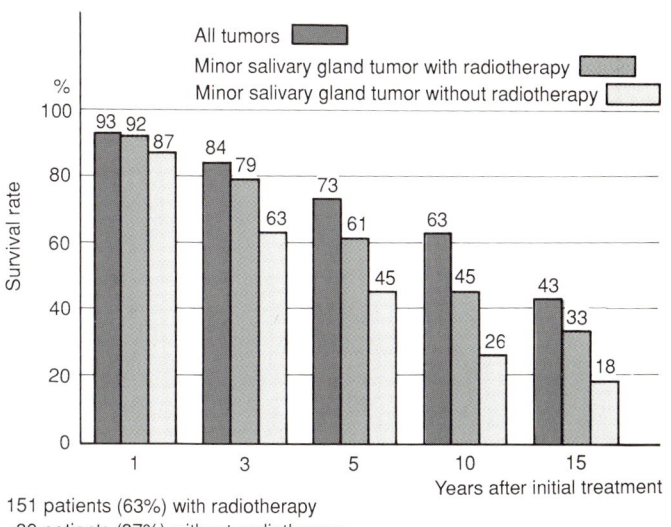

151 patients (63%) with radiotherapy
89 patients (37%) without radiotherapy

Fig. 4.17 **The survival rate for minor salivary gland tumors treated postoperatively with radiotherapy** was 33% at 15 years after surgery. Without irradiation the survival rate at this time was 18%. This evidence supports the use of irradiation postoperatively in many of these cases

5
Diagnosis

Signs and Symptoms

As the vast majority of these neoplasms are positioned submucosally in a minor salivary gland or are contained within the parenchyma of a major salivary gland, there is nothing to see and nothing to feel in the early stages.

The site of origin of the neoplasm naturally influences the appearance of signs and symptoms. The hundreds of minor salivary glands scattered throughout the aerodigestive system in the head and neck present multitudes of opportunities for varieties of signs and symptoms. A microscopic or macroscopic tumor focus in any of these glands cannot be diagnosed clinically. Patients must wait until there is some type of gross abnormality before they can respond. There is, of course, the rare, early diagnosis when a patient can see or feel a small lump in the lip, buccal, or palatal areas. A doctor or dentist may also be fortunate enough to discover a small lump in these areas and follow through with a diagnosis. In the majority of cases the neoplasm grows to a recognizable size, extends beyond the capsule of the minor salivary gland into soft areolar tissue, muscle, nerves, periosteum, and bone. Only 5–7% of these have regional metastasis at the initial examination. At this stage, however, about 20% had some type of pain or discomfort, which indicated that a sensory nerve was being involved by the neoplasm. About 5% of these tumors became ulcerated, which may cause bleeding or pain. As these tumors enlarge in the nasal cavity, they block breathing and drainage and may invade adjacent bone, branches of the trigeminal cranial nerve, the orbit, or base of the skull. By this time, the tumor is probably incurable. In the pharyngeal cavities, floor of the mouth, and larynx, these neoplasms of the minor salivary gland form a small mass under the mucosa and then subsequently expand into the areolar tissue and muscle and bone, causing obstruction and difficulty with swallowing and speaking. At this stage, there is usually some discomfort. The vagus and hypoglossal cranial nerves are the most frequently involved, but the tumor has usually been present for over ten years before this occurs.

The same biological process of expansion goes on with neoplasias in the major salivary glands, with the exception that it takes place in the early stages of development within a large volume of the parenchyma of the gland. Minor salivary glands are only 1–3 mm in diameter, and any malignant neoplastic process expanding in them invades the surrounding tissues within a short period of time. In the major salivary glands, these tumors are usually contained within the gland itself until they have grown beyond the small and medium sizes. Only highly advanced tumors in the major salivary glands invade adjacent structures. It is not possible to palpate a small tumor positioned in the center of the parotid or submandibular glands because of the overlying parenchyma. Tumors in the deep lobe of the parotid gland are particularly difficult to diagnose in the early stages. It is possible to palpate and to see medium-sized tumors in these glands if they are situated on the periphery of the gland and expand centrifugally. They hardly ever ulcerate or bleed, but about 20% do cause discomfort or pain. In advanced cases in the parotid gland, they grow into the mastoid bone, masseter muscle, deep lobe, mesopharynx, and into the facial nerve in about 13% of the cases. Advanced cases in the submandibular and sublingual glands invade the lingual and hypoglossal nerves, mandible, tongue, palate, and neck.

There is no rule regulating early diagnosis, as most tumors are first discovered by the patient and then confirmed by the doctor. It is logical to inform the patient regarding the early danger signals of neoplasia. This has been successfully carried out with melanoma and cancer of the breast. Unfortunately, the patient has little opportunity to apply this information, if indeed the information is known, with respect to early diagnosis in salivary gland tumors, because of submucosal position and containment within a larger salivary gland and because of the possibility of their being positioned in inaccessible areas. It is indeed fortunate that CT scanning and MRI techniques are available to assist diagnosis in many of these cases.

Age, Sex, Incidence, and Sites

This tumor can occur in any decade of life; however, in this series of 406 cases, it occurred in only one patient younger than 10 years of age, and in three additional patients under 20 years of age. There were 25 cases of ACC in patients older than 70. The great bulk of the tumors (83%) occurred between 30 and 70 years of age, with a peak of 27% between 50 and 60 years of age.

Female patients made up 56% of the cases, and 44% were males.

Tumors of the minor salivary gland composed 59% of the group. There were 26% in the parotid gland, 9% in the submandibular gland, 4% in the sublingual gland, and 2% at other sites of the aerodigestive system in the head and neck. It is paradoxical that the systems that contain the smallest amount of parenchymal tissue had the highest incidence of malignancy. Within this group of minor salivary glands, certain regions with a high percentage of minor salivary gland structures had a low incidence of malignant neoplasia. This was demonstrated in the tongue and pharynx. The reasons for this relative immunity are not known, but most likely these areas have a singular, protective genetic coding.

Biopsy

The diagnosis of adenoid cystic carcinoma may be immediately apparent or provokingly obscure. No clinician and no scientific test can diagnose an incipient adenoid cystic carcinoma. It must be positioned close to the surface in an accessible portion of a major or minor salivary gland to be available for inspection or palpation. It must be approximately 1 cm in diameter to be discovered through imaging or scanning techniques. There are circumstances when it may be discovered fortuitously. A small enlargement in an accessible minor salivary gland or a small mass in the sinus or nasal cavity should be removed for diagnostic purposes. A malignancy rate of 65% in minor salivary glands certainly emphasizes the importance of microscopic diagnosis in these early cases. The advent of microsurgical techniques in intranasal diagnosis and treatment should facilitate early diagnosis to a certain degree in those areas, but it will probably take one or two decades of experience to establish its criteria.

In view of the fact that the vast majority of diagnoses are made on the basis of the presentation of symptoms and signs first recognized by the patient and subsequently diagnosed by the physician, the interval of delay of the discovery may be two to six months on the part of the patient. A certain delay is justified in the medical management program if the initial clinical examination is negative for neoplasm and there are other possible contributory factors requiring other treatments. When the original symptom, however, persists, the primary physician will order additional tests or refer the patient to a specialist in that field. Certainly routine annual examination will diagnose some of the early lesions, but these routine check-ups are usually more oriented toward general health factors and do not emphasize the possibility of early salivary gland neoplasia. It is rational to believe that the majority of these cases will be moderately or well advanced when first seen.

In the end, the final diagnosis is made by biopsy of the suspicious lesion. Because of the intricate anatomy adjacent to these tumors, biopsy may be complex. As the vast majority of these tumors develop in the submucosal elements of the minor salivary glands and the intraglandular tissues in major salivary glands, the technique of punch biopsy is not as readily applicable as it would be in an ulcerating squamous cell cancer of these areas. Therefore, excisional biopsy of the accessory minor salivary gland tumors, fine-needle aspiration biopsy in certain major salivary gland tumors, and formal open surgical approach for the less accessible neoplasm are satisfactory in the majority of cases. There are exceptions, where the approach to the tumor requires a preparatory procedure of exposure, such as in parotidectomy and blind biopsy in certain instances, by microsurgical sinus techniques, and by direct sinus exposure.

There is always the question concerning fine-needle aspiration biopsy and frozen-section diagnosis as a basis for proceeding with the definitive surgical extirpation. Fine-needle aspiration biopsy can have a

95% accuracy rate in the diagnosis of these salivary gland tumors; however, it must be recognized that this is an optimal figure and does not represent a universal level of accuracy. Frozen-section technique presents the pathologist with a larger volume of cells to be studied and should be more secure than fine-needle aspiration under optimal conditions. Frozen-section technique can usually be done immediately, whereas fine-needle aspiration often requires an interval of days prior to planned surgical treatment. Both of these methods of diagnosis have validity and can be used effectively under highly controlled circumstances, but it is also appropriate to recognize their potential weaknesses and to incorporate every other safeguard of confirmation and support before carrying out a major resection. If the contemplated procedure is a mutilating one, it is wise to have the patient evaluate all aspects of the operation and then sign the appropriate documents before proceeding. It may be efficient, tempting, and intelligent to attempt to organize the treatment in a single composite procedure, but these are special events with certain risks that must be assessed carefully beforehand with each surgeon and each patient.

Pain and Nerve Involvement

Pain was associated with this type of tumor in approximately 20% of the cases. Pain must be analyzed as an ache, a sharp intermittent sensation, or a sense of discomfort. It may be associated with hypoesthesia or anesthesia or referred to another site. It may only be present in connection with a physiological function, such as when swallowing. It may be mild or very severe. These variations depend on the size of the tumor, the special nerve involved, and the type of tissue affected by the tumor.

Ordinarily, pain is not expected in T1 tumors. The neoplasm must expand beyond its capsule and first invade parenchymal tissue before encountering sensory nerves and proprioceptors. This neoplasm is universally recognized as having an affinity for perineural spaces and, ultimately, axons. It is a slow process whose length depends on the proximity of neural tissues. It may take three to ten years for this invasion to occur. In most instances, growth in the nerve is centripetal. Pain is more common in recurrent adenoid cystic carcinoma, most likely due to the extensions into adjacent tissues and the longer historical time interval, allowing involvement of a sensory nerve.

There are multiple nerves in the head and neck area that can be involved by this tumor and can produce pain. In this series, each separate region of the head and neck had a different incidence of pain, depending on the proximity of the cancer to a sensory nerve and the extent of involvement of that nerve. It is interesting that almost half of the patients had some type of nerve invasion upon microscopy, but only about 20% complained of pain as a presenting symptom or developed it with recurrences. These figures are general baseline figures and after more exacting microscopic examinations and a more detailed history, one would most likely discover that the correlation of nerve involvement and the sensation of pain or discomfort would be somewhat higher.

The nerve elements which are most susceptible are the inframaxillary branches of the trigeminal nerve in adenoid cystic carcinoma of the maxilla. The sensory branches of this exceptional nerve also innervate the lips, the alveolus, the floor of the mouth, and the buccal areas. Adenoid cystic carcinoma in the minor salivary glands, the sublingual gland, and the submandibular gland invade the branches of this nerve at those specific regions and then spread centripetally toward the gasserian ganglion. As this affliction progresses, there may be tingling, "pins-and-needles" sensation, numbness, hypoesthesia, and, ultimately, total anesthesia. At this stage there is usually no pain.

Adenoid cystic cancer in the parotid gland may cause pain by involving the sensory elements of the facial nerve, the great auricular nerve, or auriculotemporal nerves. The lingual, alveolar, and hypoglossal nerves may be involved with adenoid cystic carcinoma in the floor of the mouth, alveolus, and tongue. Recurrent laryngeal, glossopharyngeal, and vagus nerves may be affected by adenoid cystic carcinoma in the pharynx, paralaryngeal, and upper tracheal regions. Adenoid cystic carcinomas which have reached the base of the skull or vertebrae place all of the cranial and spinal nerves in jeopardy.

It is well recognized that nerve invasion is an extremely serious prognostic sign in dealing with all types of cancer in the head and neck. This is particularly so with adenoid cystic carcinoma. It is essential, therefore, to obtain a negative frozen section on the proximal segment of any involved nerve, if it is technically possible. This is additional insurance against recurrence in that nerve, however, this advantage is almost always lost through recurrences in regional tissues and systemic metastases. In dealing with an essential nerve, such as the facial nerve, it is justified to carry out immediate nerve grafting as a rehabilitative technique.

Prognosis

There are no absolute rules that can define the prognosis in all of its aspects; however, there are at least 12 factors that can influence the progress of the disease. These features play a role in deductive thinking, but cannot control or predict all aspects of the biological process, as these are unknown. In a very general way, these factors can be used to make some predictions regarding prognosis.

Staging of the disease indicates the general gravity of the problem. Only 27% of the tumors in the series were classified as T1 lesions, 66% were represented in T2 and T3, and 7% in T4. These ominous figures create a baseline for the overall gravity of the disease.

The *volume of cancer cells* in the tumor is important in evaluating the burden and risks of controlling or curing it. It is reasonable to state that the volume of cancer cells is usually underestimated in almost every instance. The gravity of the prognosis exists in almost direct proportion to the volume of cancer cells.

Ulceration occurred in just less than 5% of the cases. It is an ominous sign because these tumors begin within a glandular structure and are either submucosal or intraglandular in the early stages. Ulceration represents advanced disease and classifies the neoplasm as T4.

Position of the neoplasm has a bearing on the prognosis. If the tumor is close to a vital structure or if the tumor is close to nerves, bone, or fascial spaces, the outlook is certainly more serious.

Histology of the tumor is now recognized as germane to prognosis. Of these cases, 78% were either tubular or cribriform in histological presentation. Both of these types are low-grade and have the best prognosis for cure. However, 22% were of the basaloid small-cell type, which proved to be more aggressive.

The *gland of origin* must also be considered. Adenoid cystic carcinoma in the minor salivary glands has a more serious prognosis than in the major salivary glands. This is an unfavorable situation, because the majority of these cancers originate in the minor salivary glands. The reason for this worsening of the prognosis is elucidated in this chapter under "staging."

Sex: The majority of adenoid cystic cancers occur in women and the overall outlook is slightly better in women than in men.

Age: Younger patients have in general a better prognosis than older patients.

Perineural invasion is an extremely serious prognostic sign. Of the patients in this series, 46% are reported to have had perineural invasion, but it is reasonable to state that the actual percentage is somewhat higher.

Local recurrence is an ominous sign; in this group, 74% of the patients were subject to at least one local recurrence. Local recurrence not only signifies failure of control of the primary tumor, but establishes the possibility of extended regional growth, perineural invasion, extension well beyond the limits of the original tumor, and an increased time interval that facilitates the possibility of systemic metastases.

Regional metastasis is uncommon with adenoid cystic carcinoma. Only 5% presented it at the initial examination and ultimately 12% developed it as the decades went by. It is, however, an additional, serious impediment to cure.

Systemic metastasis was present in only 3% initially, but ultimately over 50% of the patients manifested it in some organ or region of the body, 24% occurring within five years. The lung, the brain, and bone were the most common areas of occurrence, and the metatasis rarely assumed the form of a single, solid mass, but appeared more often in multiples and was rarely of the miliary type. These distant spreads appeared 15, 20, and even 30 years after the initial treatment of the primary tumor. This is a grave prognostic sign. Although metastases lend themselves to temporary control and palliation in many instances, they rarely facilitate permanent cure.

All of these clinical factors are combined in each case and are modified by immunological factors that can regulate the tempo of the disease process. It is therefore not possible to make accurate predictions in the early stages and usually not necessary to make them in the later stages of this disease.

Staging

In 1980, the American Joint Committee on Cancer Staging (AJCCS) published guidelines for the staging of tumors of the major salivary glands. Their classification, however, does not include cancers of the minor salivary glands, which make up the majority of the cases of adenoid cystic carcinoma. T1 in the major salivary gland includes tumors with a measurement of 2 cm or less. T2 includes those between 2 and 4 cm, T3 those between 4 and 6 cm, and T4A and T4B those over 6 cm without significant local extension, as well as tumors of any size with significant local extension. The AJCCS has also presented a classification of postsurgical residual tumor and a classification of tumor grade. These criteria are suitable for the major salivary glands, but unfortunately one of the very important aspects of adenoid cystic carcinoma arising in a minor salivary gland is not included. The staging of salivary gland tumors usually includes all types across the board, but it is obvious that those occurring in the minor salivary glands do not fit comfortably into these numerical measurements.

It is logical that staging be established on the basis of the size of the primary tumor and the presence or absence or regional and systemic metastases. This method is quite satisfactory for "surface" cancers, such as epitheliomas, but even here the measurements are made in centimeters from a horizontal and vertical axis. Although this can establish the size of the surface of the tumor, it does not indicate the depth or the volume of the cancer cells. Both of these latter features are very significant in evaluating prognosis. Nor does it take into account the real size of the cancer with respect to the tissue or organ that contains it. This is particularly true in the case of tumors of the salivary glands, among which there is a great variation in size. For example, an adenoid cystic carcinoma in the parotid gland is quite different from one in a minor salivary gland. The tumor beginning in the parotid gland may take years to be discovered and to reach a size that can be measured clinically, and still never transgress the boundaries of the gland. Its growth is contained within that gland, within its restricting architecture and biologic forces. The tumor has not gone beyond its site of origin. However, when a tumor arises in a minor salivary gland which measures only a few millimeters in diameter, it becomes greater than the size of the gland in a short period of time and spreads beyond its capsule into the adjacent soft tissues or bone into a new architecture and biologic environment. None of these factors are taken into consideration when staging these different cancers; however, it is recognized that the prognosis for minor salivary gland tumors is more serious than for major salivary gland tumors. This may be explained by the fact that a T1 or T2 adenoid cystic carcinoma in a minor salivary gland is more advanced biologically and physically than a T1 or T2 adenoid cystic carcinoma in the parotid gland or submandibular gland. This point illustrates that clinical staging can never be made scientifically accurate and that modifications and perhaps ultimately a completely new concept of staging are needed.

Of the tumors in this series, 66% were staged T2 and T3; only 27% were classified as T1, and 4% were T4. It is likely that all of these primary tumor measurements were lower than the tumors' actual dimensions. Before imaging techniques were available, the assessment of the size of many of these tumors was difficult and inaccurate. CT scanning and MRI have greatly enhanced the accuracy of this estimation. Nevertheless, it is still reasonable to state that a large percentage of these neoplasms are understaged.

Imaging
(Figs. 5.1–5.11)

There is no radiologic imaging technique that is capable of diagnosing a histologic neoplastic process. Some images are strongly suggestive of certain pathologic entities, and a process may be developed in the future that will eliminate the need for a histologic diagnosis, but at the present time, histologic diagnosis is a sine qua non. However, this in no way diminishes the amazing value of the new imaging techniques. In fact, it has been proposed that a system of classification be developed from these images.

Radiologic evaluation of adenoid cystic carcinoma is multifaceted. Various diagnostic imaging techniques are required to detect the presence of the disease, to define the extent of the tumor, and to depict involvement or destruction of adjacent structures. Radiologic techniques are also used in surveillance of tumor recurrence, detecting metastatic spread, and monitoring the efficacy of therapeutic modalities.

Adenoid cystic carcinoma has no specific radiologic features that lead to a definitive X-ray diagnosis; however, a variety of radiologic findings may give indirect evidence of the tumor's presence, although infection or inflammatory processes may be enhanced in the image and may create inaccuracies in interpretation.

Plain film radiography was the primary radiologic tool in early management of this disease; however, its inability to detect or assess early lesions has limited its role.

Polytomography offered definite advantages over plain X-ray, but has been surpassed in recent years by the high definition offered by CT scanning and MRI techniques. The latter two modalities offer distinct advantages in management of this disease process. Their ability to define soft tissue and bone changes has given the clinician a more accurate assessment of the dimension and location of the primary tumor even in its early stages.

Plain radiography takes advantage of subtle footprints left by the tumor progression and may give some estimates as to the extent and aggressiveness of the disease. The techniques are limited, in that they are neither specific nor particularly sensitive. Plain films are said to show evidence of orbital involvement by ACC in 30–40% of cases (Forbes et al., 1980). The growth of adenoid cystic carcinomas is characterized by slowly progressive infiltration. This may be manifested by sinus opacification, widening of neural foramina, as well as bony expansion or destruction or both. Evidence of maxillary nerve invasion may be seen through widening of the infraorbital foramen or foramen rotundum. Perineural spread along the mandibular branch of the trigeminal nerve may be evidenced in expansion of the mental foramen or the foramen ovale. Spread through other foramina is more difficult to visualize using plain film techniques.

It should be mentioned that the existence of perineural lymphatics has been questioned by several investigators (Dodd et al., 1970). Some authors, noting the relative resistance of nerve fibers to tumor invasion, have proposed that adenoid cystic carcinomas spread by following the path of least resistance along nerve sheaths.

Depending on the location in which they arise, adenoid cystic carcinomas may be visualized as soft tissue masses in plain film radiography or complex motion tomography. Tumors arising in the nasopharynx may be seen as submucosal masses arising from the posterior-superior or lateral walls. The lesions may extend toward the clivus, even manifesting bony erosion of that structure. ACC in the larynx may be detected as a soft tissue mass which may erode cartilaginous structures. Findings of ACC in the paranasal sinuses may include a soft tissue mass, pressure erosion of bone from slow growth, destruction of bone indicating invasion associated with malignancy, and invasion of surrounding structures. When examining potential lesions of the paranasal sinuses with plain X-rays, one must pay particular attention to the medial wall of the antrum, the orbital floor, the ethmomaxillary plate, and the lateral wall of the olfactory fossa. This latter finding is said to have a 95% accuracy rate in detecting anterior fossa spread from nasal cavity or paranasal sinus tumors, according to Pagani et al. (1979).

Weber and Stanton (1984) present an algorithm for the radiologic evaluation of tumors in the nasal cavity and the paranasal sinuses. Changes in the contour of thickness of bony boundaries, enlargement of bony foramina, unilateral obstruction of the nasal cavity, and opacification of a sinus not responding to appropriate antibiotic therapy should all arouse the clinician's suspicion. In addition to the plain film signs, clinical presentation of persistent facial pain, paresthesia, ocular signs of exophthalmos, diploplia, decreased vision, cheek and periorbital swelling, and bloody nasal discharge should prompt further investigation with CT scanning or MRI. If none of these signs or symptoms are evident, the clincian should continue with conservative medical management, provided adequate resolution is demonstrated on follow-up plain films. Osborn and McIff (1982) suggest angiography to rule out a vascular lesion if a tumor shows marked enhancement upon administration of contrast material.

CT scanning has increased exponentially the ability of the clinician to evaluate and manage salivary gland lesions of the head and neck. This is particularly true in the case of adenoid cystic carcinoma, where information about both bone and soft tissues is required. Axial and coronal imaging is often quite helpful in evaluating tumors of the orbit and paranasal sinuses.

CT findings in orbital adenoid cystic carcinomas have been described in many publications. Spencer described in 1986 the appearance of lacrimal gland lesions. The lesions are located primarily in the superior temporal quadrant. He noted that ACC usually showed irregular and serrated borders. Of these tumors, 80% show CT evidence of adjacent bone changes, either destruction or sclerosis. Extension posteriorly in the orbit is more typical with adenoid cystic carcinomas than with benign mixed tumors. Envelopment of the lateral rectus muscle by tumor may be demonstrated in certain cases. Hesselink et al. (1978) note the ability of computed tomography to delineate grossly cystic or solid areas of lacrimal tumors. Calcification of the lesions may also be noted. This may help differentiate ACC from other tumors, as calcification is unusual in this neoplasm.

CT scanning may be helpful in detecting orbital invasion by adenoid cystic carcinomas originating in adjacent paranasal sinuses or the nasal cavity. Hesselink and Weber (1982) state that "CT is the most definite imaging procedure for the evaluation of secondary involvement of the orbit by neoplasms." Malignant lesions generally invade the orbit directly through destruction of adjacent bone. Spread may also occur through the inferior orbital fissure or through the nasolacrimal duct. Access to the orbit via the inferior orbital fissure may also be gained by lesions involving the pterygopalatine fossa or the infratemporal fossa.

One must also be aware that orbital ACC may itself invade adjacent structures. This would include intracranial spread, invasion of the paranasal sinuses, the pterygopalatine fossa, and so on. CT can be of great value in detecting early involvement of these areas. It must be realized, however, that ACC may extend beyond the macroscopic tumor boundaries so that CT may not detect early microscopic invasion, especially along perineural routes (Mafee et al.).

As in the case of plain film imaging, there are a set of CT findings that give evidence of perineural spread in adenoid cystic carcinoma. Lee et al. (1985) describe three cases of intracranial perineural spread. The lesions consisted of hyperdense, extradural masses that mimicked meningiomas. Curtin et al. (1984) emphasize the importance of the pterygopalatine fossa (PPF) as a key crossroad in the extension of the tumor along the trigeminal nerve. Obliteration of fat in this region is said to be a sensitive indicator of perineural spread. Spread of tumors into this area may occur even if there has been no evidence of bone destruction. This is referred to as the "resurfacing" phenomenon, where a tumor spreads silently from one area through a bony canal and reappears in the relatively loose confines of a fossa at the other end of the bony canal. Tumors of the palate can track through the greater and lesser palatine foramen into the PPF. Tumors in the maxillary sinus may invade this space by following the infraorbital nerve, the superior alveolar nerve, or by direct bone erosion posteriorly into the PPF. The fat of this fossa can be followed into the apex of the orbit. Other signs of perineural invasion include enlargement of neural foramina, increased enhancement in the region of Meckel's cavity (gasserian ganglion), and atrophy of the muscles innervated by the trigeminal nerve. It must be emphasized that perineural spread may occur in a retrograde or antegrade fashion. Adenoid cystic carcinoma may also spread through marrow spaces or along the periosteum.

Maffee et al. state that CT scanning may be the imaging modality of choice in the evaluation of temporal bone tumors. Its ability to delineate fine bone detail and to show intracranial extension offers many advantages over other radiologic techniques. Curtin, Wolfe, and Snyderman (1983) note the ability of CT to identify the facial nerve between its exit from the stylomastoid foramen and its entrance into the parotid gland. Alteration of the fat surrounding the nerve allows for the study of it in pathologic processes.

Evaluation of tracheal ACC reveals some of the shortcomings of CT imaging. While it accurately shows extratracheal extension of the tumor in axial cuts, CT tends to underestimate the longitudinal extension of the lesion. This is due to volume-averaging in the axial mode. It is difficult to obtain direct coronal images in this region, and sagittal reconstructions from axial cuts are subject to the same volume-averaging limitations. CT also fails to identify pathologic adenopathy of less than 1.5 cm. In addition, CT is felt by Spizarny et al. (1986) to underestimate invasion of adjacent organs. Evaluation of tracheal lesions is one area where complex motion tomography in coronal and sagittal planes may remain the procedure of choice. MRI of the trachea has yet to overcome the motion artifact during respiration and requires further refinement.

ACC of the parotid gland is well visualized using CT techniques. Isodense lesions may be delinated using CT sialography. It is in the arena of the evaluation of tumors of the parotid gland that *magnetic resonance imaging* (MRI) first proved itself as an invaluable tool in the management of salivary gland neoplasms. Several reports have compared the two techniques in imaging parotid gland tumors. Both modalities are capable of demonstrating medium-sized and large-sized tumors. Teresi et al. (1987) describe the MRI characteristics of parotid neoplasms. They showed intermediate to high signal on T1-weighted images, slightly more than muscle but less than fat. T2-weighted sequences showed more obvious tissue differences. Schaefer et al. (1985) feel that MRI is equal to or better than CT scanning in several aspects. MRI does not expose the patient to radiation, nor does it require contrast injection. Direct coronal or sagittal images are obtainable without repositioning the patient. There is no artifactual degradation of magnetic resonance images from dental fillings. The internal architecture of the parotid gland and the tumor mass is felt to be visualized better with MRI. Schaefer et al. see only the lengthy processing time required for MRI as a limitation to the technique. Mandelblatt et al. (1987) feel that the "conspicuity" of parotid gland tumors in MRI was superior to imaging done with CT scanning in seven cases, that both techniques were equal in six cases, and that MRI was inferior in one case. In this report, one tumor was visualized on MRI that was not shown in CT scanning. The facial nerve could be visualized within the parotid gland on thin sectioning with sagittal MRI. The relation of small-sized and medium-sized tumors to the facial nerve is consistently demonstrated on MRI in Teresi et al.'s report. Mandelblatt et al. feel that tumor margins may be better evaluated with MRI. Parotid gland tissue was also thought to be distinguished more easily from surrounding structures with MRI.

There have been attempts at using magnetic resonance images to discern whether tumors are benign or malignant. Tumor margination, apparent infiltration, and intralesional characteristics have all been tested for their predictive value in determining malignancy. To date, there are no reliable characteristics in MRI or CT scanning that will make that determination.

MRI may offer some clues as to the relative vascularity of various neoplasms. Som et al. (1987) describe 40 neoplasms of the parapharyngeal space. Although ACC was not included in the series, it is possible to extrapolate as to how MRI can be of value in managing ACC in this region. Most tumors had an intermediate signal on T1 imaging and a high signal on T2-weighted imaging. Vascular tumors, such as paragangliomas, showed a "salt and pepper" configuration of high-flow and low-flow states. Salivary gland lesions tended to show a more homogeneous appearance. Some larger lesions showed focal areas of low signal intensity, however, corresponding to dystrophic calcification or fibrosis.

On occasion, it may not be clear whether the location of a lesion in the parapharyngeal space is intraparotid or extraparotid. MRI is often able to make that distinction on the basis of the integrity of a fat pad surrounding the gland. Infiltrating tumors in Som's series were most likely malignant, but a zone of inflammation around a benign tumor may give the same appearance.

Metastatic spread of ACC to neck nodes is not common, occurring in 10% or less of cases. Its detection will have an impact on therapeutic planning for the patient. CT scanning and MRI techniques give the clinician the ability to detect pathologic nodes in certain circumstances. Lymph nodes in levels 1, 2, and upper level 3 are considered pathologic when they exceed 1.5 cm in diameter. Nodes in the remaining levels greater than 1 cm are likewise deemed abnormal. Nodal necrosis may be visualized equally in CT or MRI. High signal intensity on T2 imaging within a lymph node corresponds to sites of tumor necrosis. There are some guidelines which may be used to separate malignant nodes from inflammatory nodes. A thick, irregular zone of enhancement around a necrotic central area indicates inflammation (for example, tuberculosis or infected branchial cleft cyst). A thin enhancing rim with some nodularity is consistent with a malignant metastasis. A node which enhances upon administration of intravenous contrast material is most likely inflammatory. Whith the exception of spread from papillary carcinoma of the thyroid, calcification within a lymph node is most often a result of inflammatory or granulomatous disease. While CT has been shown to demonstrate extranodal spread even in a small node, neither CT nor MRI is capable at this point of detecting microscopic involvement in a normal-sized non-cavitating node.

Radiologic investigation is essential in the early detection of recurrent disease or metastatic spread. A program of routine radiologic surveillance should be established for each patient following initial treatment of his or her adenoid cystic carcinoma. This would include CT scanning or MRI of the primary site. The interval of scanning will depend on the location of the primary tumor and its accessibility to physical examination, the aggressiveness of the initial lesion, the size of the lesion, and the form of initial therapy (surgery vs. radiotherapy). Scans are usually obtained every 6 to 18 months. A high percentage of ACC spreads to the lungs. Yearly chest X-ray is recommended to detect its occurrence.

It is hoped that, as imaging techniques continue to develop, diagnosis of adenoid cystic carcinoma and other head and neck malignancies may be made in earlier stages. Furthermore, it is hoped that advances in radiologic investigation will detect minute spread of diseases such as adenoid cystic carcinoma so as to enhance treatment planning.

Imaging 35

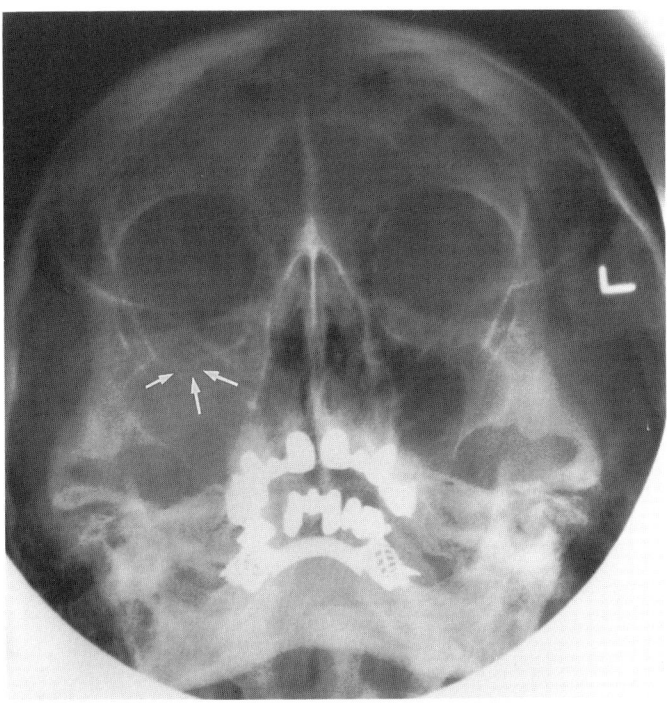

Fig. 5.**1** **Plain film radiograph** (Waters view) showing opacification of the right maxillary sinus and widening of the right infraorbital foramen (arrows) by a massive adenoid cystic carcinoma

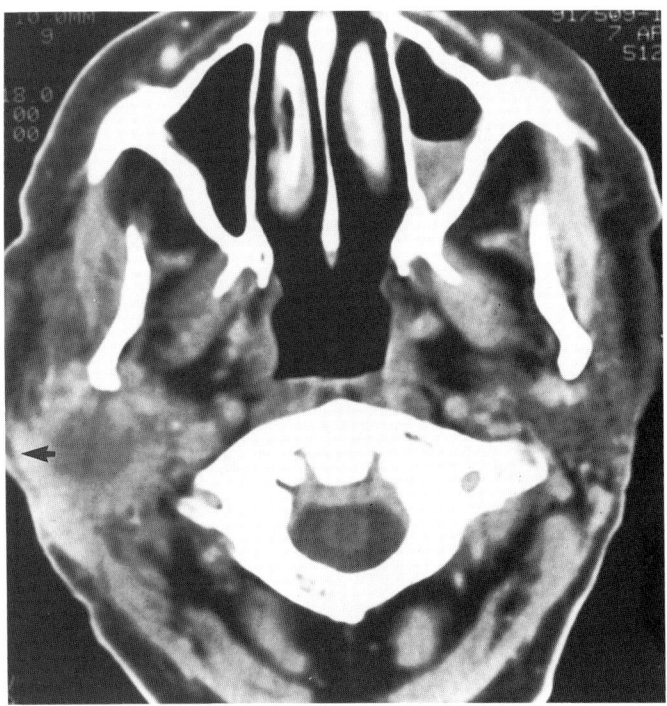

Fig. 5.**2** **Large adenoid cystic carcinoma (arrow) in the right parotid** (axial CT scan). The patient had facial nerve weakness on the involved side. (Courtesy of Dr. Joseph Castro, Radiation Oncology Department, Lawerence–Berkeley Laboratory, University of California at Berkeley)

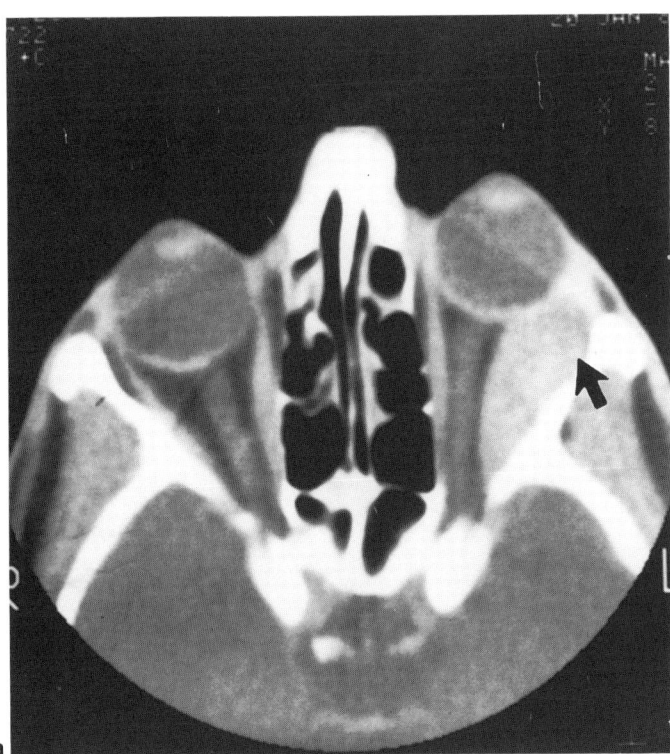

Fig. 5.**3a, b** **Adenoid cystic carcinoma (arrow) originating in the lacrimal gland, showing proptosis. a** Coronal view, **b** axial view. (Courtesy of Dr. Joseph Castro, Radiation Oncology

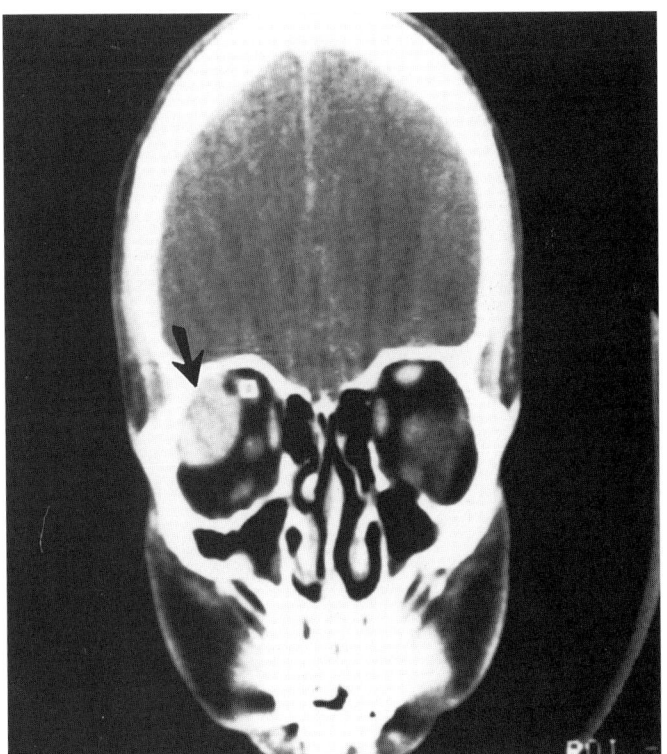

Department, Lawrence–Berkeley Laboratory, University of California at Berkeley)

36   5 Diagnosis

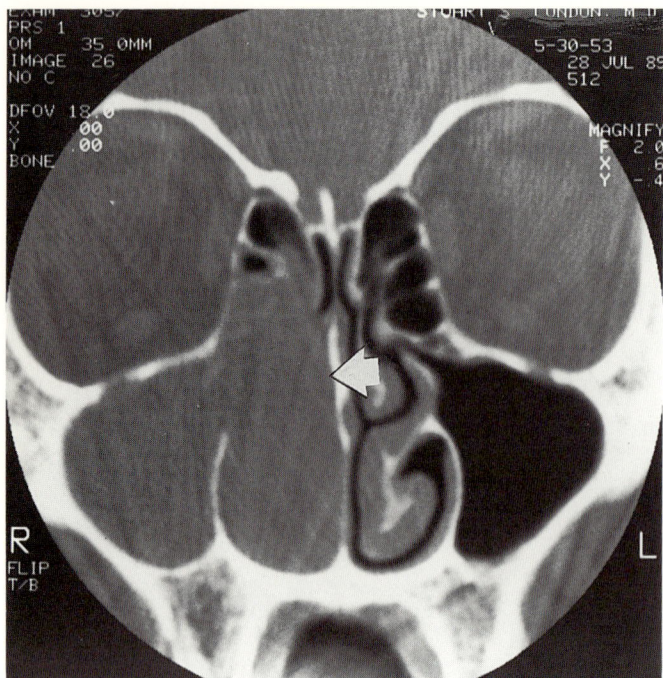

Fig. 5.**4 Bony erosion caused by a large adenoid cystic carcinoma (arrow) originating in the ethmoidal region.** (Coronal CT scan, courtesy of Dr. Joseph Castro, Radiation Oncology Department, Lawrence–Berkeley Laboratory, University of California at Berkeley)

Fig. 5.**5 a–c Large adenoid cystic carcinoma (arrow) involving the left maxillary sinus and nasal cavity. a, b** MRI, **c** CT scan. (Courtesy of Dr. Joseph Castro, Radiation Oncology Department, Lawrence–Berkeley Laboratory, University of California at Berkeley)

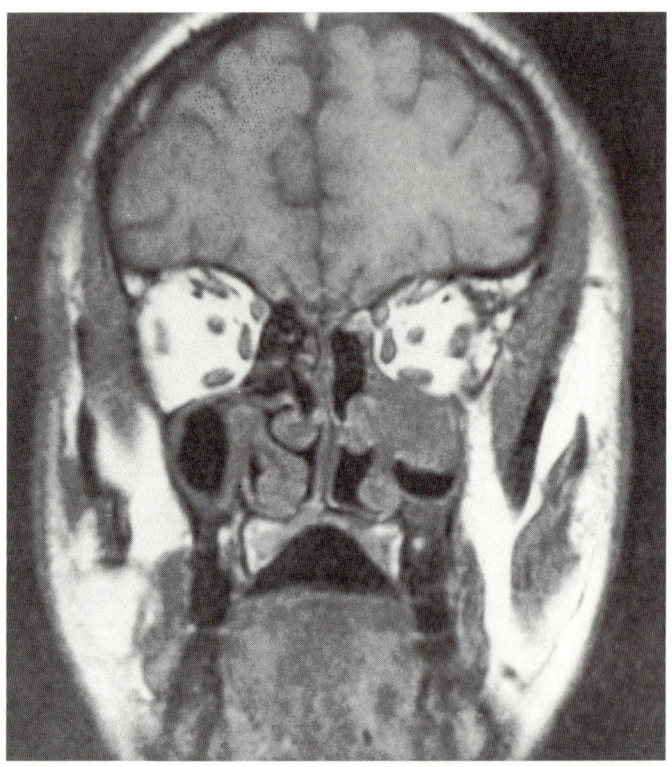

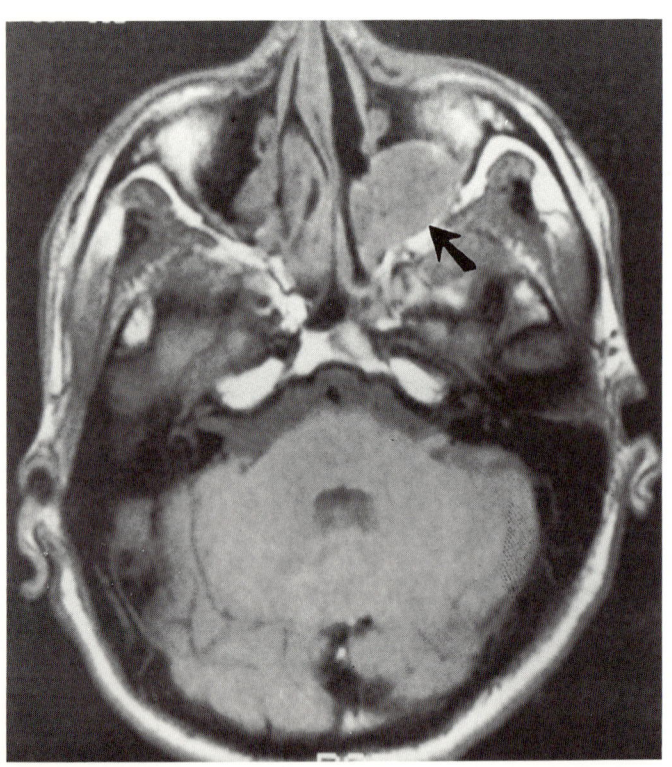

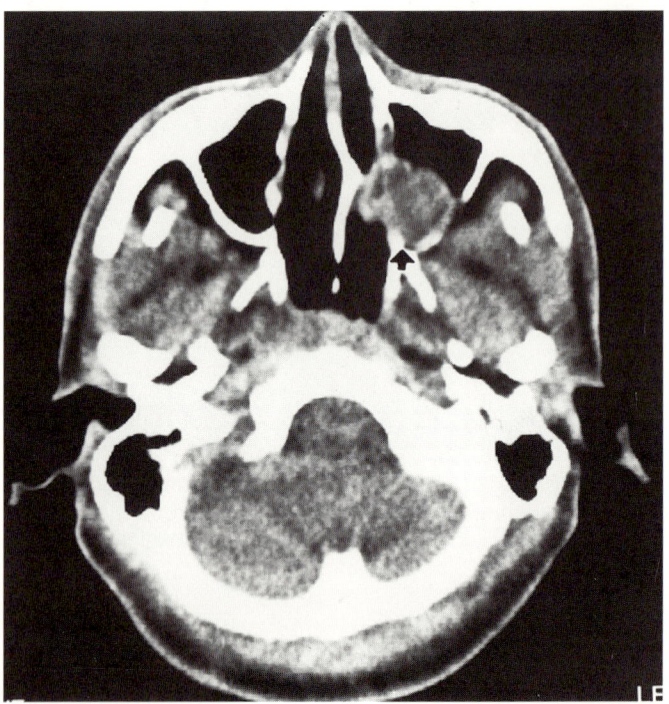

Imaging 37

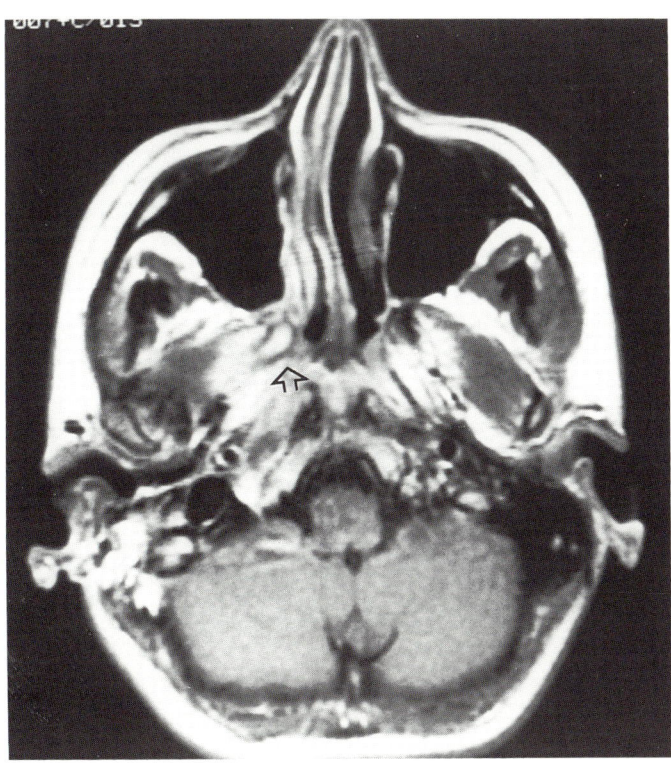

Fig. 5.**6a** **Subtle adenoid cystic carcinoma (arrow) which originated in the nasopharynx** (CT scan). The tumor arose in Rosenmüller's fossa and extended posteriorly into the cavernous sinus region

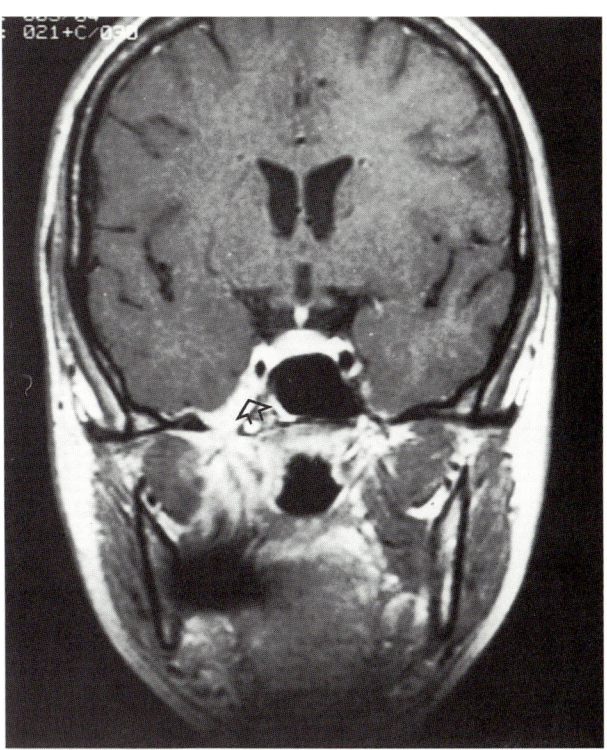

Fig. 5.**6b** The tumor (arrow) may also be seen extending inferiorly into the pterygopalatine fossa

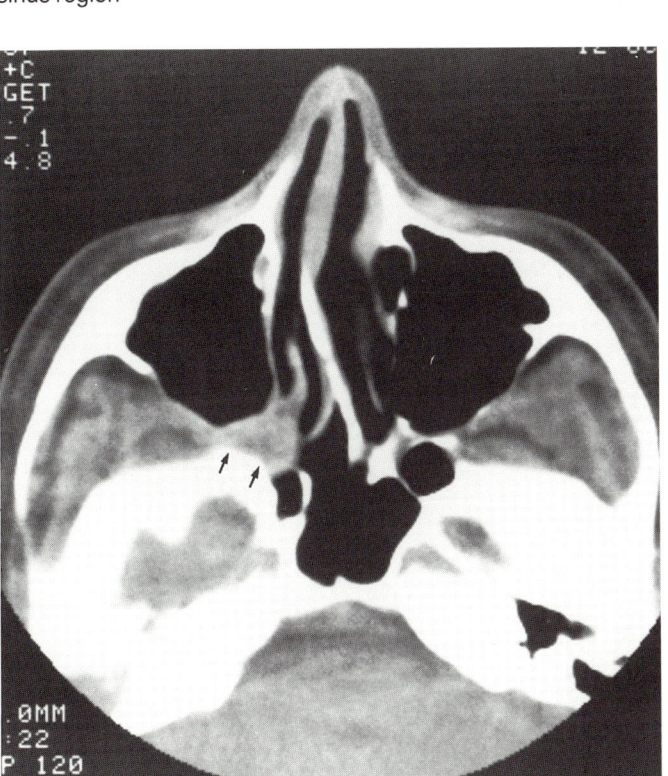

Fig. 5.**6c** MRI scan. The patient had presented with unilateral serous otitis. The lesion (arrow) was only apparent after radiologic examination

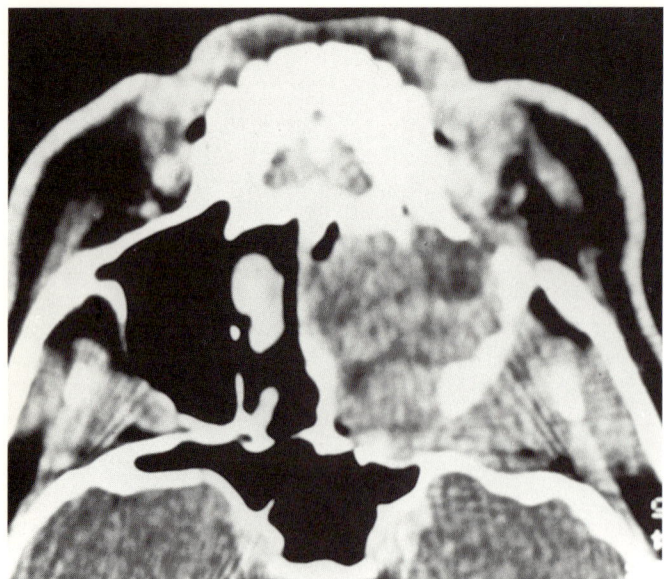

Fig. 5.**7a** Extensive adenoid cystic cancer involving a major portion of the nasal cavity and antrum, and extending posteriorly toward the base of the skull

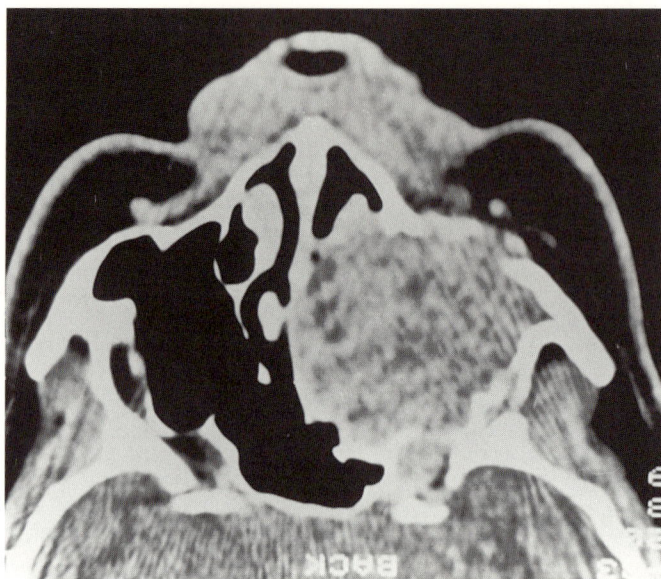

Fig. 5.**7b** It is seen extending into the area of the hard and soft palates

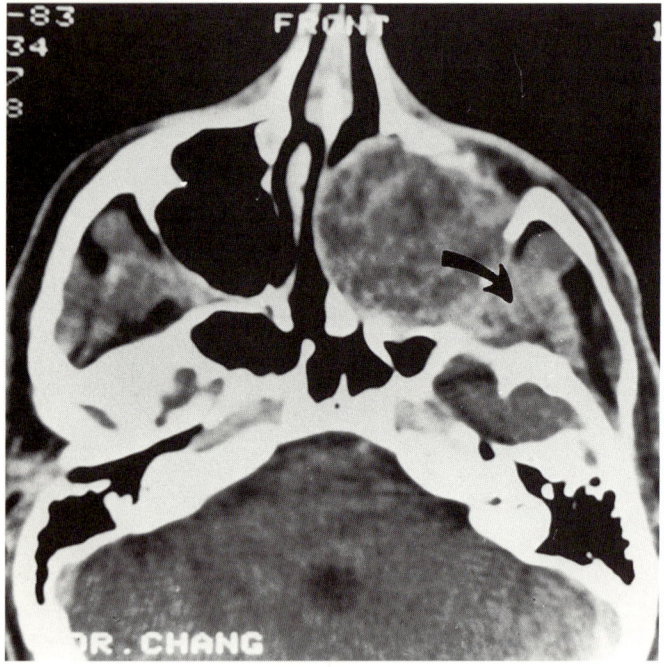

Fig. 5.**7c** It is also extending into the infratemporal fossa (arrow)

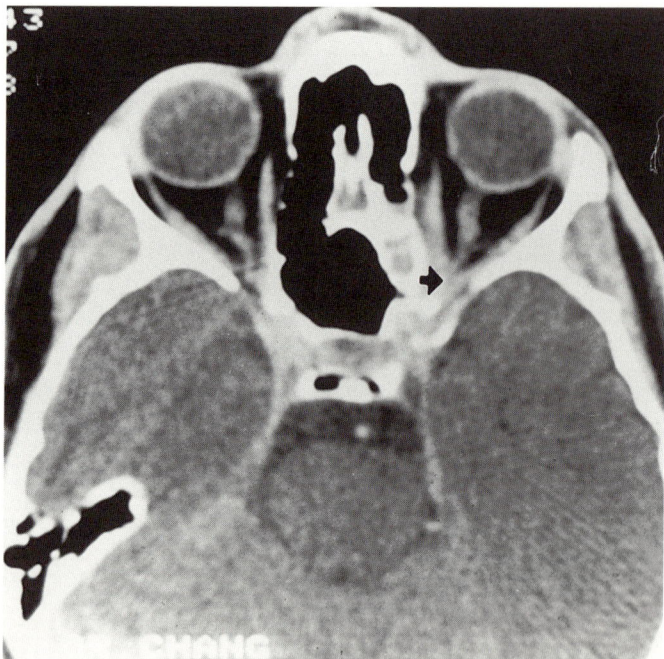

Fig. 5.**7d** The cancer is compromising the apex of the orbit (arrow)

Imaging 39

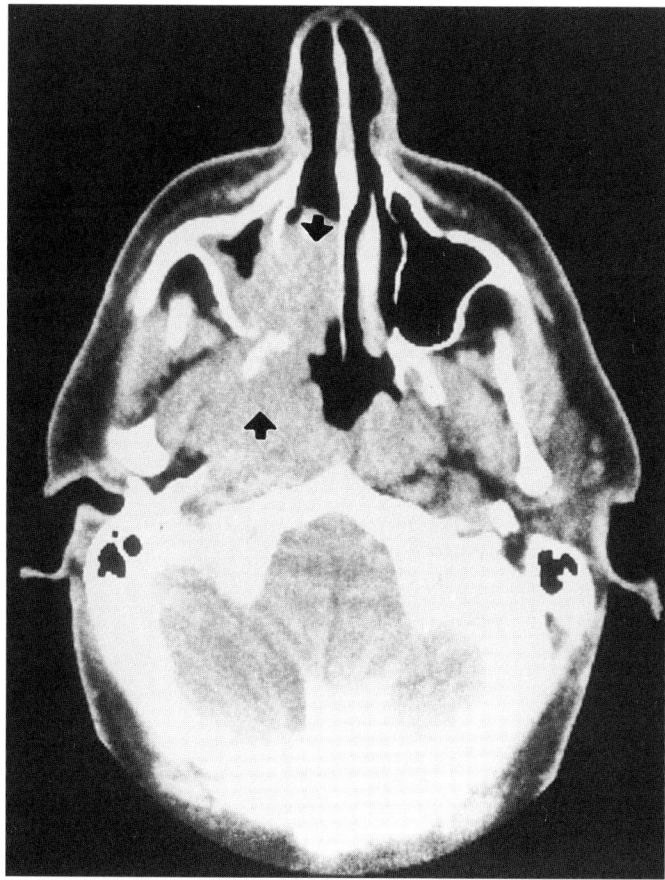

Fig. 5.8a **Adenoid cystic cancer involves the nasal cavity, antrum, and posterior nasopharynx (arrows)**

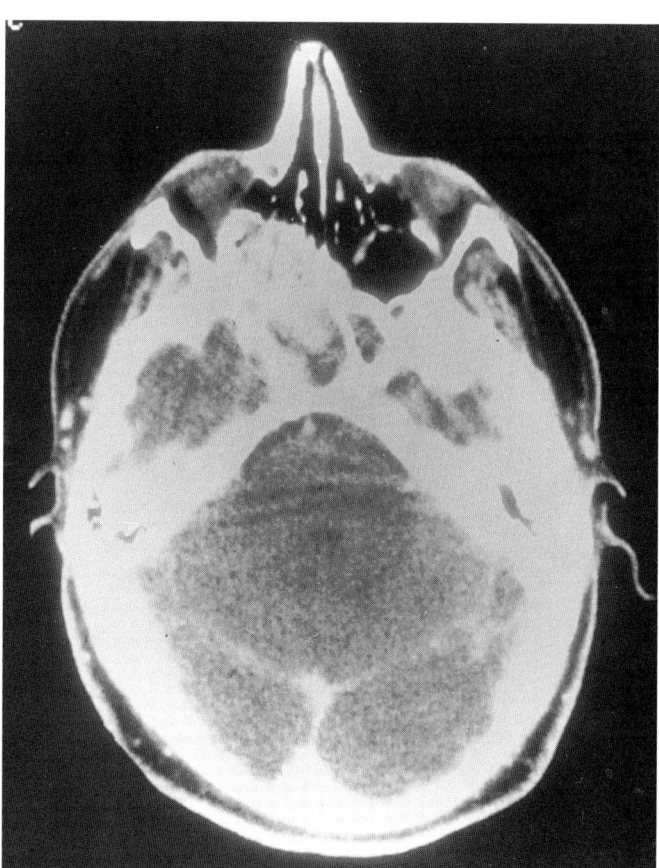

Fig. 5.8b It also extends into the sphenoid

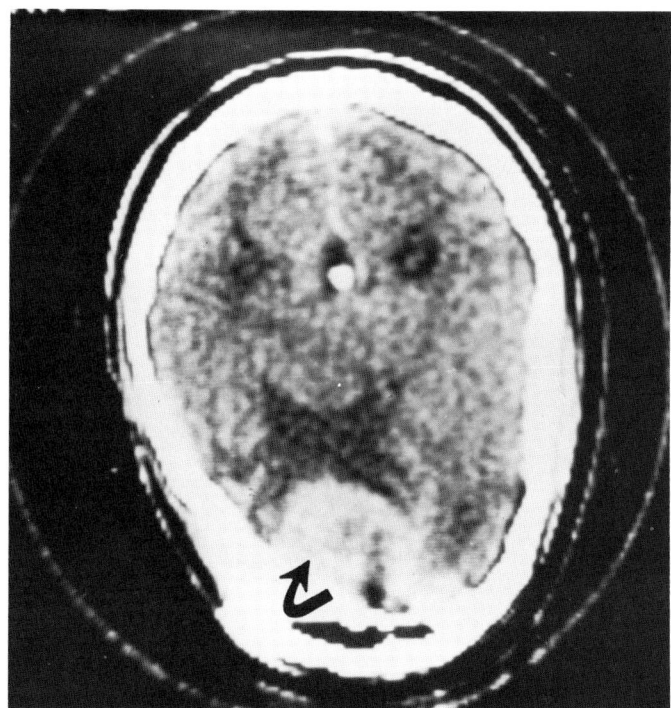

Fig. 5.9a **Adenoid cystic cancer of the ethmoids** has invaded the base of the skull and the brain (arrow)

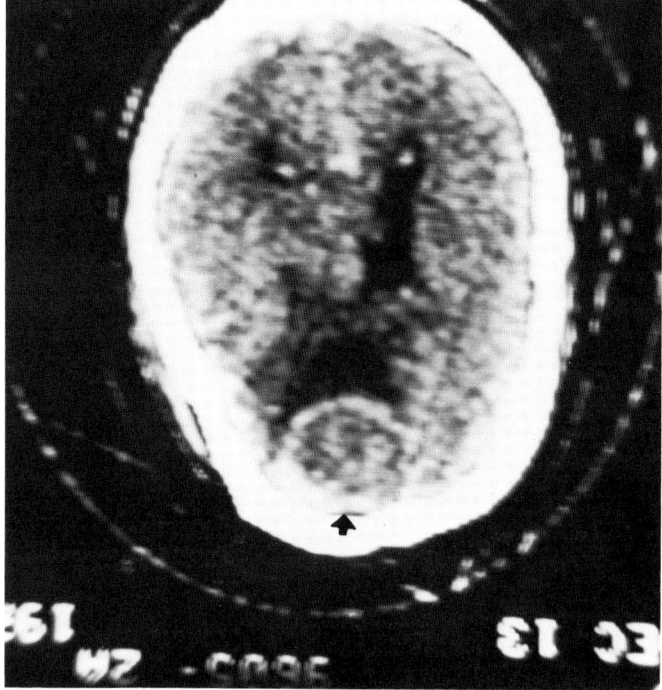

Fig. 5.9b It has also compromised the frontal sinus. The patient had no intracranial symptoms and this most likely would not have been diagnosed without CT scanning

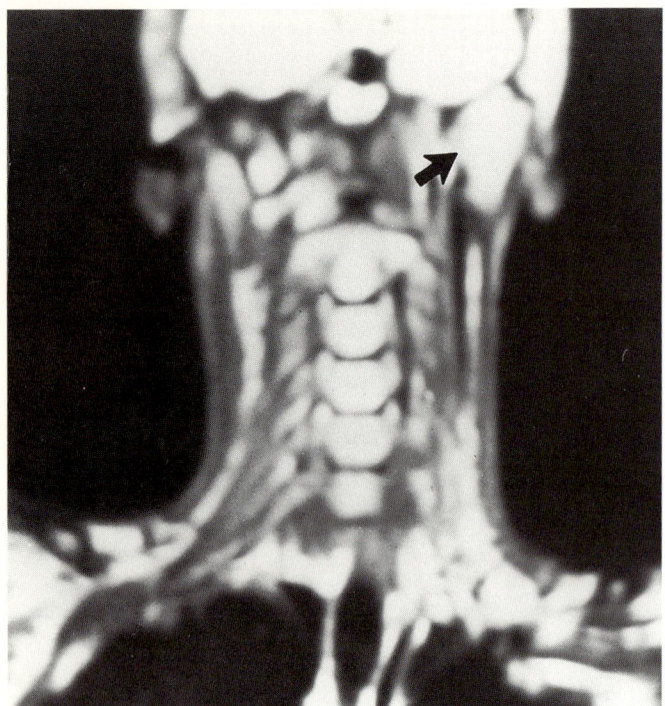
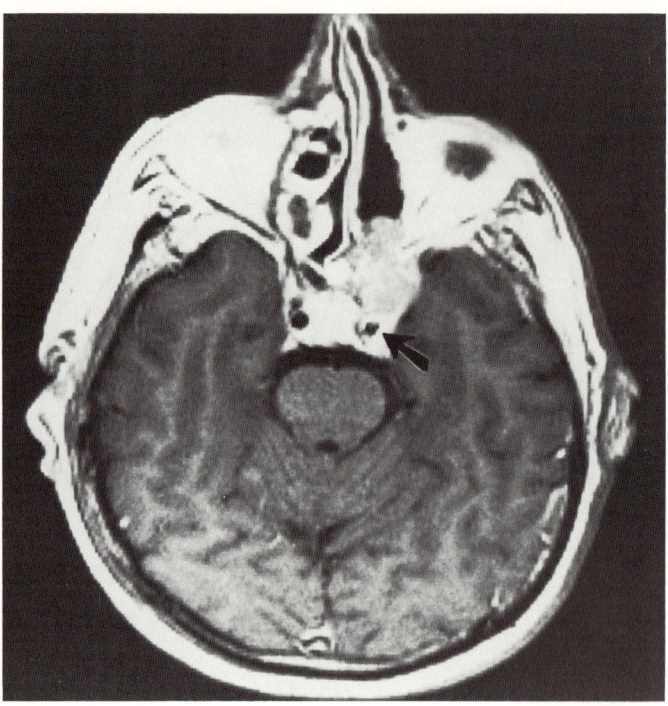

Fig. 5.**10 Adenoid cystic cancer of the tail of the left parotid gland,** showing extent and position (arrow)

Fig. 5.**11 Recurrent adenoid cystic carcinoma (12 years) of posterior nasal cavity, sphenoid, and base of skull,** showing also involvement of the cavernous sinus, internal carotid artery, and intracranium (arrow)

6
Tumor Behavior

Predictables

This tumor covers a broad range of predictables and unpredictables. The predictables are distilled from tumor behavior observed in the vast majortity of the cases, and the strategy of management has been developed on the basis of these predictables. This outline of biological behavior is, of course, modified according to the actual clinical behavior of the disease in each individual case.

The overriding predictable is that approximately 60–70% of patients with adenoid cystic carcinomas in the major salivary glands and 80–90% of those with ACC of the minor salivary glands will ultimately die of the disease. These data are very discouraging, but there are other predictable factors that are less so. Only a very small percentage of patients die within the first three years. The vast majority die between five and ten years after initial treatment. The exceptions to this general rule are those individuals who have delayed their treatment for three years or more, and those who almost show a tolerance for their disease postoperatively and who go on for 10, 20, even 30 years.

The tumor's location, its volume or staging, and its histology influence the predictables. Minor salivary glands have a more serious prognosis than major salivary glands; some reasons for this are stated in chapter 10, under "Morbidity and Mutilation." The small, compact, basaloid histologic type of adenoid cystic carcinoma is more serious than the cylindromatous or cribriform types. Tumors located in inaccessible regions are usually not diagnosed early, contain a large volume of cancer cells, and are more difficult to operate on than those in major salivary glands. The vast majority of cases are treated within these biological perimeters, and are either cured or ultimately develop a local recurrence.

This presents us with another predictable: 70–80% of these cases will develop one or more local recurrences. This is an ominous sign and usually means incurability. It is not imminently fatal, however, as local recurrence can usually be treated and rarely compromises a vital structure for an indefinite length of time. 17% of patients were living with disease and 13% were free of disease after the treatment of a local recurrence. Obviously, these 30% of patients will be in and out of a treatment program until their cancer has compromised a vital organ system.

Another predictable factor is the high probability of systemic metastases. Approximately 8% of the patients in this series of 406 cases had metastases at the initial examination. Only 5% of these metastases were in the regional lymph nodes. Between 5 and 10 years later, however, the lung became the primary location of metastases. Brain and bone were also sites for a small percentage in this unique process of systemic metastases which extends over a period of 20 to 30 years. There is an axiom which states that patients who continuously have local recurrences ultimately develop metastases to the lung. The therapeutic program chosen to treat systemic metastases is very important, as it marks the beginning of the dying process which may extend over 5 or 10 years.

There are other predictables, such as the incidence and gravity of perineural invasion, the free margins at the first operation, and the beneficial effects of irradiation given either for palliation or to improve the chances of cure. Although this disease is more common in women, there is no significant difference in curability between the sexes. All of these predictables and their counterpoint unpredictables create a composite picture of a low grade, but very pernicious cancer that can involve from 3 to 30 years of your life with local recurrences and, ultimately, systemic metastases. However, if all of the predictables are used in an optimal manner toward a cure, for example, adequate resection and complementary radiotherapy, one can hope to have done the best for the patient.

Unexplained Clinical Behavior and Unusual Cases

It is appropriate to discuss this subject to expose the broad gamut of clinical behavior a small percentage of these neoplasms has, and to emphasize that we actually know very little about the fundamental aspects of tumor biology. This not only applies to adenoid cystic carcinoma, but all malignant tumors. Perhaps adenoid cystic carcinoma is more unique in this respect, in that it was initially considered to be a benign tumor with a histologic picture that not only overlapped with other tumors, but also defied accurate microscopic documentation and classification in relation to its clinical behavior for over one hundred years. Many of these misconceptions have been clarified, but there remain enigmas and unpredictables that amaze the clinician and unsettle the treatment program.

A short discussion of four unusual cases will demonstrate the broad spectrum of behavior this tumor is capable of. These four cases present a range of unpredictable clinical behavior that lends itself to considerable speculation but no specific conclusion.

Case 1. This case presents low-grade chronicity of untreated adenoid cystic carcinoma for a quarter of a century and then overwhelming systemic metastases and regional recurrence following an aggressive ablative surgical procedure. Up to this time, the tumor had been a local, clinical problem without microscopic diagnosis and not seriously interfering with the patient's day-to-day activities. It was gradually extending and invading all regional tissues, however, increasing the number of cancer cells until their number was out of proportion to that of the host, at which point it then behaved as an uncontrollable aggressive cancer (Fig. 6.1). The fundamental question is whether in this case, this mass should have been excised 25 years before, and whether this would have presented a possibility for cure at that time, or if

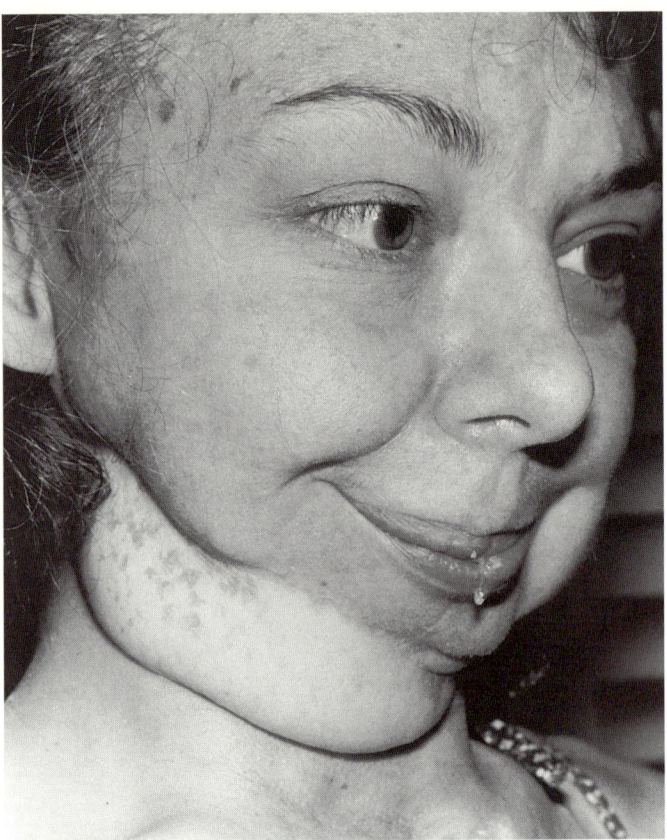

Fig. 6.1a **This patient had untreated adenoid cystic carcinoma of the submandibular gland for 25 years.** At the time of surgery it had involved the mandible, floor of the mouth, tongue, neck, and had extended toward the base of the skull

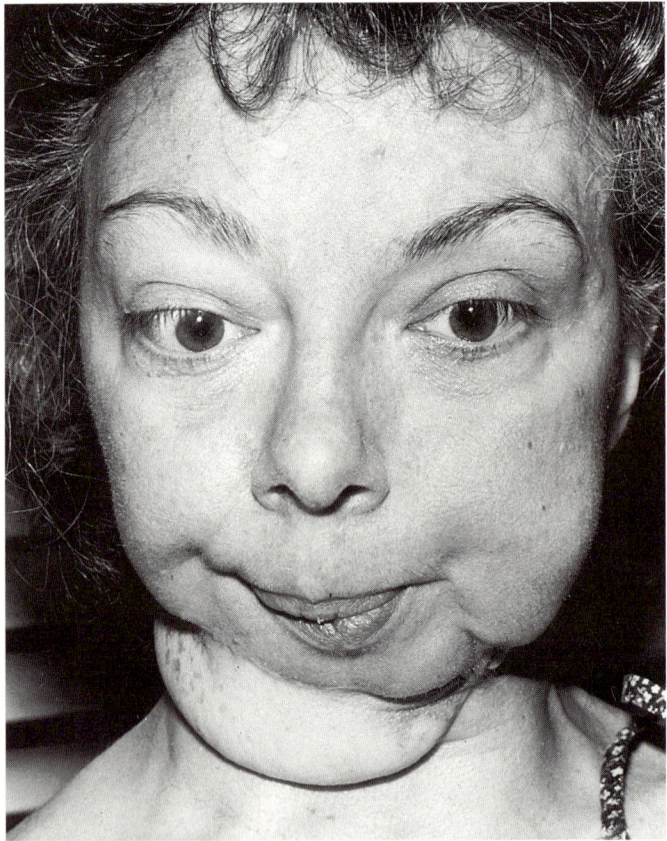

Fig. 6.1b It was treated with a gemini pectoralis major myocutaneous flap with an internal and external lining. The patient developed pulmonary metastases and was dead within a year

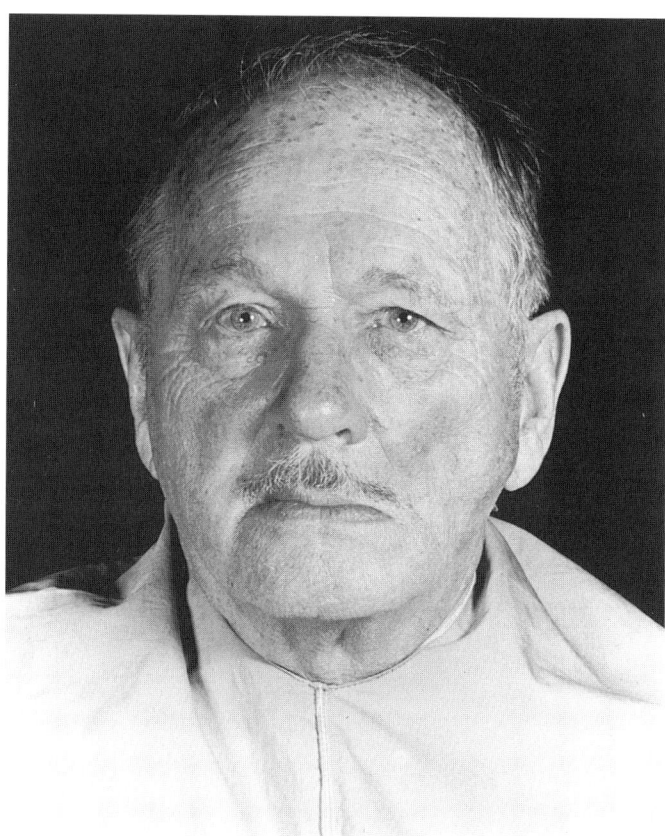

Fig. 6.2a **This patient had had an adenoid cystic cancer of the left buccal area removed 16 years prior to this recurrence.** He had never been treated with radiotherapy. On the original slides, there had been a misdiagnosis of benign mixed tumor

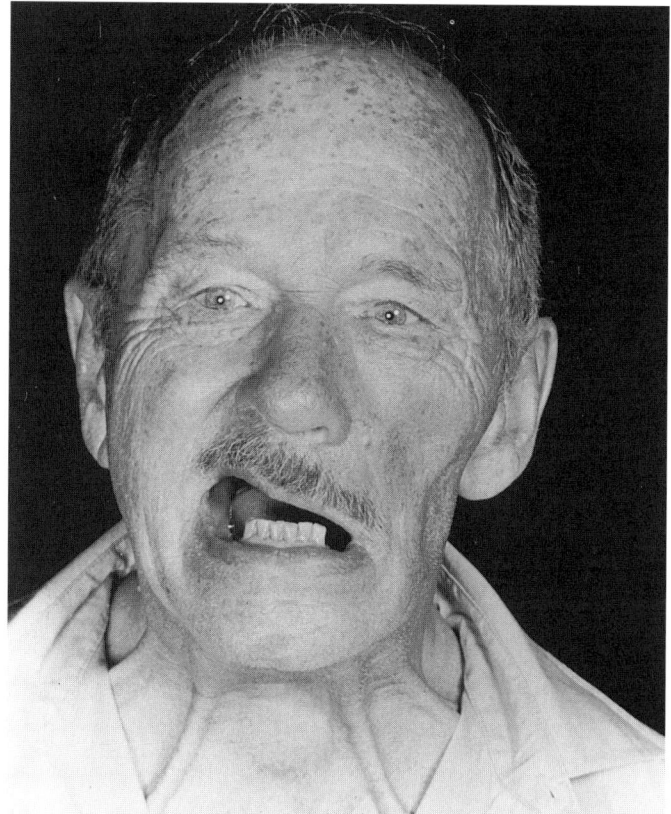

Fig. 6.2b The patient developed two more local recurrences and a proven metastatic solitary focus in the lung. These were treated by surgical resections. The patient had been free of disease for over five years without local recurrence in the buccal area or in the pulmonary area and without regional metastases. The entire history of his adenoid cystic carcinoma extended over 41 years and he died of old age, free of gross disease

indeed the patient's life might have been shortened and her travail increased by such an operation. No one knows the answer, but that would certainly be the accepted plan of management today. It is conceivable, therefore, that the rationale of unpredictable and unexpected protracted morbidity without treatment could be used as an unguaranteed substitute solution in cases involving the elderly and with those who resist surgical intervention. This has been termed the philosophy of "the strategic retreat." These are nebulous factors in a therapeutic program of observation that, at the best, hopes for an indefinite period of palliation.

The highlights of this case are its chronicity without treatment for 25 years, the minimum symptomatology until the last six months before a major operation, a tumor which had invaded bone, soft tissue, tongue, and nerves. This tumor did not respond to radiotherapy as a palliative measure in the end. Some of the questions that arise in this case are: Was this mass always an adenoid cystic carcinoma, or was it an infection or another type of salivary gland tumor in the beginning, such as a benign mixed tumor? Was the pulmonary metastasis secondary to the operation or primarily an aspect of the biology of the disease? Did the massive surgical ablation and radiotherapy hasten death?

Case 2. Mr. A. G. became aware of a painful mass in the left buccal region in 1935. On August 10, 1937, through an intraoral incision, a cribriform type of adenoid cystic carcinoma in a minor salivary gland was excised. The procedure was described by that surgeon as a gross subtotal resection; the base of the wound was curetted and packed with iodoform gauze.

The patient remained well until May, 1953, at which time a recurrence measuring 3 × 2 cm was noted in the cheek, extending just below the malar prominence to the level of the angle of the mouth. This recurrence was excised by the same surgeon on May 20, 1953, through an external melolabial incision, removing the specimen in two separate pieces. A lower facial paralysis was noted following that operation. The tumors removed in 1937 and in 1953 were originally described pathologically as benign mixed tumor. In 1971, however, these slides were reviewed by Dr. Karl Perzin in the Department of Pathology at Columbia–Presbyterian Medical Center, and a diagnosis of adenoid cystic carcinoma of the cribriform type was established (Fig. 6.2a).

Om May 29, 1968, following a negative metastatic work-up, a resection of a 6 × 8-cm recurrent tumor was performed using an inferior face-flap approach and en bloc dissection of all tissues from the oral commissure back to the ascending ramus to the mandible. Pathology indicated that all lines of resection were free, and the tumor was identified as a cribriform type of adenoid cystic carcinoma.

The patient developed a third recurrence on March 29, 1971, in the left cheek and associated with the parotid gland, measuring 3 × 4 cm; the mass was mobile. This was removed through a standard parotid approach and a total parotidectomy was accomplished with preservation of the upper division of the facial nerve. Again, pathology reported that all margins were free of tumor and that there was no evidence of perineural invasion or metastasis.

On June 30, 1971, a solitary 1-cm mass was noted in the upper lobe of the right lung and was removed by thoracotomy. The tumor was described as fragmented during the enucleation procedure and as being consistent with a metastatic adenoid cystic carcinoma of the cribriform type.

In October, 1976, five years following the pulmonary resection, the patient died of a myocardial infarct, free of discoverable disease, with a negative chest X-ray three months prior to his death and no evidence of local recurrence in the cheek 41 years after initial discovery of the tumor. This patient never had postoperative radiotherapy (Fig. 6.**2b**).

This case highlights several points and also poses several questions. It is interesting that, after 15 years, there was a change in diagnosis from benign mixed tumor to adenoid cystic carcinoma. This patient had three local recurrences, one tumor was 6 × 8 cm, and spillage and fragmentation was noted in the first operation, but there was no recognized recurrence for 18 years. There was no regional metastasis and no perineural involvement. A single metastatic node to the lungs is unusual; the question is whether this was influenced by surgical interventions or whether it was purely associated with the biological activity of the disease. This man lived for 41 years with his disease with 4 major local operations and one thoracotomy for metastasis, and he died free of disease five years after the thoracotomy.

Case 3. Mr. G. P. presented on July 28, 1965, at the age of 68 with complaints of left-sided nasal congestion, epiphora, and occasional epistaxis for one year. Physical examination revealed a 4 × 4-cm tumor mass obstructing the major portion of the nasal cavity on the left side, involving the ethmoids, turbinates, ascending crest of the maxilla, medial antral wall, and extending toward the nose, cheek, and upper-lip region. There was no evidence of metastasis (Fig. 6.**3a**).

On August 23, 1965, the patient underwent a radical ablative procedure, including an en bloc resection of the floor of the orbit, upper hard palate, medial nasal wall, and lamina papyracea, a pansinusectomy, and the skin in the area of the inner canthus (Figs. 6.**3b, c**). The pathology report identified the tumor as an adenoid cystic carcinoma, cribriform type, arising primarily in the ethmoids. The report explicitly stated that the tumor had violated the margins of the resection in several areas. Three months following this operation, the patient had a forehead-flap reconstruction in a separate procedure to close the opening into the nasal cavity. The patient had never had postoperative radiotherapy and had no evidence of disease for over 16 years.

Unexplained Clinical Behavior and Unusual Cases   45

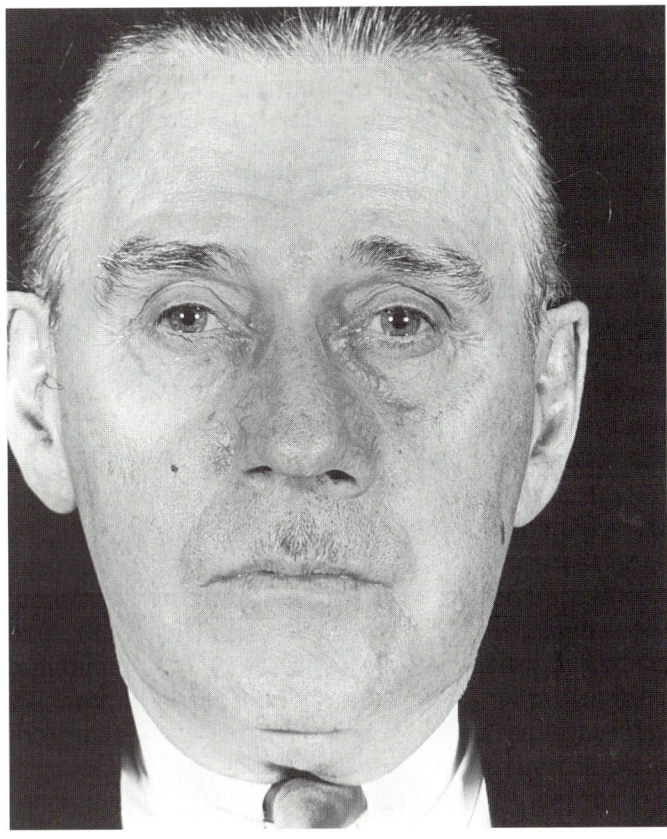

Fig. 6.3 a This patient had nasal congestion and a mass filling the left nasal cavity for a period of one year

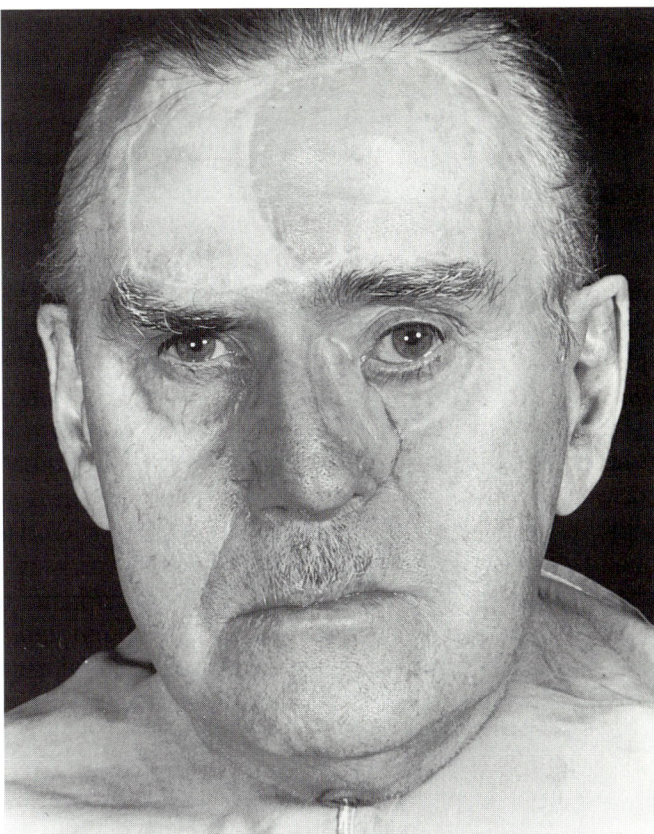

Fig. 6.3 b He underwent a radical ethmoidectomy, including the skin of the lateral nose and inner canthus, along with all of the tissues in the nasal cavity and a portion of the maxilla

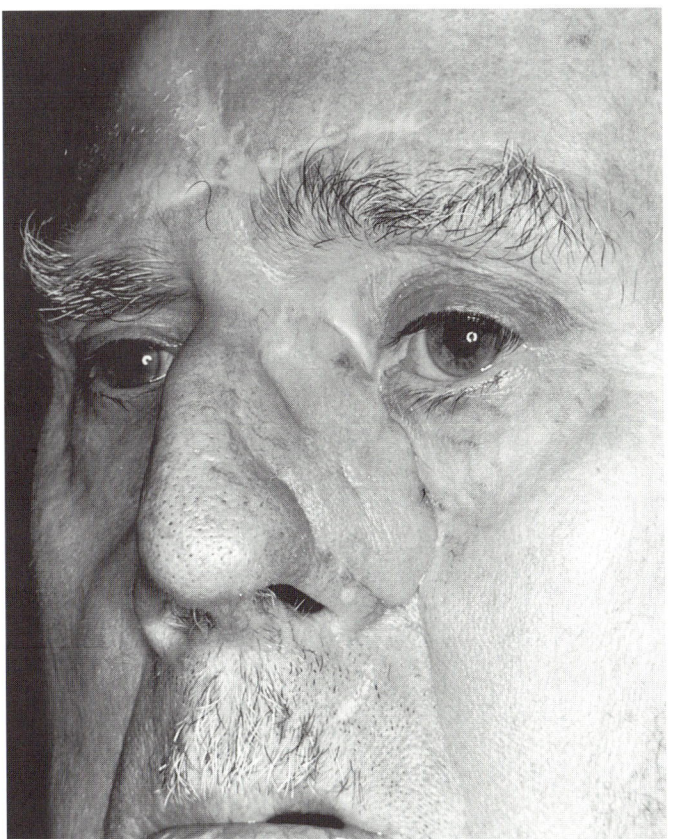

Fig. 6.3 c He did not have postoperative radiotherapy and has remained free of disease for over 16 years without local recurrence, systemic spread, or extension to the brain or to the orbit

Case 4. In 1960, Dr. M. R., age 25, noticed a lump in the left submandibular area. In 1966, two biopsies were done, one under local anesthesia which was negative, and then a second under general anesthesia which was positive for adenoid cystic carcinoma, cribriform type. He subsequently underwent a very extensive composite operation including the submandibular area, a conservative neck dissection, the adjacent mandible, the floor of the mouth, a partial glossectomy, and a conservative total parotidectomy. Special attention was directed to the lingual, alveolar, and hypoglossal nerves extending up toward the base of the skull. The wound was closed by direct approximation. There was no regional metastasis and all margins were declared free. The patient did not receive postoperative radiotherapy. He returned to an active professional life in spite of the magnitude of the operation.

After eight years of careful follow-up, the patient felt quite secure about his outcome and was checked locally thereafter. In the 13th postoperative year, he experienced pain in the hip and back. An X-ray examination revealed multiple bone metastases in the pelvis, spine, and lungs. All palliative measures were used to ameliorate this condition including irradiation, chemotherapy, interferon, and cloning. The patient survived another four years and died in 1983. He never developed a local recurrence.

This case also poses the question of whether the systemic metastases had occurred prior to the original biopsy and surgical ablation; did the biopsy or the operation cause the spread of the disease? Why were the metastases so dormant and asymptomatic for such a long period of time? Why did the metastases primarily prefer to involve osseous tissue? It also supports the theory that an "adequate" local resection will cure the primary cancer. It also demonstrates a chronicity of 23 years with good quality of life for 19 years before the clinical manifestation of systemic spread.

See Figure 6.4 for an illustration of another unusual case.

Reflections

The second case exhibits a chronicity of 41 years with three local recurrences and one pulmonary metastasis. The first surgical excision was undoubtedly subtotal, but the patient did not have a clinical recurrence for an interval of 15 years. Then, over the next 8 years, the patient had two additional local recurrences and a pulmonary resection, but was never mutilated, and died 41 years after the incipiency of his disease, having been free of clinical tumor for five years. This patient certainly benefited from his surgical intervention. There was an escalation of the activity of this tumor after a 15-year interval, but this was brought "under control." The reasons for this must be speculative but imply assistance from his own immune system and from the surgical resections. No one would believe he had been cured of his cancer, but he had no gross clinical disease at the time of his death. The capabilities of his immune system were working in his favor, but nobody knows what that means. It is not predictable or controllable, but may be a consequence of the surgical program. Such a biological boost cannot be programmed as a strategic part of the therapeutic protocol. This patient never received postoperative radiotherapy.

The third case is similar to the second in its favorable outcome, but the primary tumor was situated in a more strategically difficult position in relation to the orbit and the brain. The primary operation was a gross subtotal resection, and the patient never received postoperative radiotherapy. According to all the rules, he should have had local recurrence and possibly systemic spread, but remained free of disease for over 16 years. This remarkable situation again suggests that the gross removal of this primary tumor altered the immunological balance in his favor, and if he did not "cure himself" he at least eliminated the growth capability of the tumor for 16 years. Again, these situations are very unusual, unpredictable, and uncontrollable. Their therapeutic results are, however, attributable in part to surgical intervention.

The fourth case exhibits the chronicity of this disease, the 13-year period of silence postoperatively, and then the inadvertent discovery of wide-spread osseous metastases in the pelvis and spine, and ultimately metastases in the lung. Biological methods including chemotherapy, cloning, radiotherapy, and regional excisions had no influence on the course of the disease. There are curious questions as to the reason for such extensive metastasis, its preference for bone (and lung), its subtlety in the initial slow-growth pattern, ending in relentless fulmination. Certainly, the initial operation was effective in controlling the cancer at the primary site, as the patient never developed a local recurrence. It is possible that this also established a favorable immunological balance for the host until the volume of cancer cells in the metastases altered these factors. This certainly supports the principle of removing all of the cancer at the primary site to prevent local recurrence; if there is no distant metastasis, the patient has an optimal chance for cure. This still remains the fundamental approach to treatment in spite of all innovations.

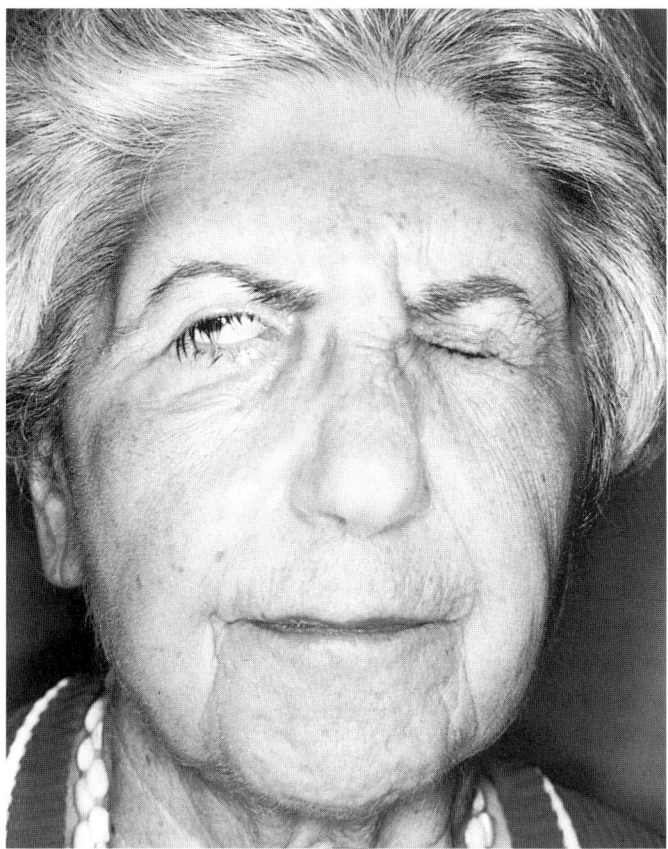

Fig. 6.4a **This patient had an adenoid cystic carcinoma of the parotid gland for 25 years.** During this period of time, she underwent six conservative operations. She finally developed involvement of the facial nerve with the seventh recurrence in 1983

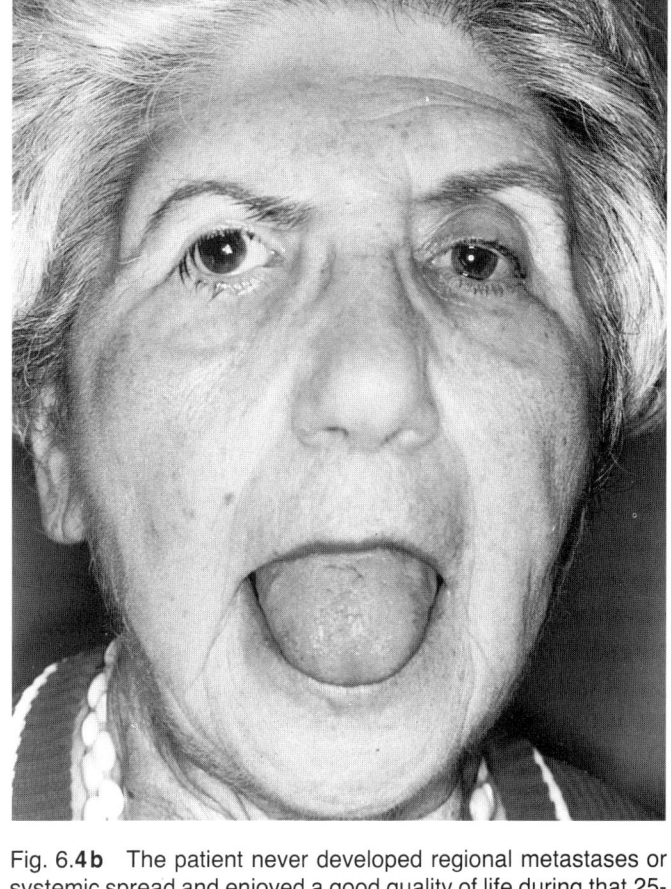

Fig. 6.4b The patient never developed regional metastases or systemic spread and enjoyed a good quality of life during that 25-year period. These situations are not predictable in advance

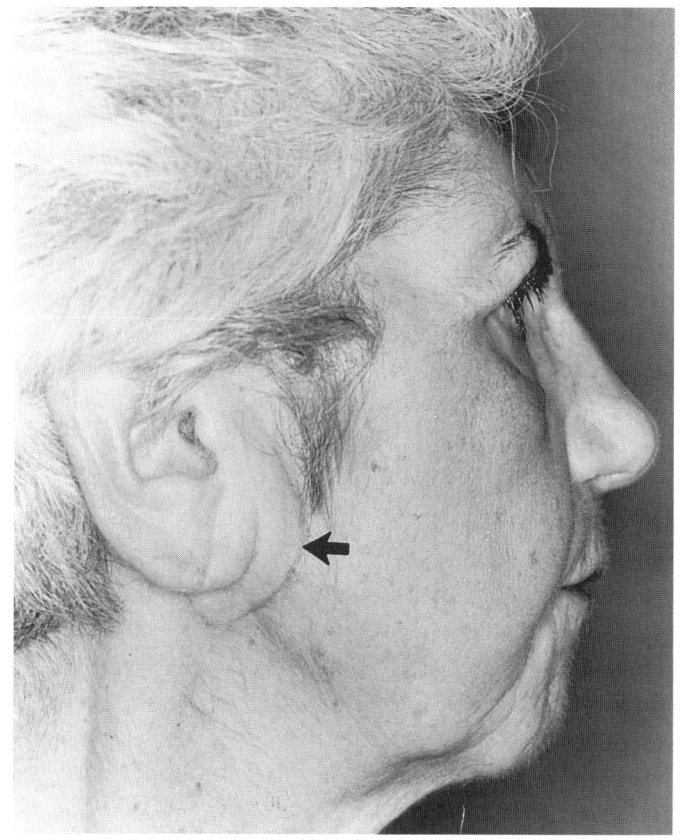

Fig. 6.4c Lateral view showing recurrence about the ear (arrow). After a radical resection, this patient underwent facial nerve graft. She has been free of disease for six additional years, making a total of 31 years from the incipiency of the tumor, and still does not have regional or pulmonary metastases

7
Management

Philosophy of Management

In some instances, management of adenoid cystic carcinoma is simple and direct. In other instances, it is very complex and in still others, it is baffling. The reasons for this variability lie in the unpredictable biological behavior of some of these neoplasms, the catholicity of their distribution in the major and minor salivary glands of the head and neck, and their chronicity and tendency to recur locally and spread distantly. Management consists of a variety of surgical procedures and irradiation. Chemotherapy has been tried in many instances, but has not been very effective, although it is still essential in the management of some advanced cases. Some of the operations are mutilating, and radiotherapy may entail serious complications. The cure rates are relatively low, and morbidity may be drawn out over 10 or 20 years. Little wonder that a combination of inopportunities can make management of these problems enigmatic.

The simplest, most favorable adenoid cystic carcinoma to treat and cure is the small, asymptomatic one in a minor salivary gland adjacent to soft tissue or muscle, which is early enough not to have gross invasion, low-grade in aggressiveness, and technically readily accessible. A similar group of conditions in a tumor in the major salivary glands with the same physical and biological factors would also be the simplest to treat. These tumors would be up to 1 cm in diameter and situated within the substance of the gland, not perforating through the capsule, and not involving the facial nerve. These ideal conditions are only rarely met, however, as the vast majority of these neoplasms have passed beyond these criteria when they are first discovered. The most complicated surgical candidates are the large tumors over 2 cm in diameter, which are associated with pain or ulceration, are high-grade, have invaded adjacent nerves or tissues, have regional or systemic metastases, and are technically inaccessible. The majority of cases are positioned between these two extremes and require variations of the ablative process.

There is also another group of cases that have systemic metastases or pernicious local extensions associated with trismus, involvement of the base of the skull, nerve paralysis, and deep invasion. They are long-standing or neglected cases in which only palliative measures can be applied.

The surgical procedures used for these various conditions may be standardized to a certain degree, but many cases require selective procedures, which are modifications on the basic theme. Regionality and the presence of vital structures, such as the facial nerve, orbit, brain, hearing system, swallowing and speaking systems, and aesthetic appearance bear considerable weight in the decision-making process. As the majority of the tumors are not cured by a surgical operation alone, the use of irradiation, either postoperatively or as a back-up to surgery, becomes a decisive factor in management.

Therapeutic Planning

Because of the unpredictable nature of this tumor, it is essential to have a strategy for the selection of the treatment of each neoplasm in each person. It is the responsibility of qualified physicians to propose a therapeutic strategy. The proposal must be accepted, however, by the patients, who should be informed of the potential behavior patterns of this tumor, so that they understand the options well. This involvement of the patients allow them to share with the therapeutic program in fighting their cancer. The patients are enabled, with medical advice and family support, to take a measure of responsibility for the treatment.

There are certain instances in which the selection procedure eliminates primary surgical treatment in favor of other modalities. There are understandably a small percentage of patients who simply refuse treatment for one reason or another. Where this obstacle does not pertain, the surgeon's first responsibility is the diagnosis by biopsy, the grading of the tumor, the classification of the primary tumor, and regional and systemic survey. If there is systemic spread, the treatment is directed toward palliation and maintaining quality of life. If the site and size of the primary tumor indicate incurability, the tumor may be declared inoperable with certain qualifications, and irradiation is the treatment of choice. In some of these instances, the radiotherapist and the medical oncologist may suggest a debulking surgical procedure. Most surgeons are reluctant to plan a partial resection in preparation for another type of therapy. But there is some biological justification for gross subtotal resection; in certain instances, irradiation and chemotherapy are more effective against a diminished volume of cancer cells than against the original total bulk. The "trade-off" here would be that the operation would not be exceptionally risky or mutilating and would have an acceptable morbidity. Resection for cure is often planned, yet not attained in a fair percentage of cases for a variety of reasons; microscopic or macroscopic neoplasm may remain in the wound, local recurrence makes its appearance. The potential sequelae are the dominant concern and must always be programmed into the primary treatment plan by the use of postoperative irradiation or chemotherapy.

After the initial selection has been made as to the type of treatment applicable for the specific case, the surgeon is confronted with selecting the best surgical procedure to cure that particular adenoid cystic carcinoma in its special position in the aerodigestive tract of a person of a certain age and disposition. Again, we aim for the goal of removal of all of the cancer cells from the patient's body when that is realistic. The chances of accomplishing this are almost inversely proportional to the size of the tumor, and influenced by its position and grade. Obviously, small tumors have the best chance for cure. This automatically poses the question of how much tissue should be excised. No one knows the answer to this enigma, but there are ways of gambling and approaching these limits with enhanced security. The undifferentiated adenoid cystic carcinomas certainly behave more aggressively than the well-differentiated ones and are consequently more threatening and require a stronger therapeutic plan. Systemic spread and gross infiltrative, local extensions are specific factors. Tumors contained within glandular tissues have the best outlook; tumors invading nerves, bone, and adjacent soft tissues have a more serious prognosis for local recurrence and systemic spread. Tumors over 4 cm in size are ominous, because they have been growing for a longer length of time or are biologically more active. Weighing all of these factors can create a dilemma with respect to the best advice and course of treatment.

There are particular instances in which the best form of management is no treatment. All specific criteria must establish this proposition and it is obviously a demoralizing situation for the patient in most instances. The cases are therefore subdivided beyond the known biological processes influencing treatment into groups according to age, sex, crippling effect, quality of life, chances for cure or amelioration. It is amazing in one sense that the professional making these judgements has limitations of his or her own in training, attitude, ability, and interest. Those who select the treatment for the patient have selected themselves, often by chance, on the basis of their professional backgrounds and yet, they are accepted heroically as potential saviors. Obviously, there is no "guarantor" in these situations concerning religious beliefs, concepts of mutilation and death, loss of lifestyle, diminishment of the living experience, unknown pain, and possible abandonment, all of which are juxtaposed to the instinct for survival. In the end, the decisions evolve from the patient, the doctor, and the family, as imperfect as they may be.

Radiotherapy

It is not possible at this time to make a definitive statement on the role of radiotherapy in the management of adenoid cystic carcinoma, but it is possible to state its role in the past and its developing role at the present time. There is no question that it has an effect on this tumor in the vast majority of cases, that it is probably not curative in advanced disease, and that it has an important role adjunctive to surgery. Palliation for local recurrence, palliation for systemic metastases is well-established and possibly the prime method of management in certain advanced cases. It is not competitive against adequate surgical excision for cure, when this is realistic. Unfortunately, this tumor does not frequently present favorable prognostic factors. The fact that adenoid cystic carcinoma occurs in major and minor salivary glands and that it may be asymptomatic and inconspicuous in its early stages of development mitigates against routine early discovery. By the time it produces symptoms, it may be T3 or T4. This obviously imposes a handicap on any form of treatment.

Before the advent of radiotherapy and the accurate microscopic identification of this tumor, the treatment consisted essentially of surgical excision. At that time, there was no classification, no definitive microscopic identification, and no fundamental understanding of the biological processes of this tumor. It was therefore unsuccessfully treated by a variety of surgical excisions. When irradiation became available in the early part of this century, it was understandably applied to this tumor with a good initial response, but never as a curative modality. Actually, at that time, the histology of this tumor had not been worked out or identified. Local recurrence and systemic metastases were inevitable. Later, it was propounded that salivary gland tumors were insensitive to radiotherapy. These statements were made primarily by surgeons, who also practiced radiotherapy, and their equipment at the time consisted of the 250-kV machine, radium needles, and radon seeds. They, however, became experts in the use of these modalities and concluded that the surgical removal of the majority of tumors in the head and neck was the preferred method of treatment and backed this opinion with impressive statistics comparing surgical and radiotherapeutic results.

After the second World War, great advancements in radiotherapy were made through those in radiophysics, radiobiology, and new technology that had never been available before. Dr. Gilbert Fletcher and Dr. Emanuel Lederman and others were the vanguard of a new therapeutic presentment in the treatment of salivary gland tumors. It became apparent in the 1960s and 1970s that new radiological treatments and new concepts in therapy were very effective in treating certain salivary gland tumors, both for cure and for palliation, and also as an adjunct to surgical excision. Its role in the past two decades has increased and is still being modified and adapted to therapeutic programs as the state of the art advances. The original negative position regarding the effect of radiotherapy has given way to a predicted initial response. This has not led to total agreement in therapy and effectiveness, but it is establishing parameters.

It is not possible to make a definite statment at this time regarding the curability of small adenoid cystic carcinomas with radiotherapy, because of the paucity of cases treated. It becomes apparent after 10 or 20 years of experience that the chances for an absolute cure of this tumor by radiotherapy approach zero in advanced lesions. It is now becoming obvious that the use of radiotherapy postoperatively has reduced the number of, and prolonged the intervals between local recurrences, and that it has prolonged life. It is also apparent that megavoltage in larger doses and larger fields are more effective than reduced dosage and smaller fields. At this time, there is no doubt about radiotherapy's effectiveness and the need for it to be incorporated into the treatment plan of many of these adenoid cystic carcinomas, either for palliation, for the repression of microscopic disease, or as an adjunct to surgical excision. The details of its use are under active study.

Chemotherapy

The role of chemotherapeutic agents in the treatment of adenoid cystic carcinoma has yet to be defined. Most reports describe the efficacy of various agents in three principle clinical situations: extensive unresectable primary disease, recurrent local or regional disease in which options of surgery of irradiation have been exhausted, and metastatic disease. Both single-agent and combination therapy have been tried in an effort to determine the most effective therapeutic regimen.

One of the earliest reports on the use of chemotherapeutic agents is by Johnson (1964). He describes his experience with intra-arterial infusion of 5−fluorouracil in two cases. One patient had extensive primary disease originating in the maxillary antrum which regressed approximately 50%, allowing a less radical surgical resection. The second patient had a large primary tumor involving the tonsil and the base of the tongue. At initial presentation, pulmonary metastases were noted, and 5−fluorouracil was infused intra-arterially to achieve local palliation. A 75% reduction in tumor size was noted, and the patient was rendered pain-free.

Sessions et al. (1982) also report on intra-arterial infusion for the treatment of adenoid cystic carcinoma. They describe the use of cisplatin in four cases. A 75% reduction in tumor mass was noted in one patient, a partial response occurred in another patient, who died of other causes two weeks later. Minimal response was noted in the other two patients, though significant symptomatic relief was obtained. The authors propose that intra-arterial infusion may allow large lesions in critical areas to become more easily resectable. The higher concentrations of the chemotherapeutic agent in an intra-arterial infusion versus intravenous administration was thought to account for the high response-rate seen in this report.

Other investigators have reported on their isolated experience with single-agent therapy in ACC. Schramm et al. (1981) report on ten patients who were treated palliatively with intravenous cisplatin. Cisplatin is known for its effectiveness on slowly growing tumors, that is, those with low growth fractions. Subjective pain relief was achieved in seven of ten cases. A partial (at least 50%) or complete response was noted in four of five patients with local recurrent disease and in one patient with regional metastases. Three of six patients with metastatic disease showed some response. Other authors have noted a higher response to local rather than distant disease. Complete responses lasting from 7 to 18 months were noted in four patients.

Vermeer and Pinedo (1979) report partial response of pulmonary metastases to single agent doxorubicin. The patient's primary lesion was in the palate. Previous treatment with 5–fluorouracil was ineffective. Unfortunately, growth of the pulmonary lesions continued after cessation of the doxorubicin.

Tannock and Sutherland (1980) describe 17 patients with adenoid cystic carcinoma who received a total of 34 trials of various forms of chemotherapy. Many of the drugs were given as single-agent therapy. In three of four patients, 5–fluorouracil produced a partial response with locoregional disease. Of eight patients with pulmonary metastases, one showed objective response, and two stabilized. Methotrexate was judged to be ineffective. This has been noted by other investigators. Cyclophosphamide, chlorambucil, vincristine, and vinblastine were all judged inferior as single agents.

Kaplan et al. (1986) review a total of 116 cases of salivary gland malignancies treated with chemotherapy. Of these patients, 106 were from three previous sources. Ten patients were new. There were 65 cases of adenoid cystic carcinoma. 50 of these received single-agent therapy. Doxorubicin, 5–fluorouracil, and cisplatin all produced response rates greater than 40% when used singly. The duration of the response was usually less than eight months. For the entire group, response rates of 59% were noted for cisplatin, 46% for 5–fluorouracil, and 43% for doxorubicin.

Various combinations have been employed in the treatment of advanced cases of ACC. Budd and Groppe (1983) report on the treatment of a 29-year-old patient with multiple recurrences over a 13-year period and metastatic spread to the lungs, to bone, and to skin. Using a combination of 5–fluorouracil, doxorubicin, and mitomycin C, the authors were able to obtain a disease-free period of 12 months after cessation of treatment. Doxorubicin was felt to be the most effective agent in the regimen. Most subsequent combinations have included doxorubicin; however, the cardiotoxicity of this drug may be a factor limiting its use. Skibba et al. (1981) report a complete response to a regimen of cyclophosphamide, doxorubicin and vincristine in a patient with metastatic disease in bone, skin, and the lungs from a primary tumor in the parotid gland. The patient died ten months later from congestive heart failure thought to be secondary to cardiomyopathy from the doxorubicin. An interesting side note on this case is the fact that this patient displayed a fulminant course of disease that may have accounted for the excellent response to chemotherapy.

Kaplan et al. (1986) describe a 60% response rate in ACC patients receiving combination therapy where doxorubicin was part of the regimen. Again, the duration of response was short, seldom more than eight months, but significant pain relief was achieved. Dreyfuss et al. (1987) report a 46% response rate in a series of 13 patients treated with cyclophosphamide, doxorubicin, and cisplatin. Nine of the patients had adenoid cystic carcinoma, four had adenocarcinoma. When broken down further, the response rate for the ACC patients was only 53%.

It is perhaps unfair (or unwise) to delineate the role of chemotherapy in ACC on the basis of its use in the worst of cases at the worst of times in their clinical courses. Perhaps there is a role for chemotherapy as an adjuvant modality in the early treatment of this disease. A study by Triozzi et al. (1987) lends some support to this notion. In this study, 21 patients were treated with a combination of 5–fluorouracil, cyclophosphamide, and vincristine. Eight of the patients were treated palliatively. Chemotherapy was received as an adjuvant to surgery and irradiation by 13 patients who had primary or locoregional recurrent disease incompletely resected, with either gross or microscopic tumor left behind, without clinical evidence of disease after postoperative radiotherapy. One partial and one complete response were seen in the palliative group. Historical controls were used to evaluate the effect of treatment on survival, recurrence, and distant metastases in the adjuvant group. No statistical difference was noted with respect to survival or recurrence. Of interest, however, was the fact that no patient in the adjuvant group had developed distant metastases at the time of writing, whereas two of the control group had developed metastases in a similar period of time. It would seem logical that chemotherapy ought to play a role in the prevention of distant metastases in this disease, in which a large percentage of patients eventually suffer that fate.

To sum up: certain chemotherapeutic agents are capable of obtaining partial or complete response under certain circumstances. Some agents (for example, doxorubicin, cisplatin, and 5–fluorouracil) show a distinct advantage over others when used singly. Combinations of the various agents are capable of achieving potentially greater responses, though this has not been demonstrated consistently.

8
Surgical Treatment

Because of the wide distributuion of adenoid cystic carcinoma in the major and minor salivary glands of the aerodigestive system, it is not possible to state a single technique for surgical excision. This situation is made more complex by the anatomical fact that some of these tumors are located in relatively inaccessible positions, some are quite large when first discovered, some have occult extensions, and some compromise vital structures. These factors create special problems in philosophy of management and surgical technique. Thus, the goal of surgically removing all of the cancer cells from the body may be thwarted and may lie beyond the capabilities of excisional techniques. Each operation must therefore be individually planned and executed within these parameters.

Minor Salivary Glands

Nasal Cavity and Sinuses
(Figs. 8.1–8)

Adenoid cystic cancer in this area poses special problems in diagnosis and treatment. This is the most common site of this tumor in minor salivary glands, however, in the early stages it is not visible and produces no significant symptoms. These two facts rarely permit an early diagnosis and this reduces the optimal chance of treatment of an early lesion. T1 lesions are in the minority and are usually discovered serendipitously. These negative factors obviously have an effect on the therapeutic program and cure rate.

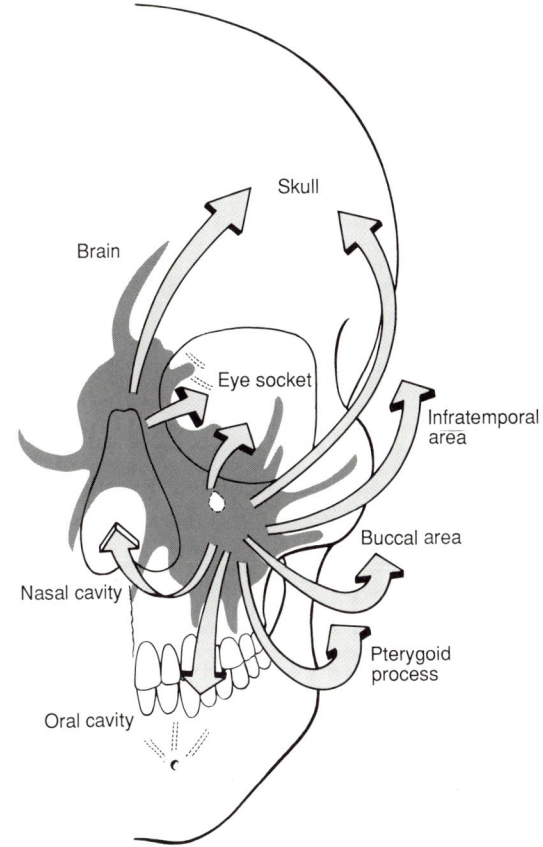

Fig. 8.1 **Primary adenoid cystic carcinoma in the sinus.** Arrows indicate areas most frequently involved by direct extension

A germane question, therefore, is how to improve on early **diagnosis.** Ideally, careful, routine ear, nose, and throat examination of every patient and the use of diagnostic assists on these lesions, CT scanning for instance would be fundamental to all diagnoses. The application of these ideals would certainly yield a few more early diagnoses of adenoid cystic carcinomas in this area, but has certain realistic disadvantages, in that they would involve a considerable amount of additional time, would be at best only marginally effective, and would be economically counterproductive. Idealism in practice is certainly to be espoused, but it cannot be expected to be more effective than realism under these circumstances. Asymptomatic patients who profess normalcy are not about to have this type of elective diagnostic researching imposed upon them, thus placing an increased responsibility on the doctor to be especially alert to minimal symptoms and to be judicious in the use of pertinent tests. Of course, this is a gray zone and may be complicated by overdoing or underdoing.

If any of these early general investigations reveal anything suggestive of a neoplasm, the doctor must make a decision to either observe it or operate on it. Each case is individual and requires a rationale that the patient is willing to conform to and that the doctor is willing to accept. All of these decisions contain the risk of delay, inconvenience, misdiagnosis, or unnecessary operations. These possibilities cannot be excluded, but the behavior should comply with the standards of normal medical practice. This means caring, follow-up, and advice on the part of the doctor, and cooperation and agreement on the part of the patient.

It is, of course, much easier to diagnose the patients who have symptoms relative to the nasal cavity, the sinuses and their environment. These comprise the vast majority of cases and are classified as T2 and T3 tumors. Those in the *nasal cavity* at this stage may be visible and cause nasal obstruction, discharge, and bleeding. As this tumor expands in the nasal cavity, there is ultimately nasal deformity, bone involvement, and pain. The tumor spreads submucosally along the nasal septum, turbinates, or floor of the nose. At first, it is obstructed by the periosteum and perichondrium, but it eventually penetrates these structures and then moves along the bone. It eventually enters the marrow space through anatomic or embryologic clefts or through the foramina of arteries and nerves. Once inside the marrow space, it may spread along vascular or neural pathways with little gross damage to the cortex and with few symptoms. This tumor may also invade the cortex of these bones directly.

Adenoid cystic tumor in the *nasal accessory sinuses* again represents a small submucosal mass that increases in vertical volume as it penetrates mucosa, periosteum and bone. There are numerous possibilities for its extensions in the sinuses. Some follow nutritional and neural routes, others spread along fascial and muscle plains, and others along congenital clefts. Some defy these "easy" opportunities and advance on a broad front, regardless of the nature of the obstruction.

The ethmoidal and maxillary sinuses are most frequently involved. Once the sinus is invaded by a sizeable tumor, there is always a concomitant infection. Infection in the sinuses causes swelling of the mucosa, purulent drainage, bleeding, pressure and pain. It is usually the combination of these symptoms that compels the patient to seek medical advice. If the tumor growth is situated such that infection does not occur at this stage, the tumor may grow to very large proportions before the symptoms are recognized as coming from the neoplasm. Symptoms directly from the neoplasm are minimal in the beginning and then present as swelling, pressure, pain, hypoesthesia, and eventually invasion into regional tissues. This latter extension may mean swelling of the cheek, nasal blockage, displacement of the eye, a bulge in the palate or temple, involvement of the base of the skull, extension to the brain, or wide dissemination. At this stage, cranial nerve involvement is common, primarily the fifth cranial nerve. All of these extensions outside the sinus are ominous signs. CT scanning or MRI provides the best opportunity to diagnose the extent of these tumors, their volume, their occult extensions, and their destructive effects on adjacent tissues. They are not exact, as they may not separate infection from neoplasm, subperiosteal and intramarrowal spread, or nerve involvement. This in no way diminishes their usefulness.

It is obvious that there is no single or simple **surgical treatment** that accommodates this vast list of possibilities in the nasal cavity and nasal sinuses. The basic surgical principle of removing all of the cancer cells requires first an estimation of how extensive the cancer really is, how much of what is shown in imaging actually represents inflammation, and how the probable occult extensions are. None of this information is accurately known preoperatively, but a working estimate may be compiled from the history and physical examination of the patient, from the imaging documentation, and from a check on nerve systems and regional tissues. Actually, it is only in the localized tumors that there is a technical reality of complete ablation. It is possible that some more advanced cancers can be cured, some symptomatically helped by debulking techniques, and some prepared for other combined ancillary modalities. Some, a very few, may be cured or controlled by changes in the "immunologic balance" of the host.

When all data points to a localized adenoid cystic carcinoma in the *nasal cavity,* it is appropriate to remove all of the tissues that enclose the cavity, along with the contents of the cavity. This means an adequate exposure, usually through a lateral rhinotomy incision with a degloving technique. The prime target is the neoplasm, and every effort is made to remove it intact. The method and the instrumentation are different for each surgeon. Instruments range from bone cutters and rongeurs to lasers. The tumor specimen is inspected after its delivery by the surgeon and the pathologist and declared either grossly adequate or violated. Areas of violation require additional surgery, which is carried out at that time, unless it is excessively mutilative, has not been explained to the patient, or has not been included in the written consent. After this has been accomplished, the encasement of this area is removed. The purpose of this is to gain additional biological security at the perimeters. This includes the nasal septum, the ethmoids, the medial wall of the maxilla, and the mucosa of the floor of the nose. These tissues are ordinarily prepared for permanent sections, unless there is something suspicious that requires immediate frozen section. Blood replacement may be necessary in this operation.

No skin graft or flap replacement is necessary in these cases. Large elements of skin graft inside the nasal cavity often create an unpleasant odor and require an active, daily cleansing process. The nasal cavity is therefore packed with an antiseptic ointment-impregnated gauze that is removed in two to five days. The cavity is then irrigated three or four times a day until healing and resurfacing has taken place by secondary intention. There are always exudates and large scabs and crusts that form during the healing process, some of which must be removed mechanically. Cleansing, however, remains very important. This aspect of healing gradually subsides over several months. Some patients continue to irrigate the nose as needed and others do not find this necessary.

Postoperative irradiation has become a favorite adjunctive treatment for this cancer. If, however, the margins of the primary specimen are negative for tumor, and all of the peripheral tissues are negative for tumor, there is a strong case for not using postoperative irradiation. This is particularly applicable in the younger age groups. If any of the margins are positive for cancer, irradiation is advised.

The same surgical principles apply in the treatment of this stage of adenoid cystic cancer occurring in a *sinus.* The technical approach is more complicated, because a conservation operation, which is adequate, is not easy to execute in all instances. Frequently some type of piecemeal resection is resorted to.

When the cancer has extended beyond these limits and has invaded adjacent structures, a broader and bolder plan of management is proposed. Radicality for its own sake has little place in medicine today. On the other hand, it has an important place when it means the possible salvation of the patient or the partial amelioration of this or her condition. These are judgments that not only stress the highest qualities of our professionality, but our deepest human qualities as well.

The planning of these extended operations is on an individual basis, depending upon the extent of the tumor, the philosophy and ability of the surgeon, and the desires of the patient. One must be prepared to realize that these plans may be found to be inadequate for the tumor in the course of the operation, or when local recurrence takes place in some phase of the postoperative course. The basic plan remains the removal of all of the gross cancer and any occult extensions that are microscopically discoverable. The final phase of this plan is to rehabilitate the wound immediately and as well as possible in order to establish an acceptable quality of life and prepare for any ancillary postoperative irradiation. All surgeons who are involved with these decisions are familiar with their complexity.

One of the most unsettling extensions of this tumor is the growth into the *orbit* from adenoid cystic cancer occurring in the ethmoidal or maxillary sinus or in the nasal cavity. Obviously, these different primary cancers take different avenues of spread toward the orbit. Adenoid cystic carcinoma of the anterior ethmoidal sinus usually passes directly through the lamina papyracea. Tumors of the posterior ethmoidal sinuses and nasal cavity often pass into the area of the apex of the orbit and frequently include the sphenoid in this involvement. The maxillary sinus tumors prefer the floor of the orbit and inframaxillary nerve as their transit passage. If it is a "pushing" neoplasm, the orbit may be preserved surgically in certain instances. This, however, puts the orbit at risk for diplopia, anophthalmia, external deformity, and the serious sequelae of postoperative irradiation in this area.

Extension of the adenoid cystic carcinoma to the *base of the skull* and *pterygoid area* also poses special problems in management. At one time, these areas were considered technically inaccessible without introducing the possibility of serious complications and an almost routinely fatal outcome. This situation has been reversed to a great degree by the spectacular advances in skull-base surgery, in which the most inaccessible and most dangerous lesions are now approached with reasonable surgical security. The overall cure rates, however, have not kept pace with the technical advances, although they have added some degree of local control, palliation, and in some instances, eradication of the disease. One would not expect a patient with an adenoid cystic carcinoma that had extended to the base of the skull or the pterygoids and required control not only of the primary cancer but also of its extensions to be saved by any operation. One must assess which operation and which approach is acceptable. Some of these techniques enter the intracranial cavity. One of the most significant advances in reducing infection, cerebral spinal fluid leak, and protracted morbidity has been the use of the epicranial, galeal, and temporalis flaps to rehabilitate these wounds. There are also cases which require regional myocutaneous flaps or free microvascular flaps for rehabilitation. Interdisciplinary cooperation with the neurosurgeon is indispensible in certain cases. The major problem is when and how surgery should be proposed to the patient as a treatment for presumed incurable disease or as a substitute for additional irradiation or trial by chemotherapy or nothing.

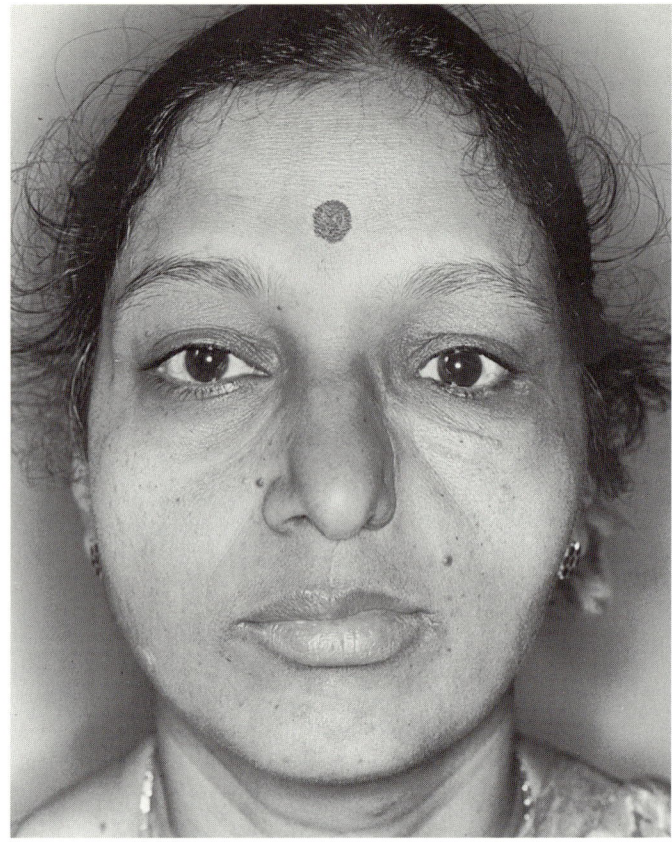

Fig. 8.2 **Patient had adenoid cystic carcinoma of the left maxilla** and underwent radical maxillectomy and skin grafting rehabilitation. She also wears a prosthesis and the orbit is intact. This is the minimal therapeutic management for adenoid cystic carcinoma of this sinus

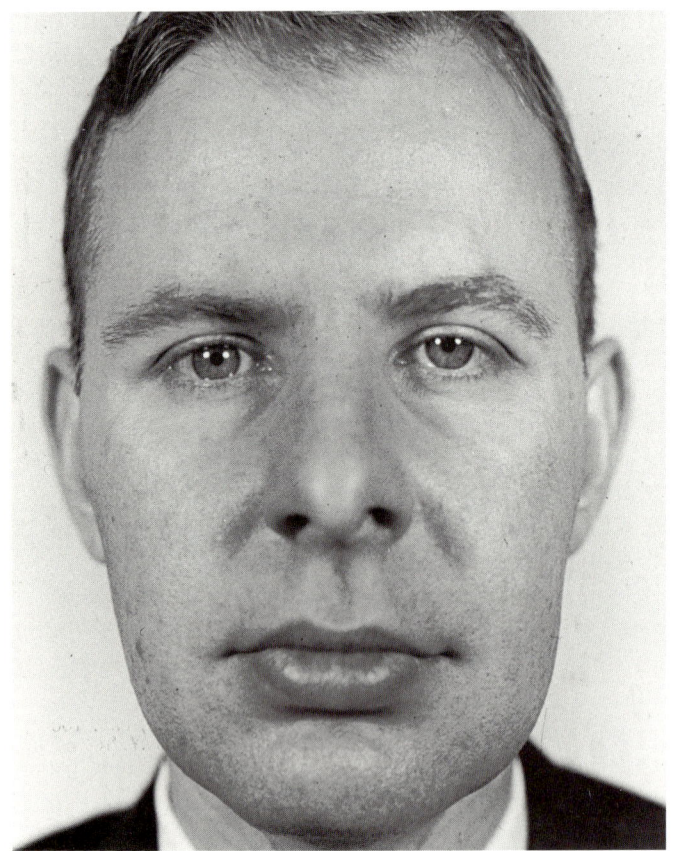

Fig. 8.3a **This patient had adenoid cystic cancer that involved the maxilla, ethmoids, and left orbit.** He had resection of all of these areas and received postoperative radiotherapy

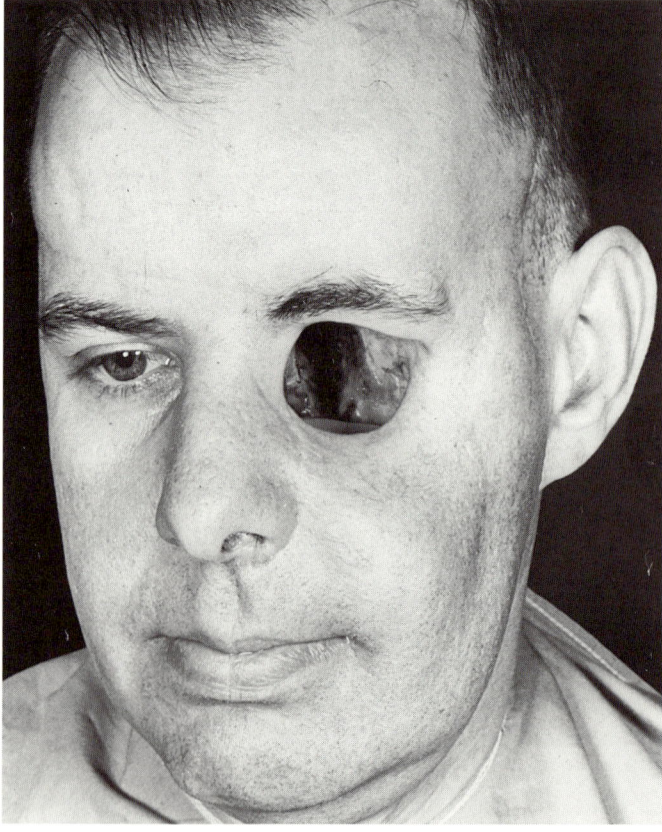

Fig. 8.3b The patient seven years after surgery. He died of recurrent local disease

Minory Salivary Glands

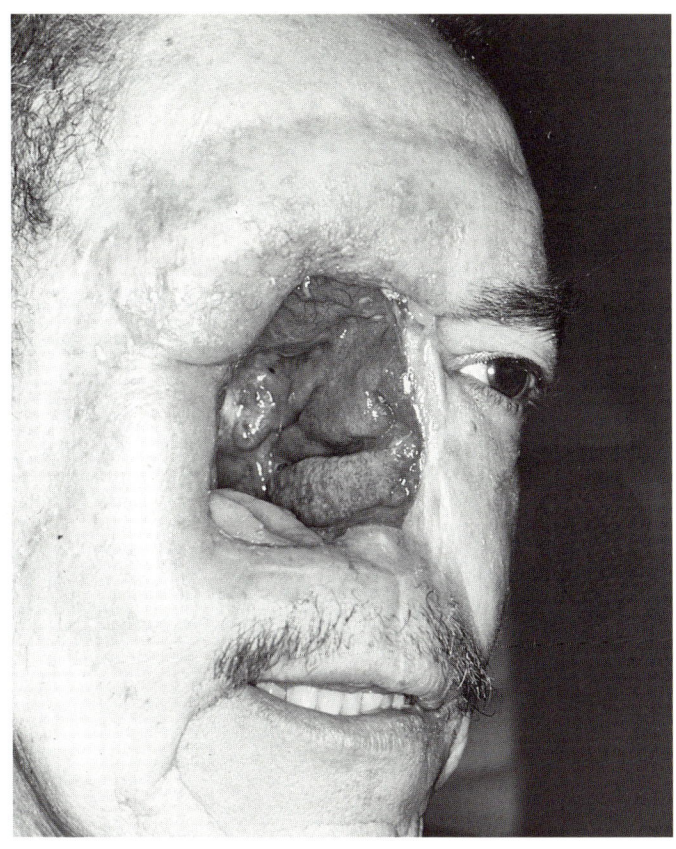

Fig. 8.4 **A maximum ablation of the orbit, nasal cavity, palate, sinuses, and nasal septum** for chronic recurring adenoid cystic cancer arising in this area. This patient lived with his disease for approximately 20 years and then died of extension to the brain and pulmonary metastases

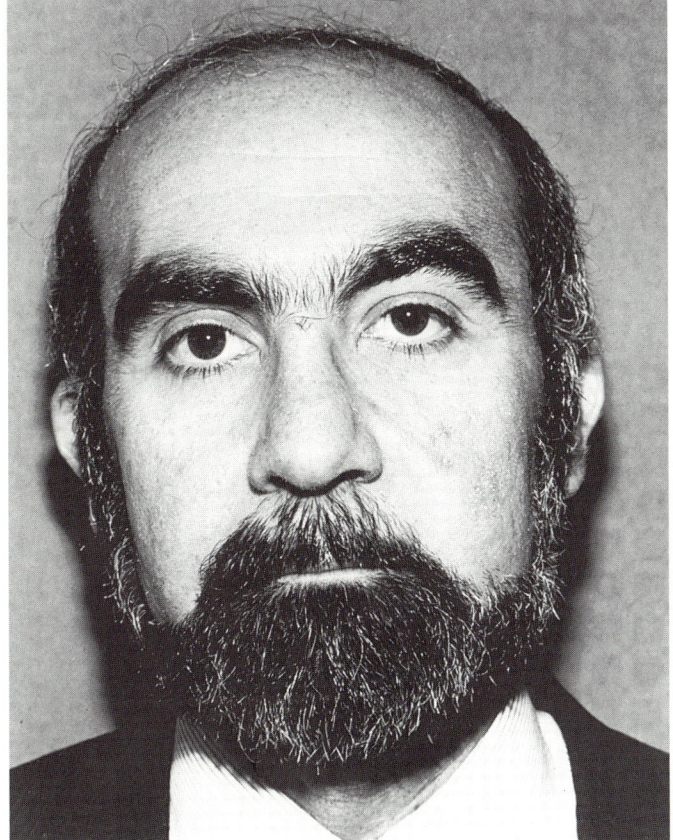

Fig. 8.5a **This patient had T4 adenoid cystic cancer involving the left maxilla, nasal cavity, ethmoids, apex of the orbit, palate, and infratemporal area.** He was treated originally by conservative gross subtotal resection of this neoplasm and then full course radiotherapy

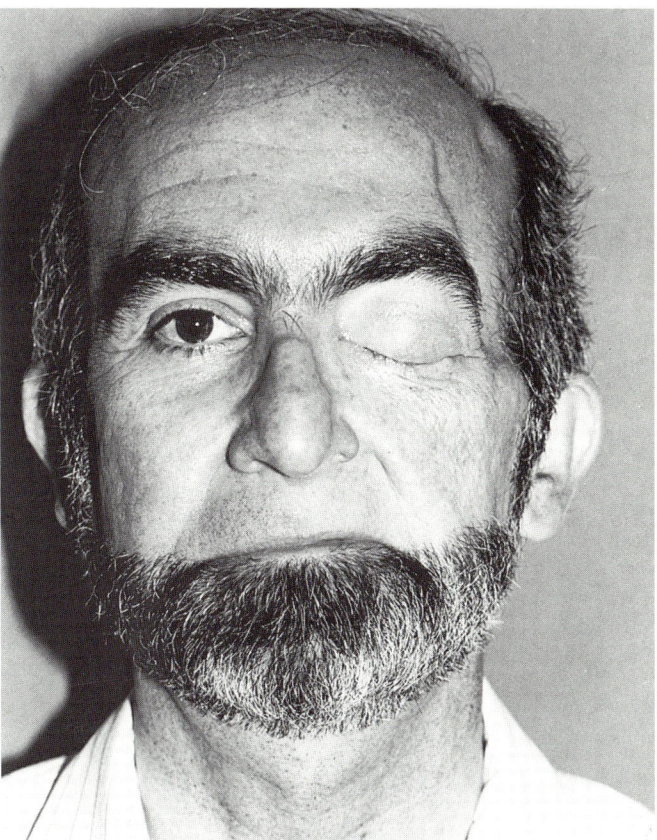

Fig. 8.5b He had three recurrences over the next eight years, had multiple courses of radiotherapy and minor surgery. He finally developed postirradiation necrosis of the temporal lobe, had that removed, and has been living for nine years without gross disease. However, there is little likelihood of cure

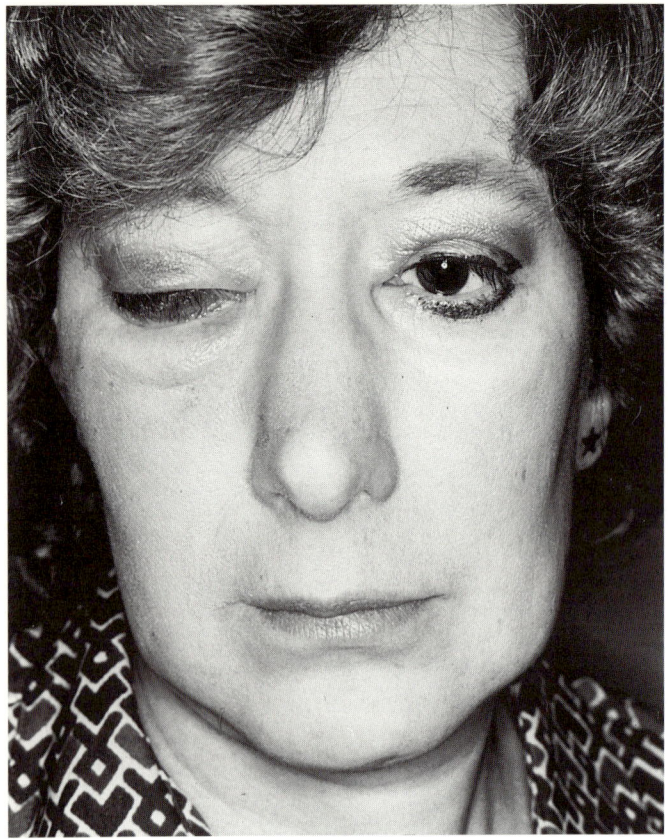

Fig. 8.6 **This patient presented with recurrent adenoid cystic cancer of the maxilla** which had recurred locally and extended to the eye. Examination revealed metastases to the lungs; she received no surgical treatment

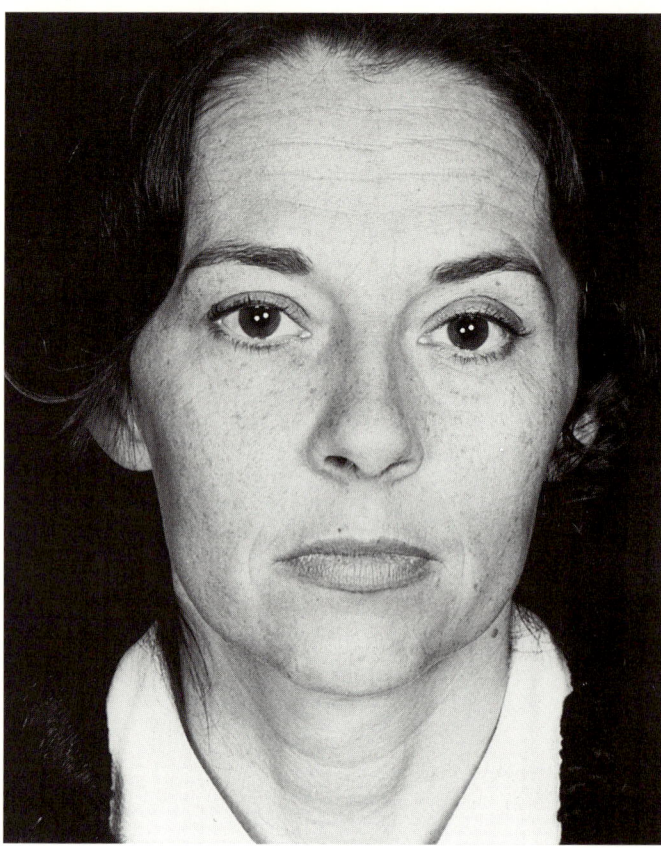

Fig. 8.7a **This patient had extensive adenoid cystic carcinoma in both nasal cavities** involving the right antrum, orbit, and turbinate, and in the contralateral ethmoids

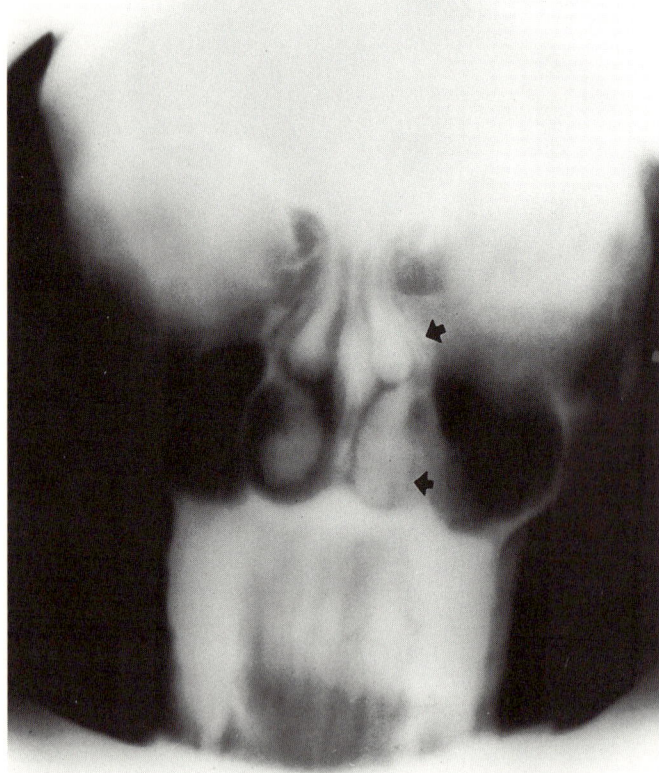

Fig. 8.7b She was completely asymptomatic. The tumor was discovered primarily upon routine X-rays of the sinuses and then biopsy. (Slide is reversed)

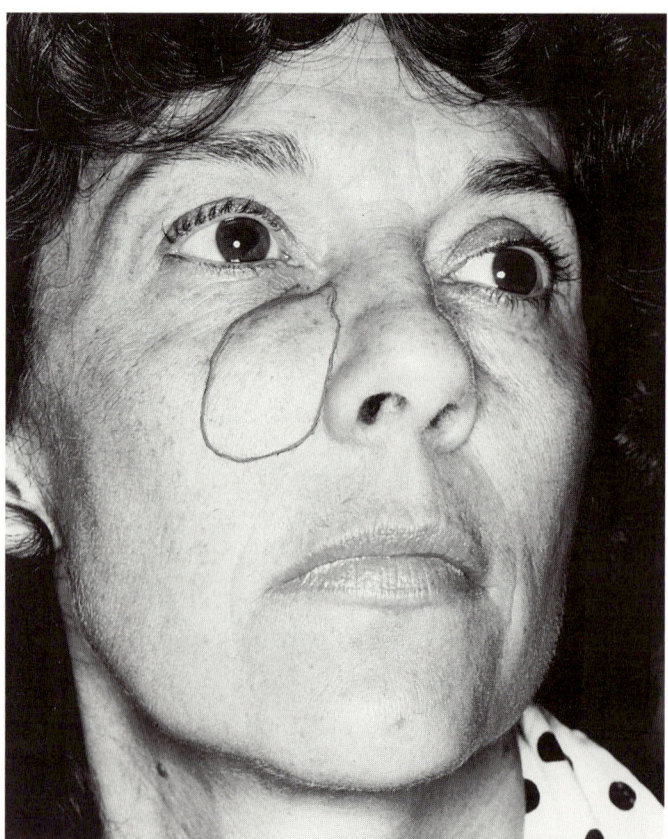

Fig. 8.7c She elected to have radiotherapy and presented with recurrence in the maxilla and right anterior cheek six years later. It was not operated

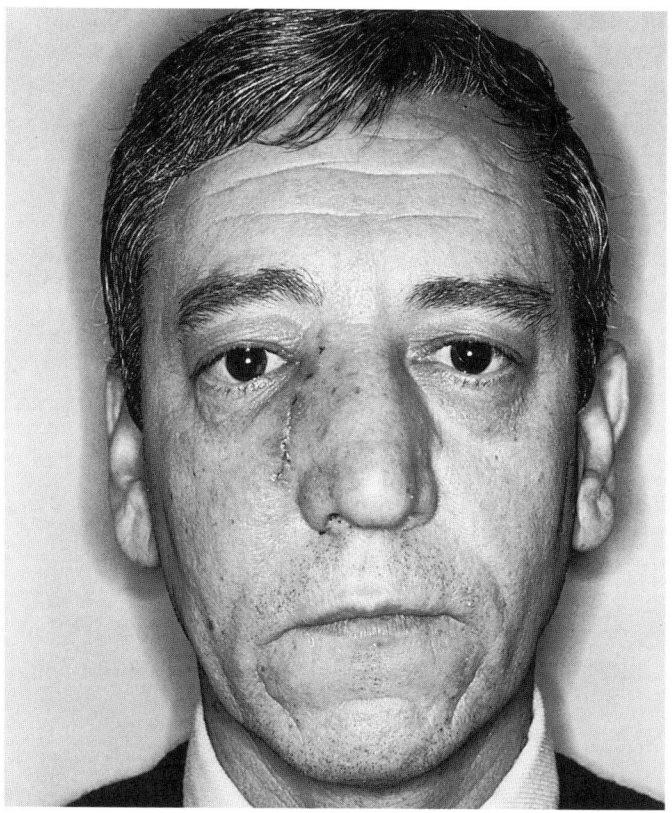

Fig. 8.8a This patient had adenoid cystic carcinoma of the ethmoids which was locally resected and irradiated

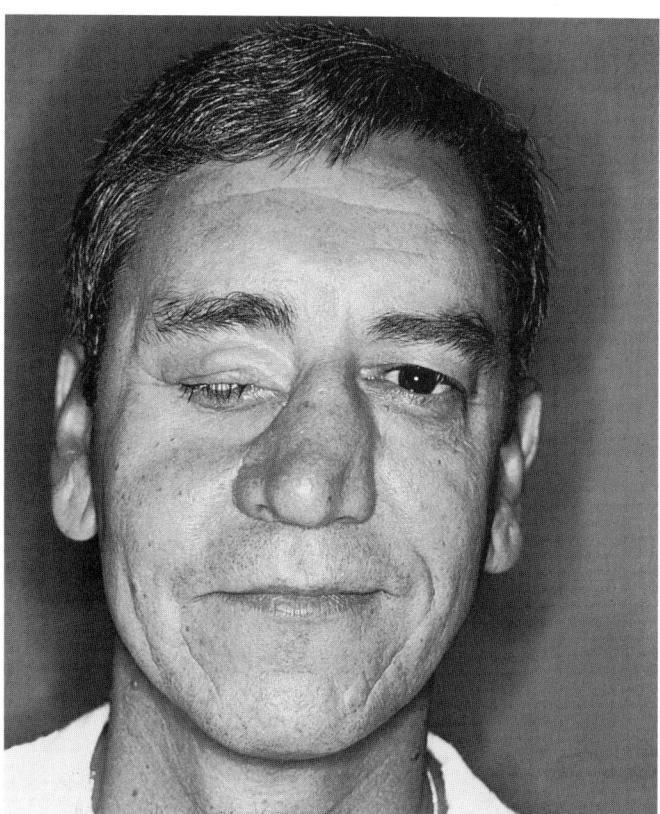

Fig. 8.8b Three years later this patient had evidence of local recurrence. Reoperation and orbital exenteration was carried out

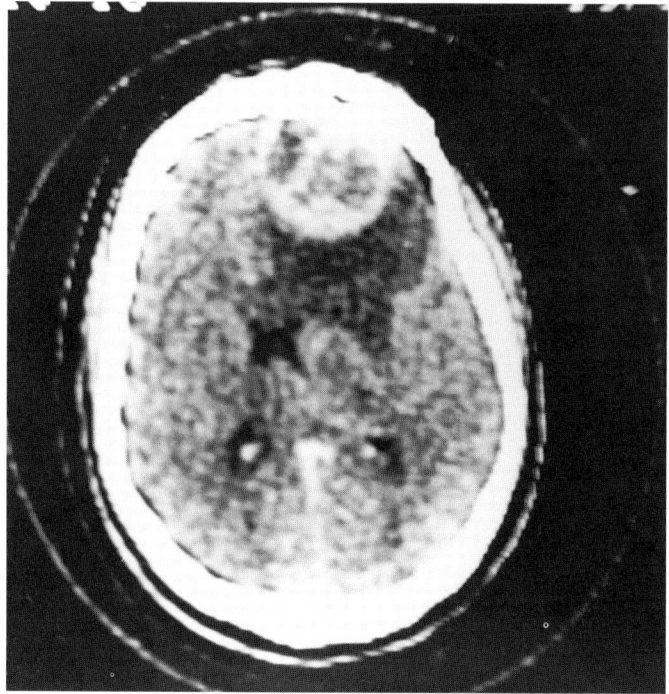

Fig. 8.8c Subsequently, CT showed extensive brain involvement

Oral Cavity

Palate
(Figs. 8.9–14)

The palate is the second most common site of adenoid cystic carcinoma of the minor salivary glands. The majority of these arise in the soft palate at its junction with the hard palate. In the early stages, the tumor is inconspicuous and asymptomatic. Discovery at this stage is accidental on the part of the patient or the patient's dentist. There is no reason not to do a conservative incisional biopsy at this stage because this is absolutely the optimal time for cure. Unfortunately, many of these tumors are not recognized at this stage, and some are not treated at this stage, because they are asymptomatic and treatment is not sought or advised. This latter position is unwise in view of a 65% incidence of malignancy in minor salivary gland neoplasias.

The surgical anatomy of this portion of the palate is bounded by mucous membrane on the oral and nasal sides, with muscle, fat, and fascia in between, and the hard palate, alveolar ridge, and pterygoid plates anteriorly and laterally. The pterygopalatine canal and greater and lesser palatine foramina with their arteries and nerves provide a ready conduit toward the base of the skull.

The **diagnosis** is made by inspection, palpation, CT scanning, MRI, and biopsy. As stated above, incisional biopsy is appropriate for the early lesions in planning treatment. This can be circumvented by excisional biopsy under general anesthesia with frozen-section diagnosis. Most patients, however, prefer to have a few days to think the situation over and to prepare for possible dental prosthesis in advance. Diagnosis in de novo large lesions is also best managed by incisional biopsy in advance of the ablative technique. Imaging of these latter lesions is very informative to delineate extensions, perimeters, and bone destruction.

The **surgical treatment** of lesions under 2 cm that have not compromised bone is basically a wide local resection which includes a large section of the soft palate and may extend into the nasal cavity. If the tumor is close to the alveolus, or to the greater or lesser palatine nerves, these sections of bone should be resected for margins and frozen section should be obtained upon the palatine nerves. It is more logical in this situation to take the grave potential of the adenoid cystic carcinoma into consideration than to be overly concerned about the size of the ablative technique. The most serious mistake that can be made at this time is to leave tumor in the wound. These surgical openings in the palate will spontaneously diminish in size over three or four months, are relatively successfully rehabilitated with a dental prosthesis, and may be closed surgically with intraoral flaps when tumor control is assured. Ten years is certainly an ample period of observation.

The surgical treatment of larger tumors requires a much more extensive resection. Removal of the entire hard and soft palates along with the dentition, pterygoid plates, and sinuses on both sides may be necessary. This formidable procedure is carried out by mandibular swing or through an upper-lip–splitting incision. It is very important to check the perimeters of the palatal specimen immediately by frozen-section examination and also to identify all borders with india ink for final inspection. The unexpected and unpredictable extensions in some tumors that have gone undiagnosed for several years and that do not reveal gross clinical disease can be shocking. The ultimate success in rehabilitation is the fabrication of a functional prosthesis, which is a highly specialized technical achievement. All patients with tumor of the palate routinely receive a full course of postoperative irradiation.

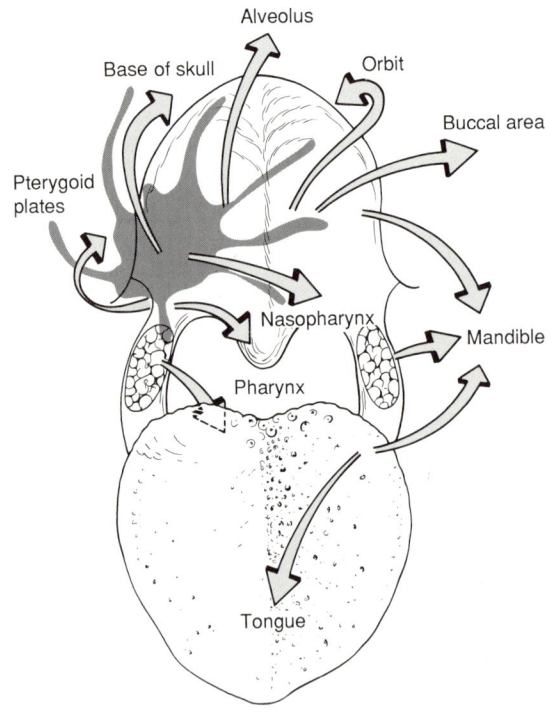

Fig. 8.9 **Primary adenoid cystic carcinoma of the palate.** Arrows indicate areas most frequently involved by direct extension

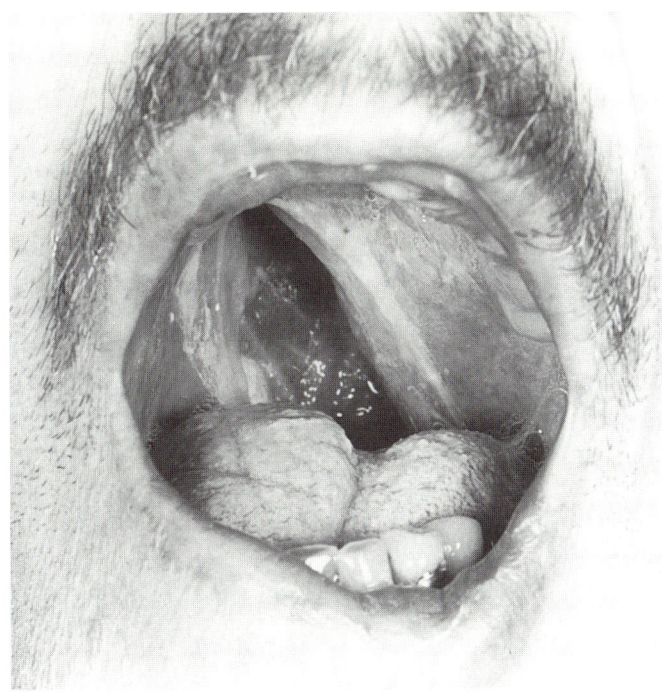

Fig. 8.10 **Adenoid cystic carcinoma of the junction of the hard and soft palates on the right side** treated by wide intraoral local resection. Prosthetic reconstruction corrects this defect

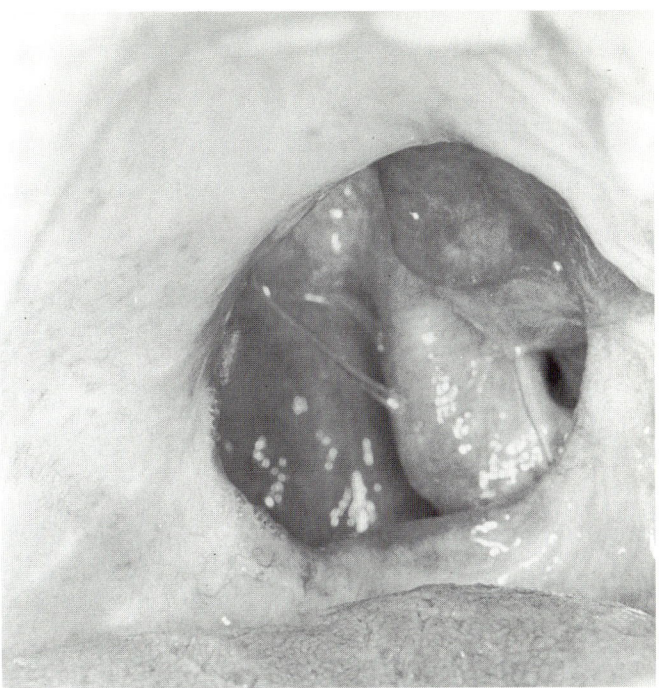

Fig. 8.11 **Somewhat larger adenoid cystic cancer on the left side at the junction of the hard and soft palates** treated by wide local resection. Prosthetic rehabilitation

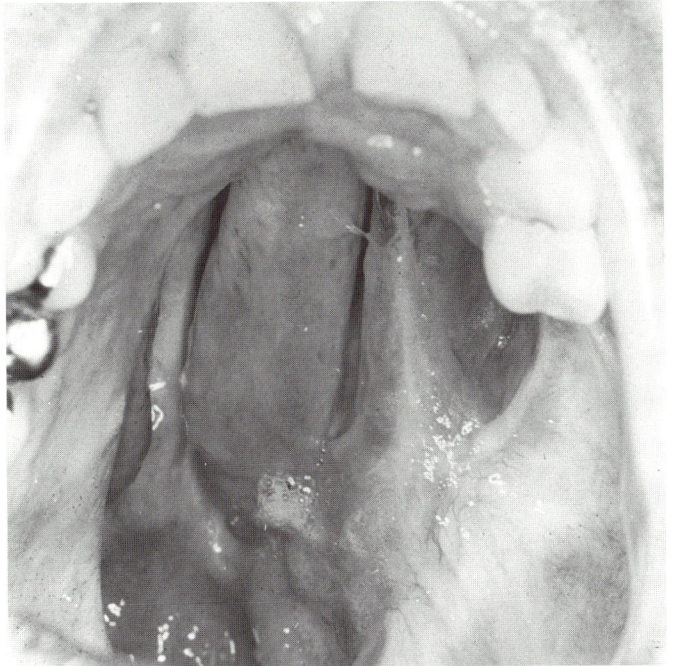

Fig. 8.12 **Total resection of the major portion of the hard and soft palates, pterygoid plate, and structures in the nasal cavity on the right side.** Prosthetic rehabilitation

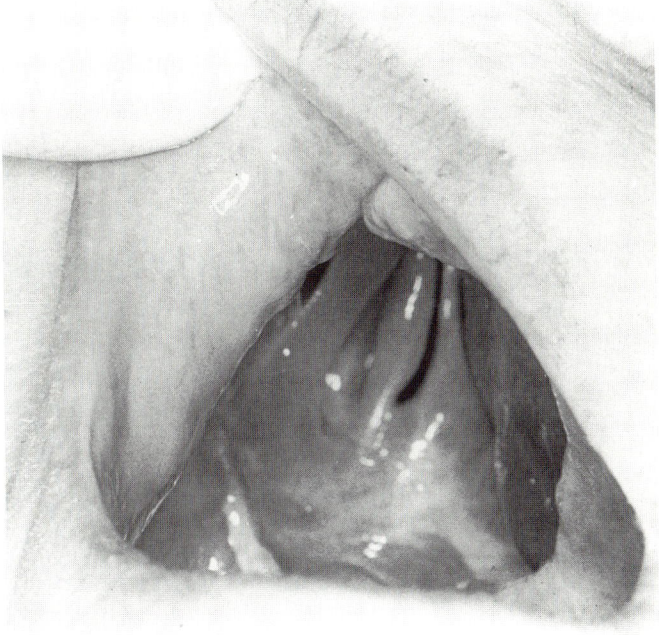

Fig. 8.13 **Total resection of the entire alveolus and hard and soft palates** with rehabilitation by prosthesis, which is much more complicated because of the absence of bone and teeth

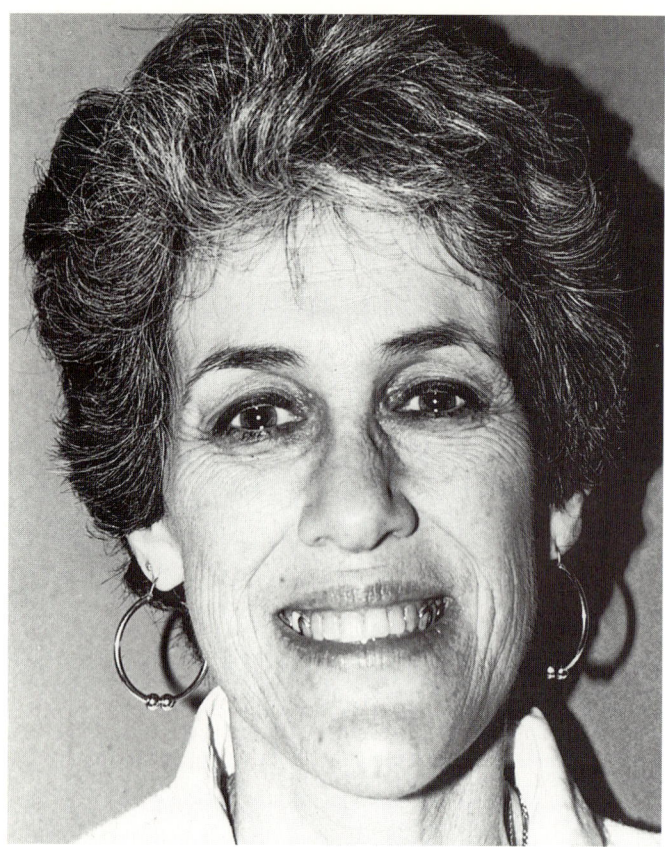

Fig. 8.**14a** **Resection of the major portion of the hard palate and soft palate**

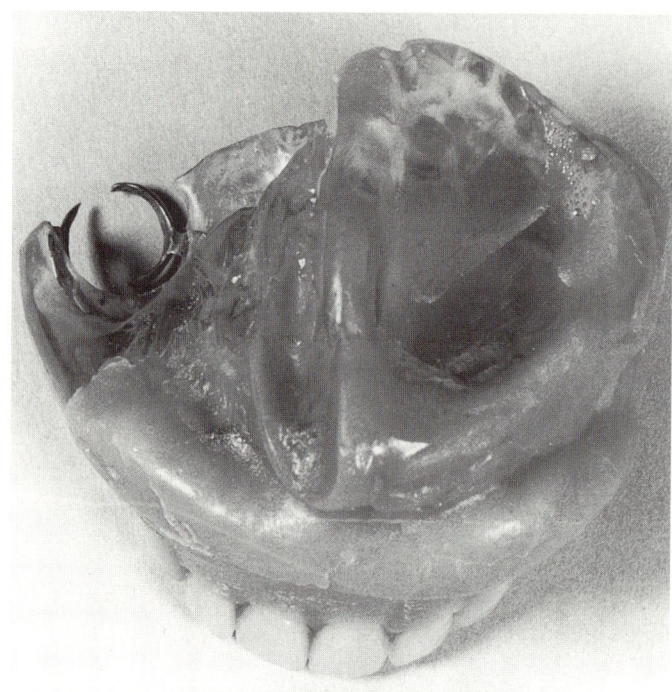

Fig. 8.**14b** Titanium implants are rarely practical. Rehabilitated by intraoral prosthesis. All of the patients in Figures 7.**10**−**14** are receiving postoperative radiotherapy

Buccal Area
(Figs. 8.**15–18**)

Adenoid cystic carcinoma in the buccal region has the third highest incidence rate of this tumor in minor salivary glands. In the cases of this study, there were no signs or symptoms in the early stages and the tumor had to reach a size that attracted the patient's or the dentist's or the doctor's attention, or it had to produce symptoms before it was diagnosed. By this time, these tumors were 1–3 cm in size.

The surgical anatomy of the buccal area presents no obstruction to the growth of this tumor. The mucous membrane is cushioned with fat and is anchored to the maxillary and mandibular sulcus above and below, to the mandibular raphe posteriorly, and blends into the mucous membrane about the lips anteriorly. The buccal fat pad and buccinator muscle give form and support to the internal part of the cheeck and the mimetic muscles and skin layer externally.

The **diagnosis** is made by an analysis of the signs and symptoms with the assistance of imaging techniques and biopsy. Tumors that are 1–2 cm in size may have an excisional biopsy under local anesthesia. This permits time for ample discussion of the problem with the patient. This can be circumvented, however, by frozen-section technique and a general anesthesia, and then a definite operation. There is no question about the efficiency of this latter program in an institution that is geared to handle it; however, on the whole, it should be carried out only with the complete sanction of the pathology department after this system of diagnosis has proved its effectiveness with the personnel involved. It would be fallacious to attempt definitive aspiration or frozen-section technique in all of the hospitals in the United States with the great variety of personnel lacking proper preparation and a clear understanding of the responsibilities involved. Preoperative incisional biopsy is also desired for the larger tumors, although they too can be managed as stated above. A misdiagnosis, change of diagnosis, alteration in the surgical technique, or a dissatisfied patient may have unhappy repercussions.

In **surgical treatment,** there is a justified instinct to want to remove small, anteriorly positioned adenoid cystic carcinomas by an intraoral approach. This is facilitated in the edentulous older patient with loose lips and no trismus. It requires an eversion of this portion of the commissure and anterior buccal area and then the removal of the neoplasm with a cuff of mucosa, fat, areolar tissue, and possibly buccal muscle and a smaller portion of mimetic muscles in this region. It is not necessary to remove skin with this lesion; the repair is accomplished by direct approximation or regional buccal-flap transposition. The cheek may be tight and depressed somewhat postoperatively, but this can be improved by massage, tissue stretching, and expansion.

Larger lesions, those situated in the posterior third of the buccal area, and those approximating the anterior wall of the maxilla or horizontal ramus of the mandible, should be approached by a lower-lip–splitting incision and lower-cheek flap. This usually means lysis of the mental nerve and resection of a large portion of the mucosa along with the buccal fat pad, proximate muscle, and, on occasion, the horizontal ramus and ascending ramus of the mandible, the anterior wall of the maxilla, the oral extension of the parotid gland, sections of the masseter muscle, and skin. These massive wounds must be rehabilitated with regional or microvascular flaps. The forehead flap is readily available and very efficient for this repair, but is not in favor today because of the defect of the donor area. Regional myocutaneous flaps and tubed cutaneous flaps can accomplish this restitution, but they are clumsy, bulky, and usually multistaged. Microvascular flaps are more convenient but require advanced technological expertise.

All patients with buccal-area tumor receive postoperative irradiation.

8 Surgical Treatment

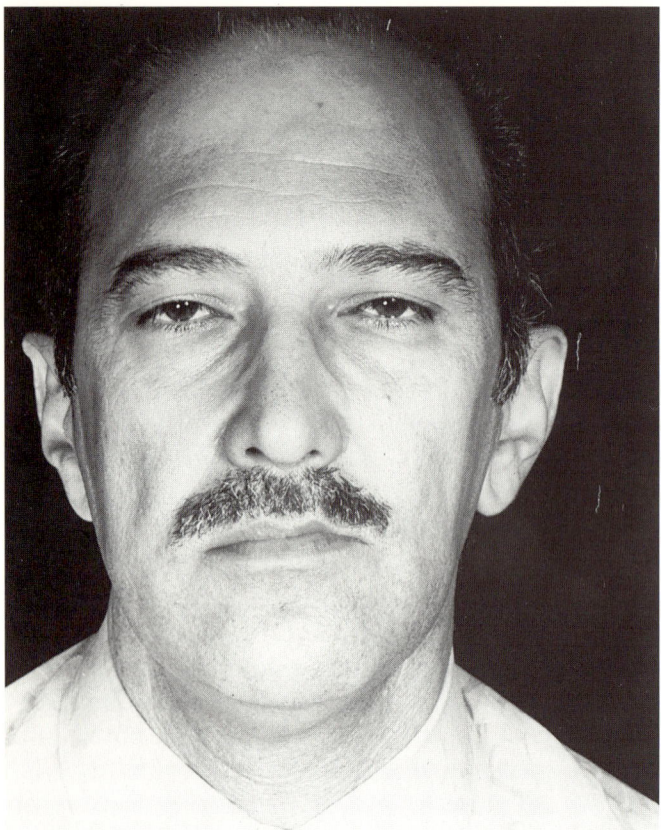

Fig. 8.**15** **Resection of small buccal adenoid cystic carcinoma on the right** including buccal mucosa, areolar tissue, and a portion of buccinator muscle, handled by skin graft repair. There is slight indentation of the right cheek

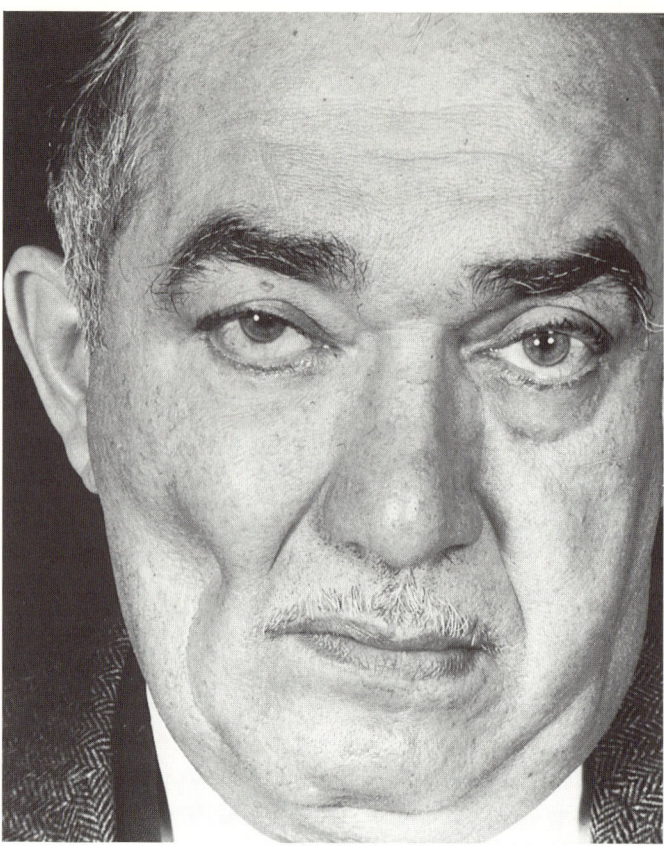

Fig. 8.**16** **A more advanced adenoid cystic carcinoma of the buccal area** treated by wide local resection intraorally and rehabilitation with skin graft. There is moderate contraction, slight trismus, and dimpling. Regional flaps are impractical at this stage

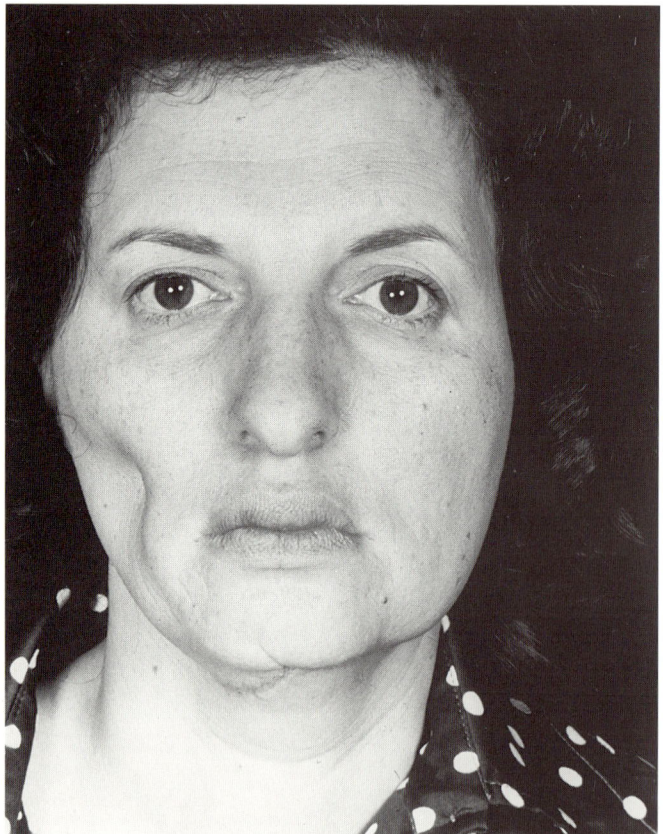

Fig. 8.**17** **Advanced adenoid cystic carcinoma of the buccal mucosa** resected by a submandibular approach and dressed with a skin graft. There is local recurrence in the region of the zygoma

Minory Salivary Glands

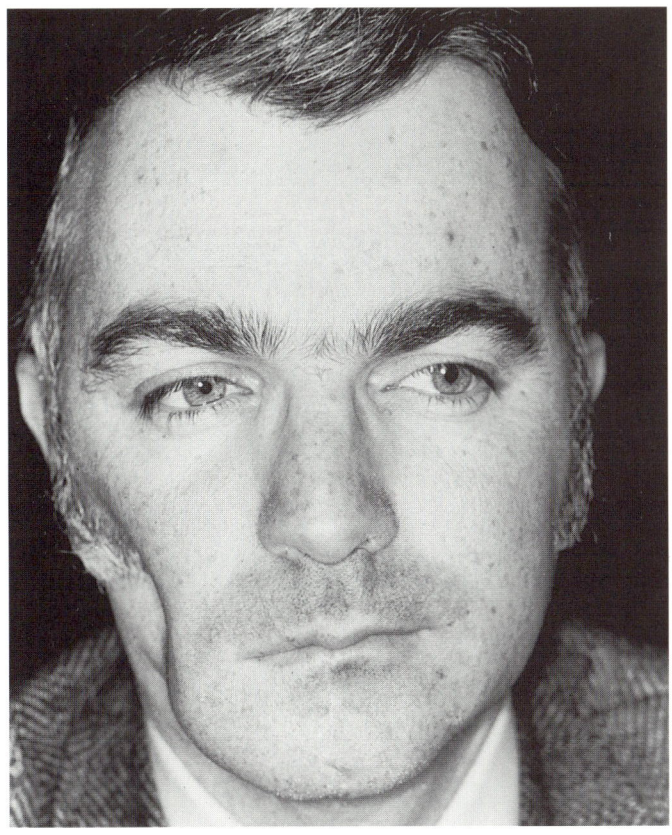

Fig. 8.**18a** **Wide resection of buccal adenoid cystic carcinoma** along with segment of ascending ramus and buccal fat pad by a lower-lip–splitting approach. There is significant cheek defect and moderate trismus.

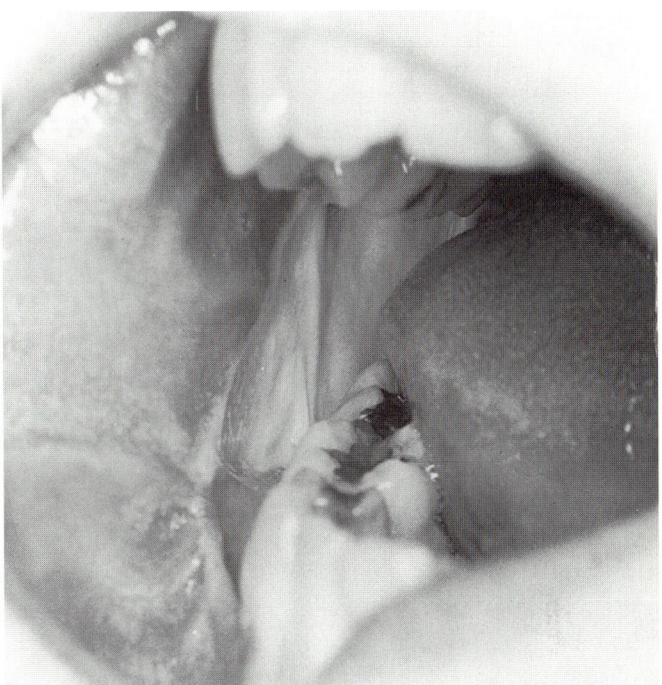

Fig. 8.**18b** This wound was corrected with a split-skin graft. Extreme radicality for buccal adenoid cystic carcinoma is difficult to apply and rarely accepted, and would incorporate regional or microvascular flaps

Tongue
(Fig. 8.**19**)

Adenoid cystic cancer is uncommon in the tongue. It is paradoxical that the anterior undersurface of the tongue has a high population of minor salivary glands and yet rarely has tumor formation in these glands. The prevalent site for this tumor in the tongue is at the base. These small, submucosal, tumors do not cause symptoms in the early stages and are invisible to routine inspection. Therefore, the incidence of T1 lesions is low. As the tumor invades the muscle of the base of the tongue, it produces alterations in swallowing and speaking. The hypoglossal nerve is at risk at this stage. Further expansion compromises the larynx, pharynx, tonsils, and palate.

The surgical anatomy of the tongue identifies this large muscular organ with supportive roles in the physiology of speaking, swallowing, breathing, and handling saliva. Its proximity to the mandible, pharynx, tonsils, and larynx make it a critical structure, and although it has a great capacity for adaption after partial glossectomy, there is a critical point between 50% and 100% ablation at which intraoral crippling can be very severe.

The **diagnosis** is made from the signs and symptoms, imaging, and biopsy. Few of these submucosal tumors are ulcerated and the biopsy must be deep enough to engage essential tissue. Some superficial lesions can be biopsied under local anesthesia, but many require general anesthesia and endoscopic techniques. Imaging is extremely valuable in assessing the extensions of these tumors.

The **surgical treatment** depends on the stage and the position of the primary tumor. Early lesions, less than 2 cm, can be managed by partial glossectomy and immediate repair. Larger lesions at the base or with lateral extension will have to include a larger portion of tongue and adjacent tissues. If the hypoglossal nerve is involved, it is a very serious prognostic sign. If the vallecula, pharynx, tonsils, or mandible are involved, cure cannot be expected and any surgical procedure would have to be classified as a massive palliative operation. Justification for this treads a delicate line and is almost always filled with some degree of frustration. Regional flaps are required to rehabilitate the large ablations. All patients with tumor in the tongue require a full course of postoperative radiotherapy.

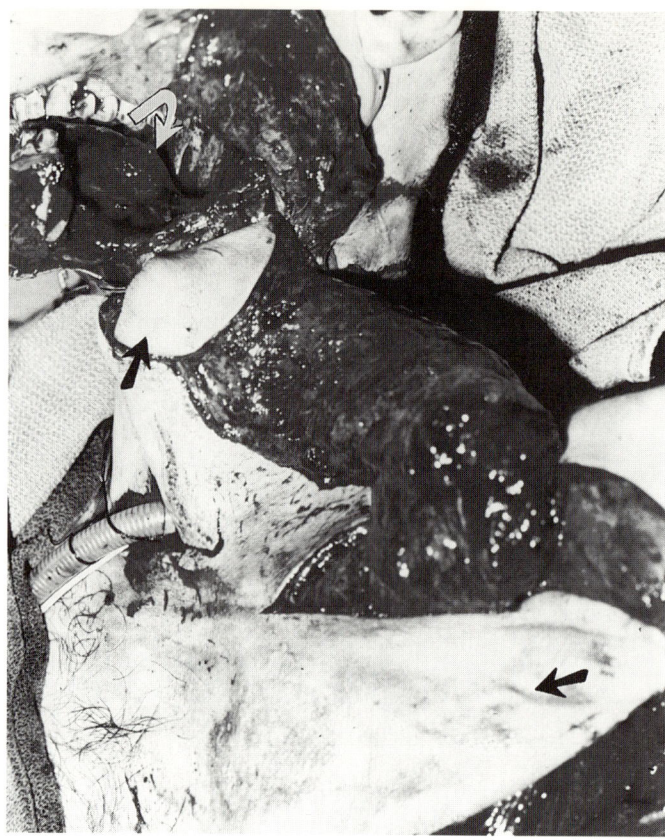

Fig. 8.**19 Adenoid cystic cancer of the base of the tongue** resected along with partial neck dissection and rehabilitation with a pectoralis major myocutaneous flap with salvage of the deltopectoral tissue (arrows)

Lips
(Figs. 8.20–22)

Adenoid cystic cancer of the minor salivary glands of the lips is rare. Its **diagnosis** may be at an early stage of development by the elective removal of an asymptomatic small submucosal mass. This may represent infection, blockage of the duct, or tumor. If it is neoplastic, there is a 65% chance that it is malignant and approximately a 35% chance that it is an adenoid cystic cancer. The significance of this data demands that all of these specimens be sent to the pathologist for microscopic diagnosis. If the specimen is benign, this minor surgical procedure is both diagnostic and curative. If the diagnosis is a malignant tumor, then this technique is classified as a biopsy procedure only, and a definitive reoperation is planned. If the lesion is large enough to form an ulceration in the lip mucosa, a biopsy is performed with forceps to establish the diagnosis of neoplasm and then the tumor is subsequently treated as outlined.

The upper and lower lips lend themselves well to **surgical treatment.** Small lesions of less than 2 cm in diameter are readily managed by regional cheiloplasty techniques. These tumors originate and grow in the minor salivary glands in the submucosal regions of the lips and gradually extend over a period of months and years beyond the capsule of the gland in first a microscopic and then macroscopic manner as they invade the adjacent tissues. These tissues include the proximal fascia, fat, muscle, mucosa, and ultimately, skin. The skin and mucosa are rarely involved in early lesions, but are included in the specimen to establish healthy margins. The lip anatomy ensures regional containment and accessibility. The occult extensions do not occur until the cancer has invaded a sensory or motor nerve or engaged the periosteum of the mandible or premaxilla. Regional or systemic metastasis is not to be expected in the early lesions. In advanced cases, however, the involvement of adjacent tissues may be discernable by physical examination or CT scanning. It is rare for this neoplasm to develop to this extent. It is appropriate therefore, to include a cuff of 0.5–1 cm of normal tissue on all cut margins of these small and early tumors. These margins should be checked by fast frozen-section examination and the margins of the specimen should be identified with india ink to faciliate the microscopic documentation of the security of the specimen. If any of the fast frozen-section specimens are positive for cancer, the dissection is extended until they are securely negative. It is also appropriate to investigate any major nerve systems in the vicinity of the tumor, such as the inframaxillary nerve in upper-lip lesions and the mental nerve in lower-lip lesions. This, again, may not be necessary or realistic in small and early lesions. It is important to realize, however, that these nerves may appear grossly normal and present no clinical signs of involvement, yet may contain cancer in the perineural spaces or in an axonal sheath. This can only be determined by a small biopsy of the nerve sheath. Injury to the nerve under these circumstances is minimal. A positive report requires extension of the resection and a negative report augments a favorable prognosis.

The technique of excision is governed by the site and size of the tumor. As stated previously, very few of these tumors are excessively large. The small lesions on either lip are managed basically by wedge resection and direct approximation. As much as one-half of the lip may be resected without serious aesthetic or functional deficit. If the lip is tight postoperatively, it may be expanded easily by stretching techniques that the patient can apply as desired. When more than half of the lip has been resected, a rotation of a melolabial flap or a sliding cheek flap augments the lip and supplies aesthetics and function. Inactive forehead, neck, and chest flaps are unsatisfactory, unnecessary replacements and have never been used by the author for this tumor.

Alveolus and the Floor of the Mouth

Adenoid cystic cancer is very rare at these sites. It would present as a small, firm mass on the alveolus, compacted between the mucosa and the bone. In the floor of the mouth, a small, moveable submucosal mass would be present and would be inconspicuous.

The surgical anatomy of the *alveolus* places the adenoid cystic carcinoma in intimate contact with the periosteum of the mandible and ultimately with tooth sockets or the invagination of the bony alveolar ridge in the edentulous patient. This adds the considerable danger of invasion of the mandible, the marrow space, and the alveolar nerve by the expanding adenoid cystic carcinoma. Once the tumor has engaged the nerve, it spreads centripetally toward the base of the skull.

The surgical anatomy of the *floor of the mouth* is intimately associated with the sublingual glands, as they share the same territory at different levels and also the same vital structures. Although it is possible in the early stages to separate a minor salivary gland from the sublingual gland, this becomes academic as the tumor enlarges and coalesces with the sublingual gland into a composite neoplastic mass.

The **diagnosis** of the adenoid cystic carcinoma is made by a review of the history and physical findings, imaging techniques, and biopsy. Two important diagnostic criteria are essential, specifically, the possibility of bone and nerve involvement. Biopsy is usually done under local anesthesia, either excisional or incisional, depending on the size and position of the primary tumor.

Definitive **surgical treatment** of the *alveolus* is governed by the proximity of the tumor to bone. There are early cases in which the bone can be spared, otherwise, shaving the outer or inner table, or performing a rim excision and still maintaining the continuity of the mandibular arch can be of great aesthetic and physiological assistance to the patient and are helpful in staging and evaluating prognosis. The more advanced adenoid cystic carcinomas and those that involve the alveolar nerve require hemimandibulectomy with frozen section on the proximal portion of this nerve. If the frozen section is positive, the ablation should extend to the base of the skull. Primary reconstruction of the mandible depends on the position and extent of the defect and the expertise of the surgeon. Free iliac bone or split-rib grafts may be used, and there is usually sufficient soft tissue to cover the graft without tension. When a skin paddle is required along with the bone graft, a composite microvascular graft with appropriate bony fixation is ideal.

The surgical treatment of the *floor of the mouth* is, in the main, similar to that of the sublingual gland.

All patients with tumor of the alveolus or the floor of the mouth receive postoperative irradiation.

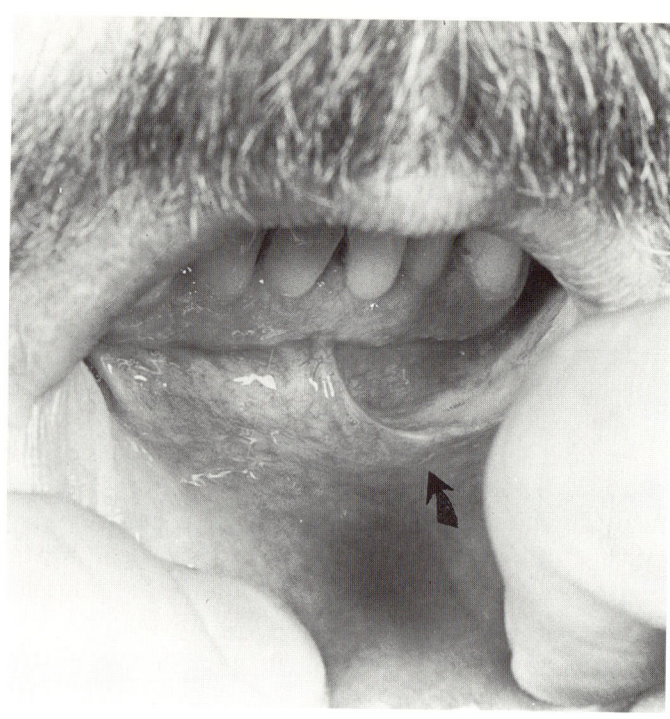

Fig. 8.**20a** **Recently biopsied adenoid cystic cancer of the deep part of the left lower lip** (arrow)

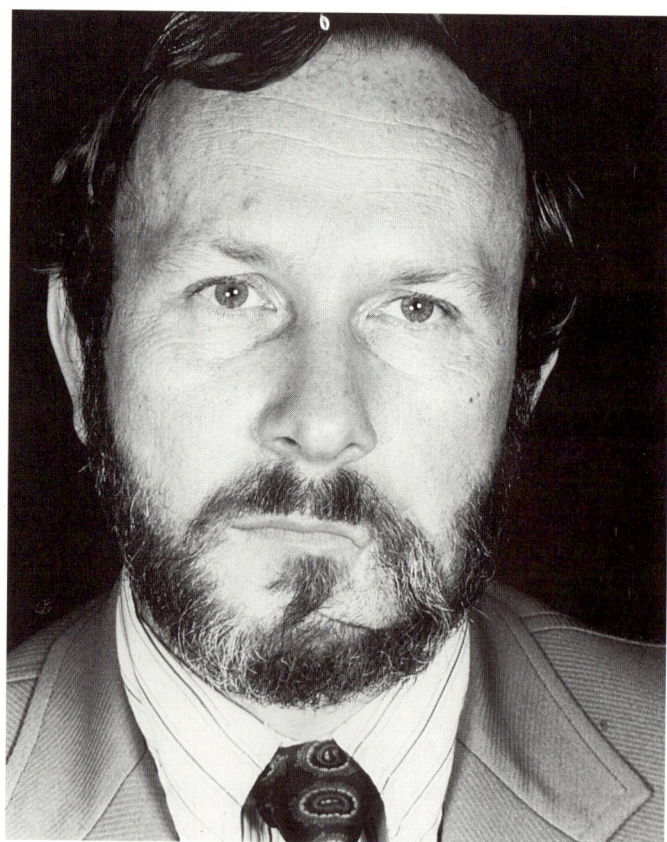

Fig. 8.**20b** This was managed by intraoral local resection with special attention to the mental nerve, periosteum of the mandible, and commissure. There was an immediate reconstruction with minimal deformity. The patient has been free of disease for ten years

Minory Salivary Glands 69

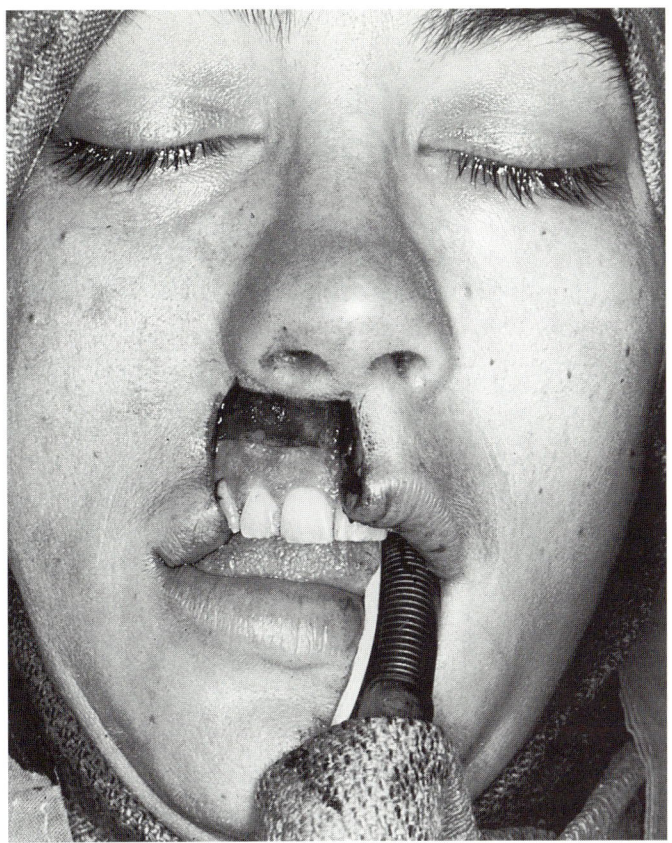

Fig. 8.21a **Carcinoma of the inner aspect of the right upper lip** treated by block resection with special attention paid to the inframaxillary nerve and its branches into this region

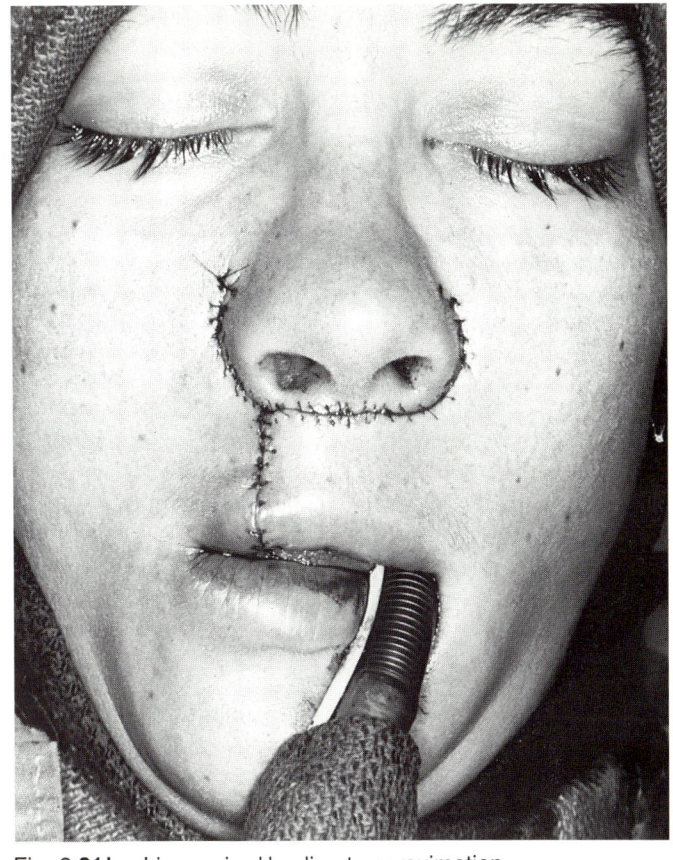

Fig. 8.21b Lip repaired by direct approximation

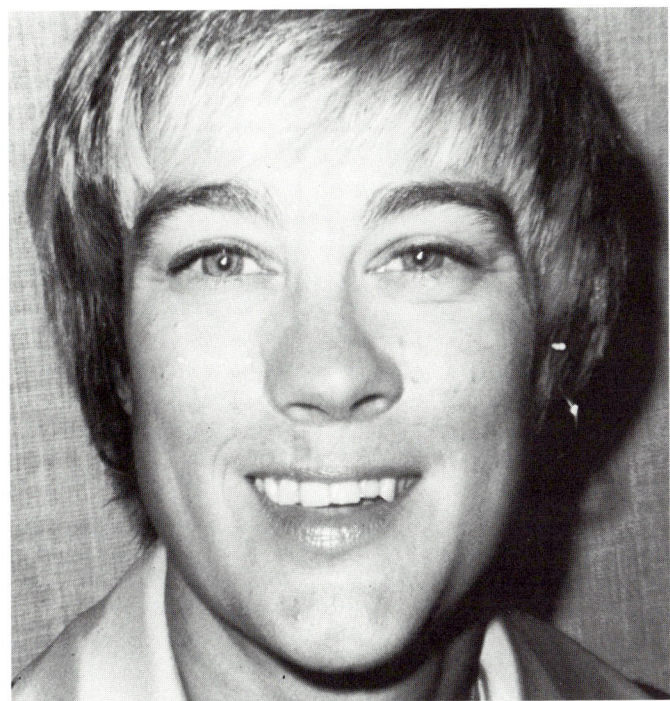

Fig. 8.21c The patient four years after surgery. She has been living free of disease for 16 years

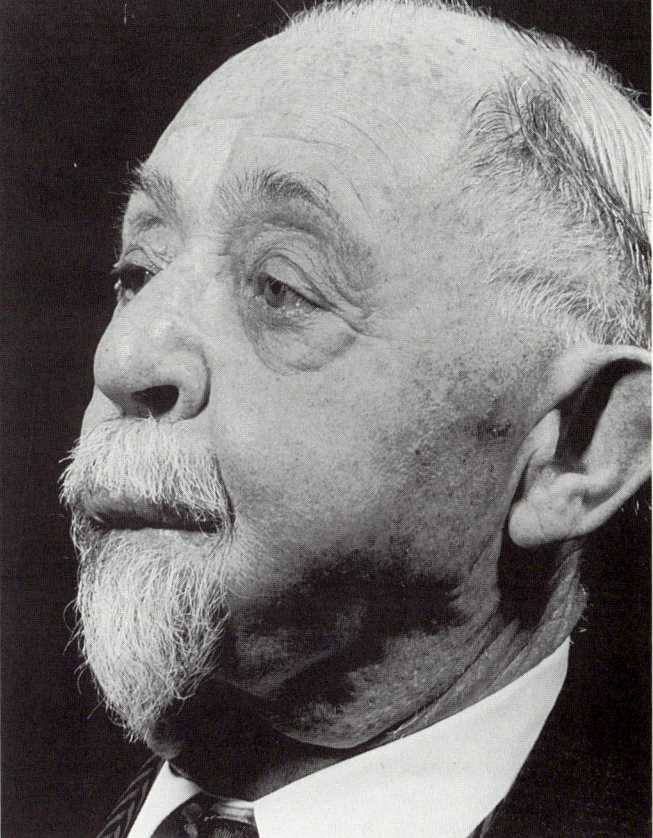

Fig. 8.22 **This patient underwent cheiloplasty of the lower lip for adenoid cystic carcinoma,** never had local recurrence, but eventually died of pulmonary metastases 16 years later

Pharynx
(Fig. 8.23)

Adenoid cystic carcinoma is not common in the hypopharynx or mesopharynx, but is somewhat more common in the *nasopharynx*. A submucosal mass in any of these areas presents no early signs or symptoms from which **diagnosis** can be made, and the patient and the doctor must wait until the volume of the tumor is great enough to recognize a lump or mass that may or may not be sensitive or painful. As this mass becomes larger in the nasopharynx, it may interfere with breathing through the nose, may compress the eustachian tube and cause serous otitis, and may ulcerate and bleed. By this time there is frequently sphenoid involvement, pain, and ultimately, cranial nerve invasion.

Because of technical difficulties in approaching this area surgically, most of the lesions have been treated with radiotherapy. Palliation by this method is initially quite good. Irradiation does not cure the tumor and the problem eventually becomes the management of incurable local recurrence. Additional irradiation is usually given without cure and the situation then has progressed to persistent cancer and often infection, ulceration, and radionecrosis.

Surgical treatment of these cases in the past has been ineffective, but this also has been changed by certain skull-base techniques. Because of the surgical anatomy of the nasopharynx and the intrinsic perniciousness of adenoid cystic carcinoma, these tumors have increased in size and produced some symptoms by the time they present for treatment. The proposition that some of these early tumors may be cured by direct anterior pterygoid, lateral, or inferior surgical approaches combined with microsurgery is certainly plausible. It still remains unlikely, however, that these innovations will save individuals with advanced disease. One might hope that new techniques in radiotherapy and a more aggressive attack would be productive; however, there is in radiobiology a point which is not predictable in every case, but beyond which serious complications are not infrequent, and no therapist is anxious to contribute to necrosis and atrophy of the brain or spinal cord, or osteomyelitis of the base of the skull. In spite of strict precautions and knowledge and experience, these sequelae can occur in the treatment of malignant lesions in this area. Some can be resolved by surgery, but some are fatal.

Adenoid cystic carcinoma of the *mesopharynx* and *hypopharynx* are more manageable because of the surgical anatomy of these regions. It presents in the early stages as a submucosal mass and does not present symptoms until its volume or invasiveness affects the surrounding tissues. In this instance, it would begin as a mass on the posterior pharyngeal wall about the tonsils, vallecula, or pyriform fossa. From these sites, it grows toward the palate, internal pterygoid muscle, mandible, pharynx, base of the tongue, and paralaryngeal structures. It is at this stage that significant signs and symptoms appear, mainly pain in the throat, trismus, difficulty in swallowing, and hoarseness.

The surgical treatment of these lesions depends upon their size and their location. The objective is the same as in all cancer operations, namely, to remove all of the neoplasm without spillage. The surgical approach is usually through the lateral cervical structures. Therapeutic neck dissection is rarely indicated because of the low incidence of regional metastasis, but in cases of certain aggressive tumors, a conservation neck dissection is appropriate. The smaller ablations are repaired by direct approximation of regional tissue or free skin grafts. Larger resections are rehabilitated with cutaneous or myocutaneous regional flaps or microvascular flap transfer.

Almost all patients with tumor in the pharynx receive a full course of radiotherapy postoperatively.

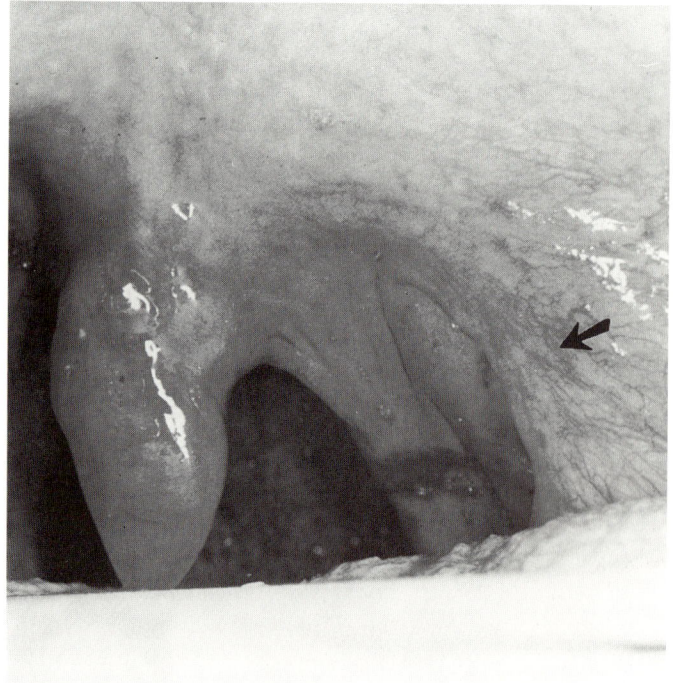

Fig. 8.23 **Adenoid cystic cancer of the left mesopharynx** (arrow) treated by surgical resection and postoperative radiotherapy

Upper Trachea and Paralaryngeal Regions
(Figs. 8.24–26).

These two sites have a very low incidence of adenoid cystic carcinoma. Both can contribute dynamically to impairment of physiological function in this area with symptoms of hoarseness, difficulty in breathing, and ultimately, difficulty in swallowing as these tumors increase in size. Adenoid cystic carcinoma does not occur on the vocal cords because of the squamous epithelial covering and the absence of glandular structures in the cord itself. When this type of cancer affects the larynx, it begins in a paralaryngeal mucosal element that is adjacent to it, such as the vallecula, supralarynx, pyriform fossa, and pharynx. As the cancer grows, it impinges on the larynx, invades the muscles and nerves in this area, and ultimately causes hoarseness and airway obstruction. There are no signs or symptoms in the early stages. When the cancer is subglottic or upper tracheal, there are no signs or symptoms until the airway is diminished and there is gradual progression to shortness of breath and stridor, sometimes associated also with a tickly cough. As these tumors enlarge, they involve the recurrent laryngeal nerves, thyroid, and cervical esophagus.

The surgical anatomy of these areas is interwoven with the physiological functions of speaking, breathing, swallowing, and coughing. Nature has provided enough of a margin of safety that at least 25% of the functional capacity of these regions must be diminished before the patient has cause to seek aid. The organs at risk are the larynx, trachea, gullet, thyroid, recurrent laryngeal nerves, and structures in the adjacent cervical area.

The **diagnosis** is made from the signs and symptoms, imaging, endoscopy, and biopsy. The preoperative endoscopic biopsy can usually be obtained, but occasionally, open biopsy may be necessary.

Imaging is again one of the most dependable diagnostic tools for evaluating occult extensions of the neoplasm.

The **surgical treatment** is often delicately balanced between adequate resection and conservation surgery for the T1 lesions. When the tumor involves the gerneral area or is recurrent, the possibility of using conservation techniques is reduced. The ablative procedures for extended carcinoma may involve the larynx and trachea and also include the thyroid and the cervical esophagus. Improvisations in rehabilitation may include regional flaps, microvascular flaps, and multistaged procedures.

All patients with tumor in the trachea or laryngeal areas receive a full course of radiotherapy postoperatively.

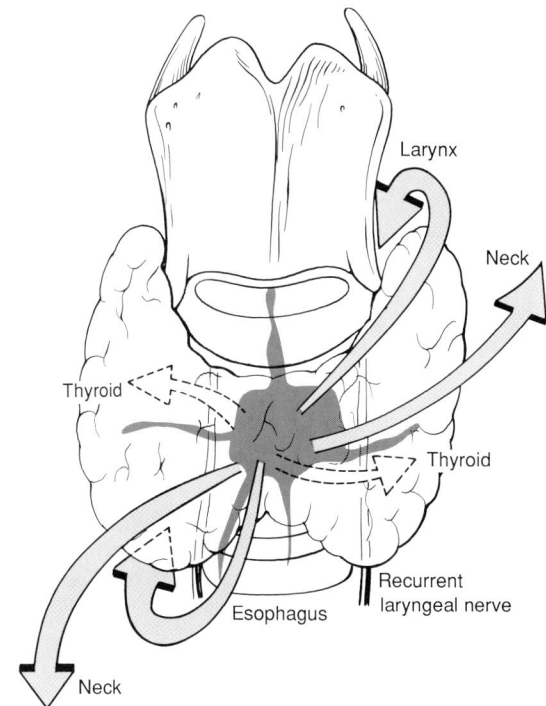

Fig. 8.24 **Primary adenoid cystic carcinoma in the trachea.** Arrows indicate areas most frequently involved by direct extension

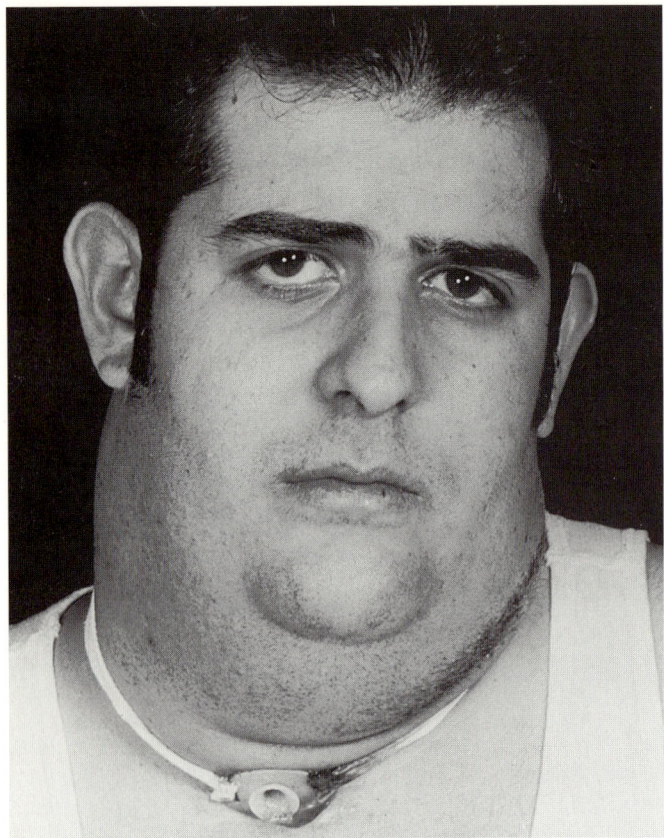 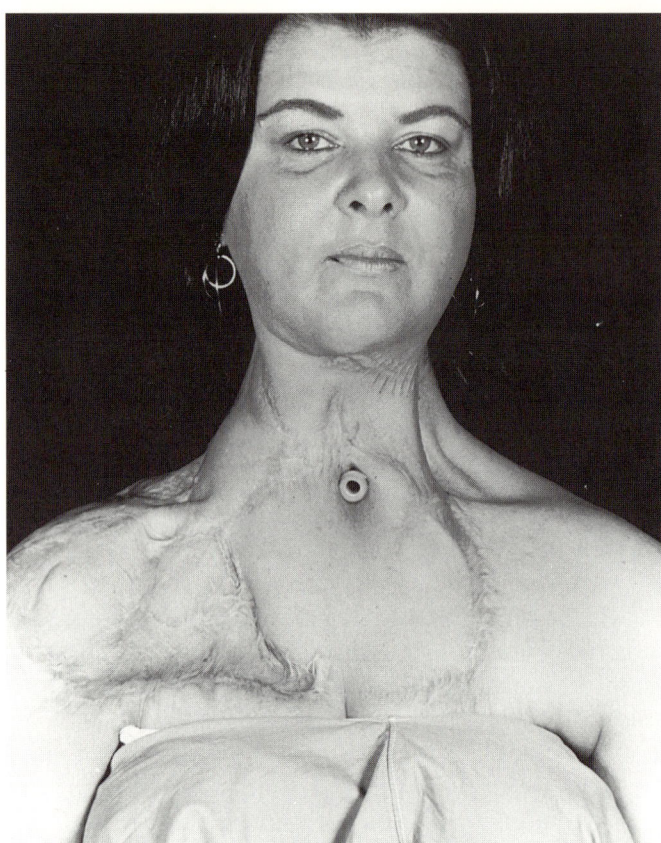

Fig. 8.**25 Undifferentiated cancer of the right supraglottis with extensive spread to the right neck.** There was controversy about the diagnosis, but it was finally declared to be a small-cell, undifferentiated type of adenoid cystic carcinoma. The patient was treated with radiotherapy palliatively. This is the only adenoid cystic carcinoma in this series that was so aggressive

Fig. 8.**26 Extensive cancer of the subglottic area affecting the larynx, thyroid, and pharynx,** rehabilitated by regional flaps. None of the patients in Figures 8.23, 8.25, and 8.26 survived their diseases

Major Salivary Glands

Parotid Gland
(Figs. 8.27—42)

Although the parotid gland contains the largest number of adenoid cystic carcinomas in this series, it does not have the highest incidence of occurrence. This is primarily due to the large number of parotid gland tumors referred for treatment; they predominate in the case load of adenoid cystic carcinomas, and this creates the impression of prevalence over tumors at other sites. The actual incidence rate of adenoid cystic carcinoma in the parotid gland is around 15%. The surgical anatomy of this gland and its relationship to the facial-nerve system make it especially critical in comparison to other regions.

This gland has parenchymal tissue encased in a capsule and surrounded by fat, fascia, muscle, bone, mucous membrane, and skin. Certain areas interdigitate with mild lobulations at the peripheral extensions. A mass of the gland is lateral to the facial nerve and a smaller portion is medial to the nerve. This is not a true embryologic or anatomic separation of these regions. They are called the lateral lobe and the medial lobe in order to identify the position of the facial nerve passing between them. It is obvious that a small adenoid cystic carcinoma in the deep lobe or in the lateral lobe cannot be identified at an early stage. If the neoplasm is at the periphery of the gland under the skin, it has an opportunity of being seen or felt at an earlier stage. In the main, however, the patient presents with advanced disease. This phenomenon is highlighted by the fact that approximately 11% of these patients had some type of preoperative facial paresis.

The **diagnosis** of this tumor begins with an analysis of its history as well as of physical and imaging techniques to detect the actual size, extensions, and possible involvements of regional structures. If there are any stigmata of malignancy, such as pain or facial paresis, fixation, anesthesia of the great auricular or auricular temporal nerves, an aspiration biopsy may be of great help. If there is ulceration of the skin, which is indeed extremely rare, a direct forceps biopsy may be sufficient. Over half of the patients in this series have had a recent operation during which cancer was unexpectedly revealed, or they had multiple operations for recurrent neoplasm. The microscopic sections of all these cases should be reviewed before proceeding with the definitive procedure because of the possibility of change in diagnosis. A formal incisional biopsy is rarely recommended today, but there are circumstances under which it might prove to be propitious for legal or personal reasons.

The variations in **surgical treatment** of the parotid gland for adenoid cystic carcinoma range from a lateral lobectomy with preservation of the facial nerve, to a total parotidectomy with preservation of the facial nerve along with a conservation neck dissection, to a total parotidectomy with sacrifice of the facial nerve and a neck dissection with possible inclusion of some part of the mandible, mastoid, or auricle. Mandibular swing technique must be considered for deep-lobe tumors that extend into the mesopharynx or palate.

The simplest operation is the lateral lobectomy, but the criteria for its application in adenoid cystic carcinoma are limited and debatable. If the neoplasm is small (less than 2 cm), is limited to the lateral lobe, is well-contained within the substance of the gland and is not involving the facial nerve, and does not present with metastasis either by CT scan or at operation, then a lateral lobectomy may be considered justified when the diagnosis is made by needle aspiration biopsy or by frozen section at the time of operation or after the permanent sections are forthcoming. The latter circumstance is rarely applicable because it is created after the fact. One might ask whether this operation is adequate for this tumor; the answer would have to be: not in every case. If the diagnosis of adenoid cystic carcinoma is made during the lateral lobectomy by frozen section, the sugeon should enhance biological control by proceeding to a total parotidectomy with preservation of the facial nerve and a conservation upper-neck dissection. This

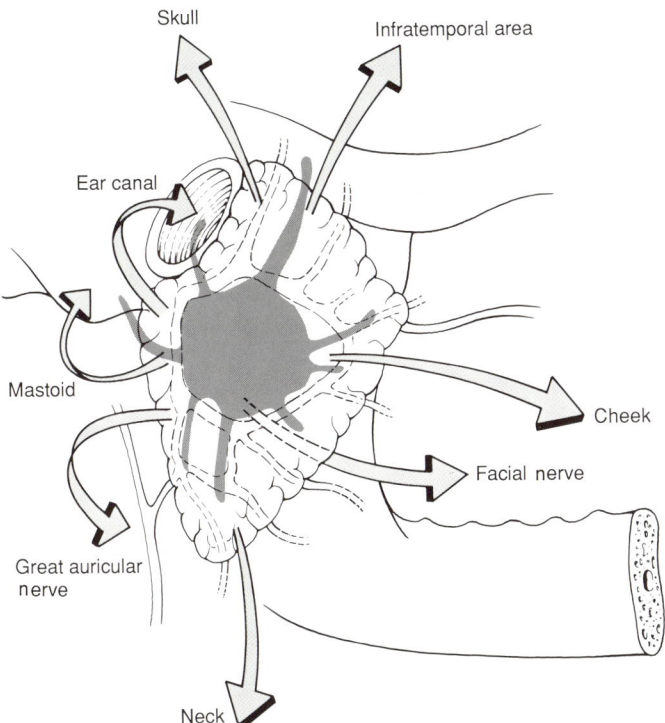

Fig. 8.27 **Primary adenoid cystic carcinoma of the parotid gland.** Arrows indicate areas most frequently involved by direct extension

technique includes the middle and upper deep jugular lymph nodes along with those in the superior spinal accessory chain, and prevascular and postvascular lymph nodes. If the tumor has a cribriform or tubular histologic pattern, one would not expect metastasis. This type of operation supplies additional information for classification, removes any possible macrometastasis or micrometastatis, and does not leave a serious wound deficit, as there is no damage to any of the cranial nerves or regional tissues.

On the other hand, a surgeon may be faced with a case in which a tumor specimen was removed in three or four segments and there is spread to a lymph node. The face is usually quite paretic at this time, but may recover movement. The size of the tumor, the histologic type, the proximity to the facial nerve, the piecemeal resection, and the proved metastasis are all grave signals, and this patient is advised to have a reoperation with total parotidectomy, resection of the facial nerve, and upper-neck dissection. The facial nerve is immediately rehabilitated with a facial-nerve autograft or masseter-muscle transfer. If this type of operation is to be executed on the basis of a frozen-section diagnosis during a routine parotidectomy, the responsible surgeon has the obligation to substantiate the microscopy with a senior pathologist and to obtain permission to resect the facial nerve at the time of the initial consultation. Some doctors do not ask for this permission and some patients will not grant it preoperatively. The surgeon must comply with this contract.

Tumors which have extended beyond the parotid gland understandably have the poorest prognosis. At the consultation, they may be de novo or recurrent extensions. Simple or limited operation will neither control the process locally nor prevent it from wide dissemination. A major ablation offers the best chance for local control, but even with this temporary success, the tumor frequently metastasizes to the lungs, bone, and other structures with a fatal outcome.

The question of postoperative irradiation comes up in the majority of these cases, regardless of the stage of the tumor. Certainly, the only patients who could avoid it would be the relatively early cases with good surgical margins and optimal biological factors. In almost all other situations it is recommended. Every tumor in this series that was exposed to therapeutic irradiation responded to it initially. The significance of this palliation can only be judged by the patient, but the effects can last for one to eight years. Unquestionably, irradiation has a very important role in management. It has been argued that postoperative irradiation minimizes the effect of a nerve graft recovery, but this has not been the experience of the author.

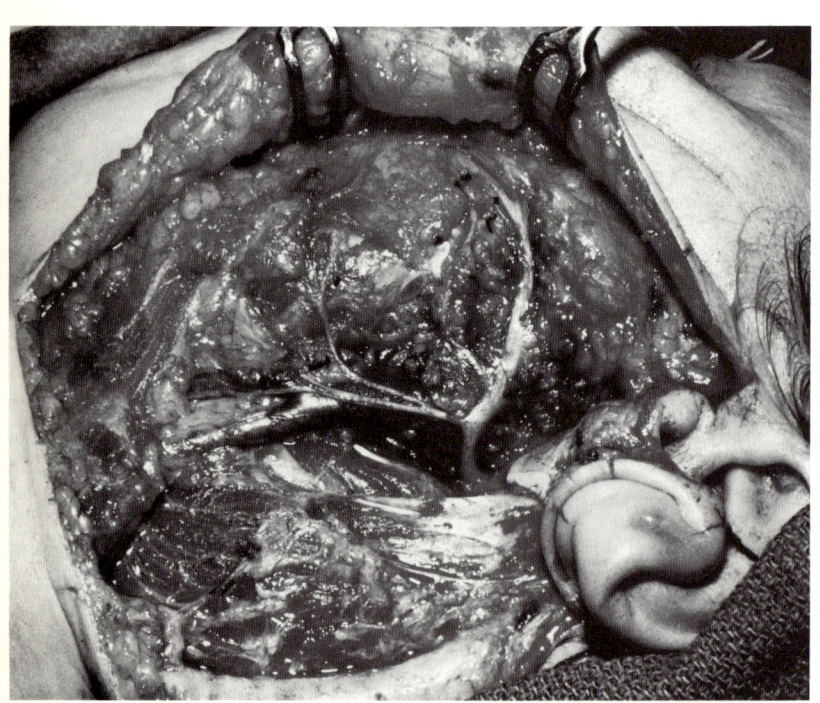

Fig. 8.28 **Total parotidectomy with preservation of facial nerve for T1 adenoid cystic carcinoma in lateral lobe**

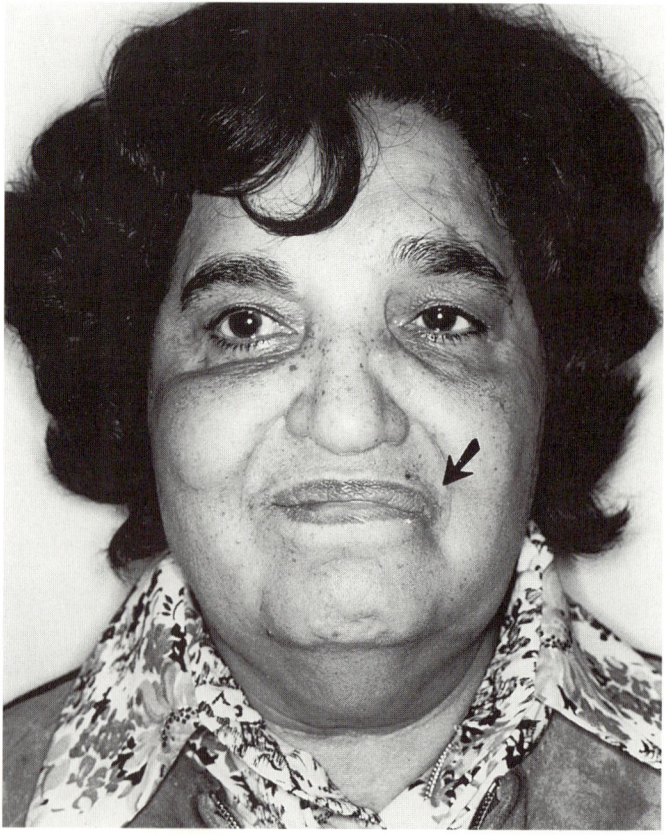

Fig. 8.29 **Selective facial nerve resection (buccal) with minimal deficit on left side of buccal branches**

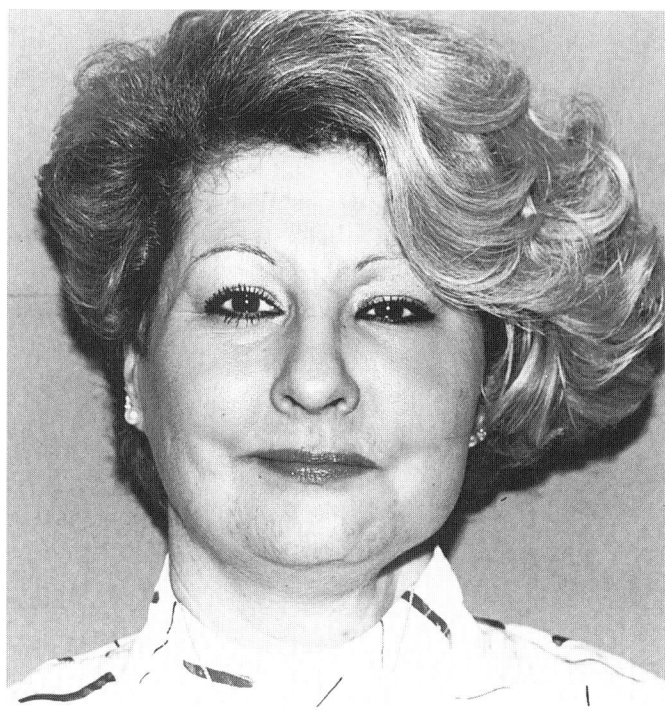

Fig. 8.**30a** **Total facial nerve graft with regionalized movement of the left side of the face** nine years after surgery

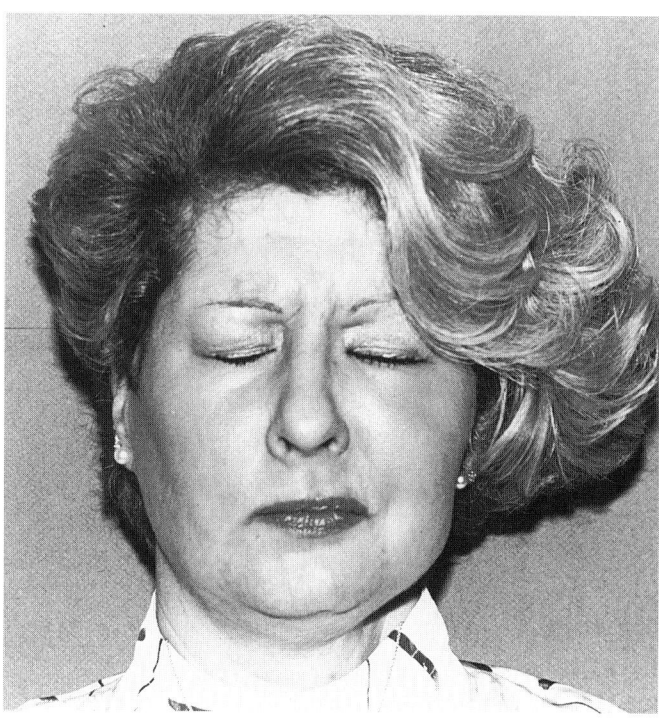

Fig. 8.**30b** Strong mass movement of the mouth, cheek, and eye

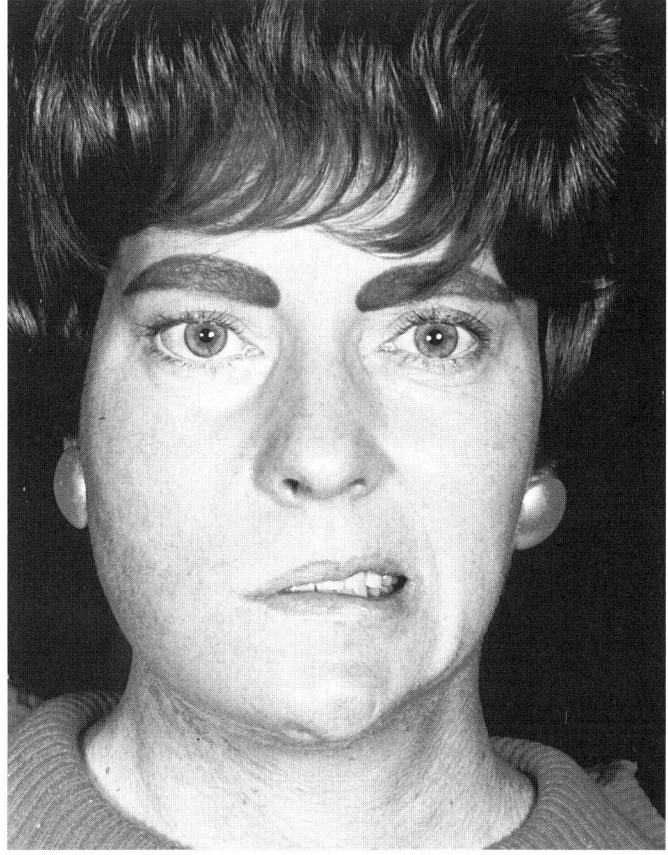

Fig. 8.**31** **This patient had progressive facial paresis on the right side from an occult adenoid cystic carcinoma of the deep lobe.** It was discovered at examination that she had preoperative metastasis to the lung. She was treated with radiotherapy only. This occult primary had been observed for 2 years with a misdiagnosis of Bell's Palsy. CT scanning reduces the likelihood of this error

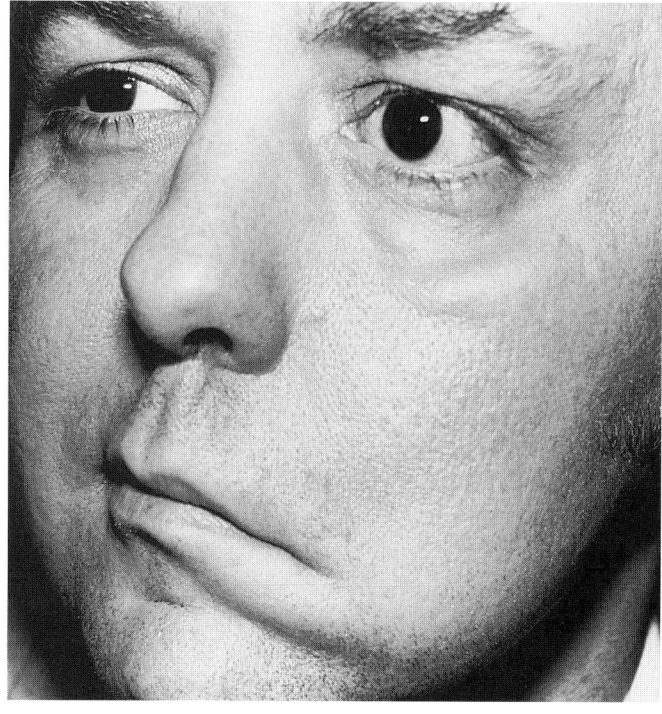

Fig. 8.**32** **This patient had a history of pain lasting over ten years and presented with complete facial paralysis** as well as involvement of the 10th, 11th, and 12th cranial nerves. The paralysis was progressive over three months

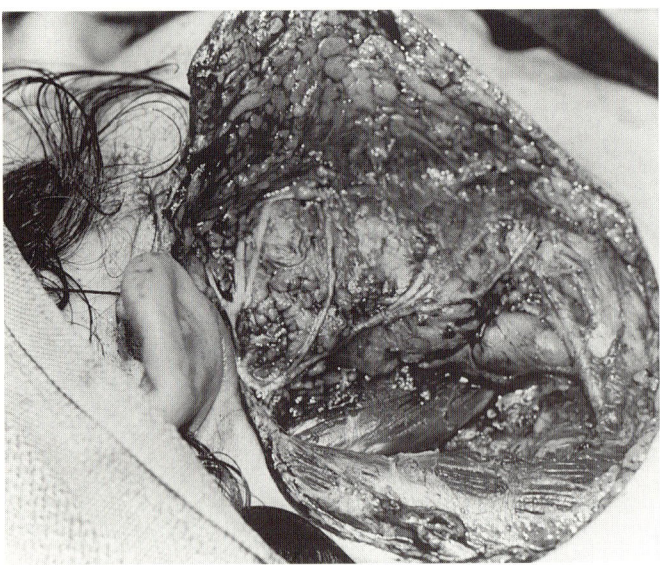

Fig. 8.33 **Total parotidectomy** including the deep lobe and the paraglandular and upper neck structures with preservation of the facial nerve for adenoid cystic carcinoma localized to the lateral lobe

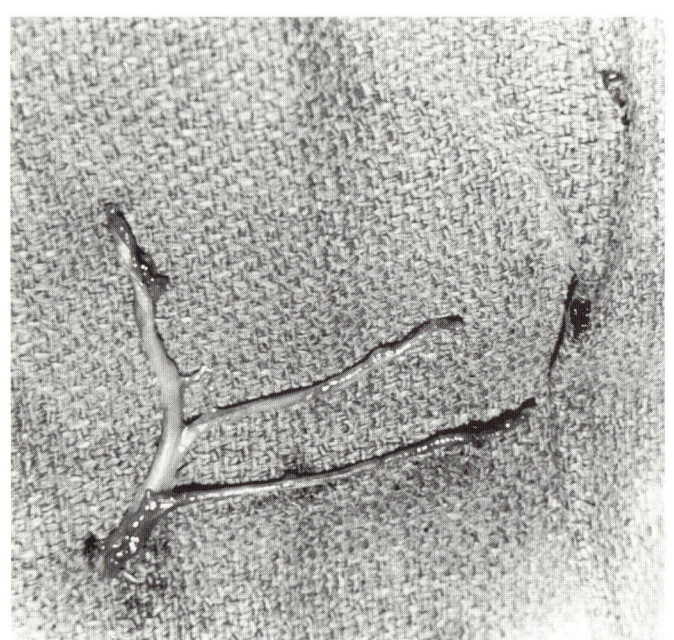

Fig. 8.34a **A great auricular nerve graft** with three branches used for nerve grafting and procured either from the ipsilateral or contralateral side

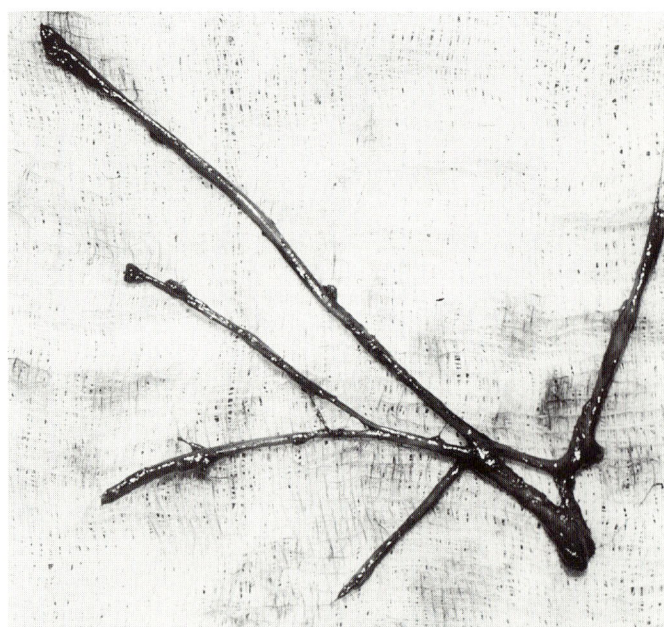

Fig. 8.34b Similar graft showing five branches

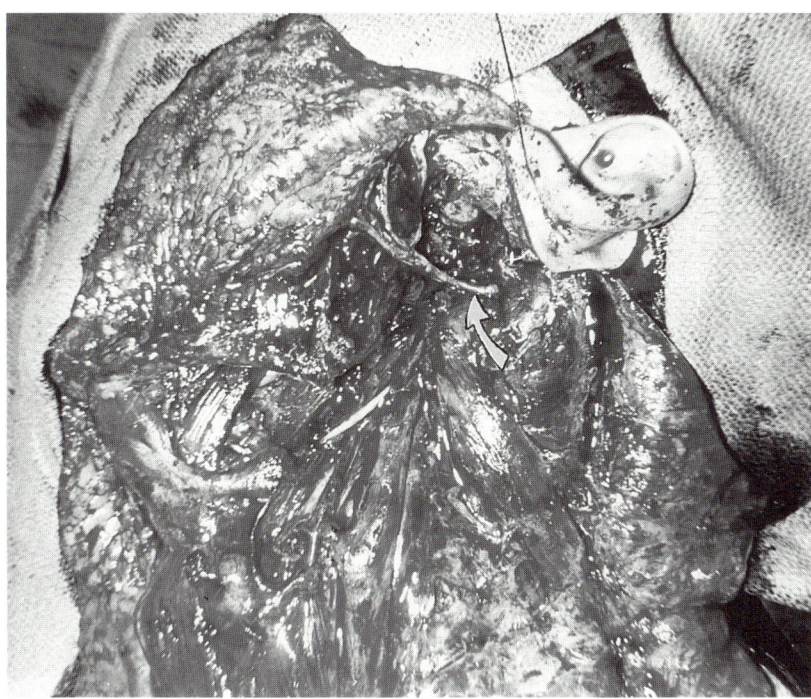

Fig. 8.35 **Total parotidectomy, partial mandibulectomy, mastoidectomy, and neck dissection with nerve graft in the fallopian canal and two branches in the face.** The primary branch goes to the zygomatic division

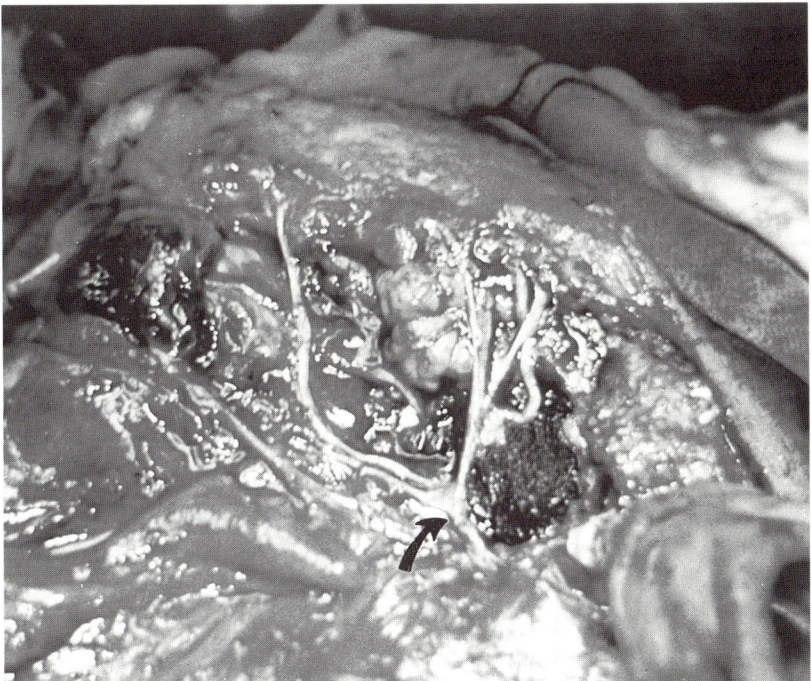

Fig. 8.36 **A five divisioned nerve graft supplying the upper and lower portions of the face**

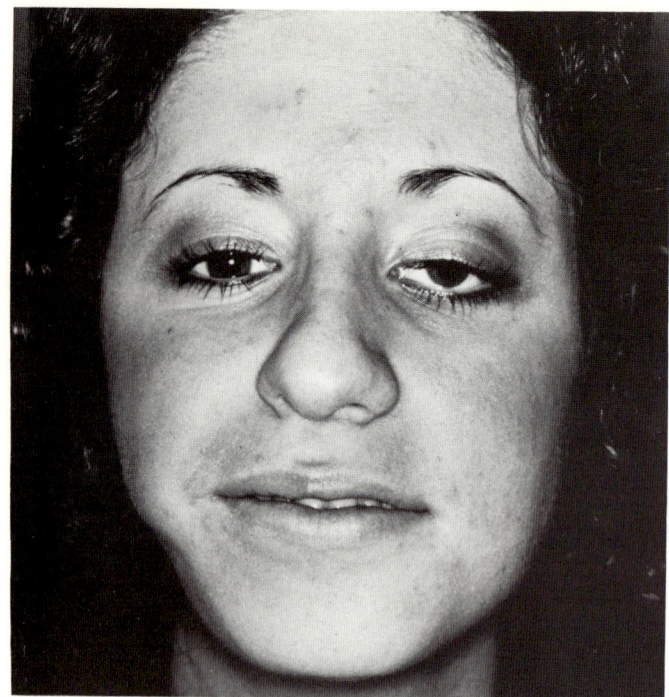

Fig. 8.**37a** **Right facial nerve graft and masseter transfer with good return of movement to face and eyelids,** three years after surgery

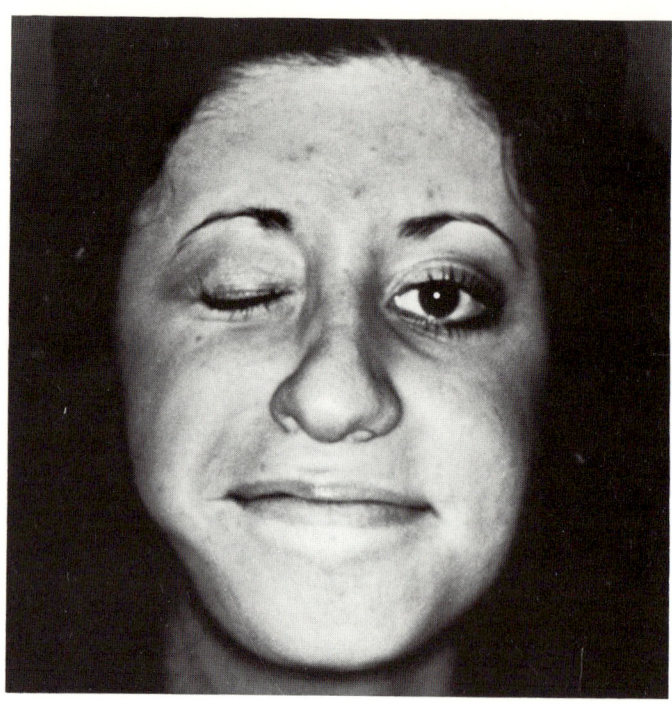

Fig. 8.**37b** Showing strong intentional contraction

These massive surgical ablations remove ulcerations, reduce pain, and create some deformity. The deformity, however, is never as bad as untreated cancer in the head and neck.

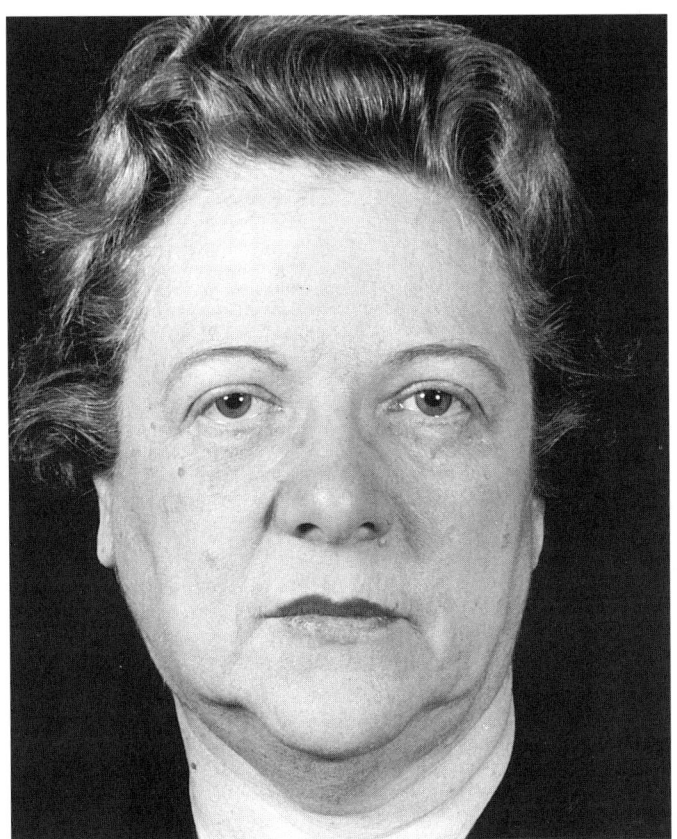

Fig. 8.**38a** **Extensive adenoid cystic carcinoma involving the right parotid gland**

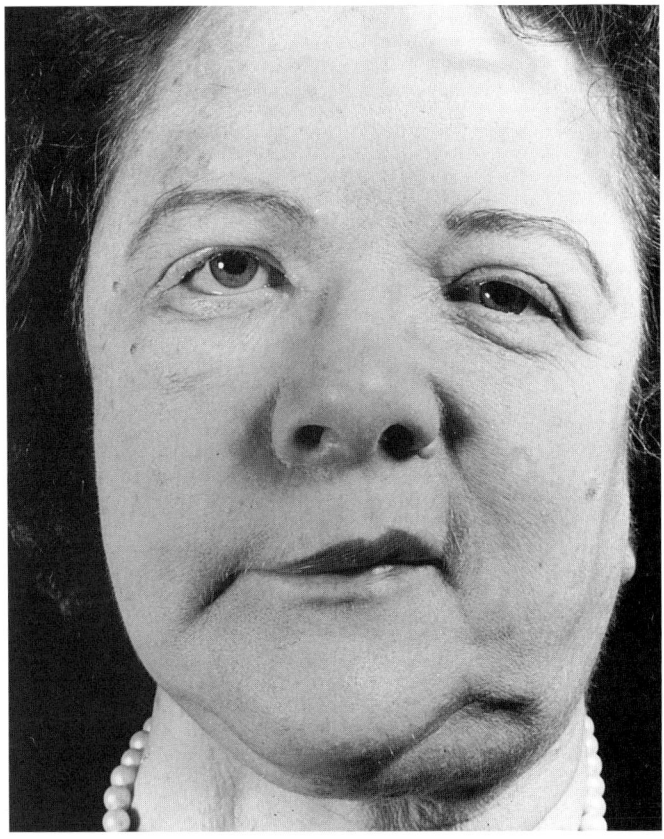

Fig. 8.**38b** The patient had metastasis to the neck and underwent radical parotidectomy and neck dissection

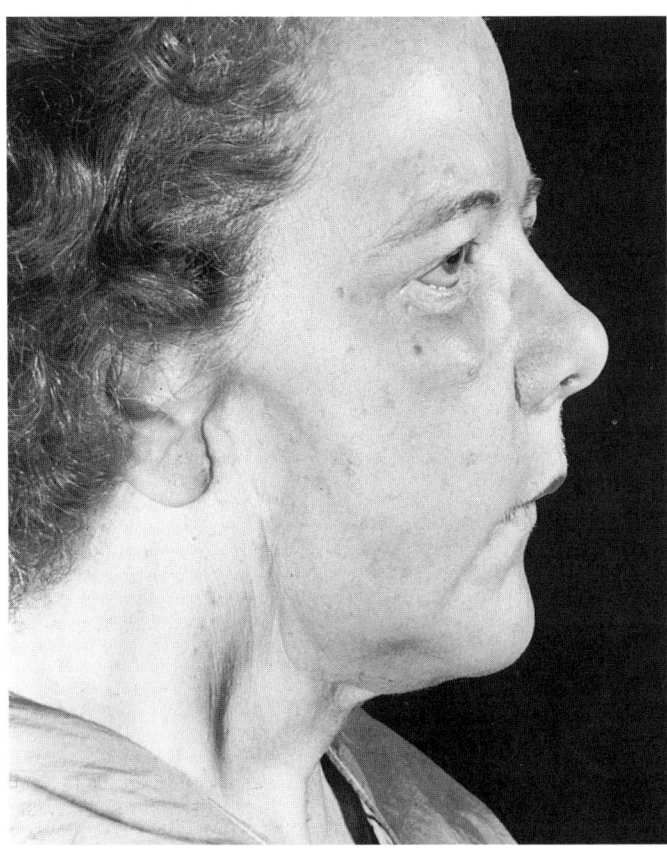

Fig. 8.**38c** Lateral view three years later

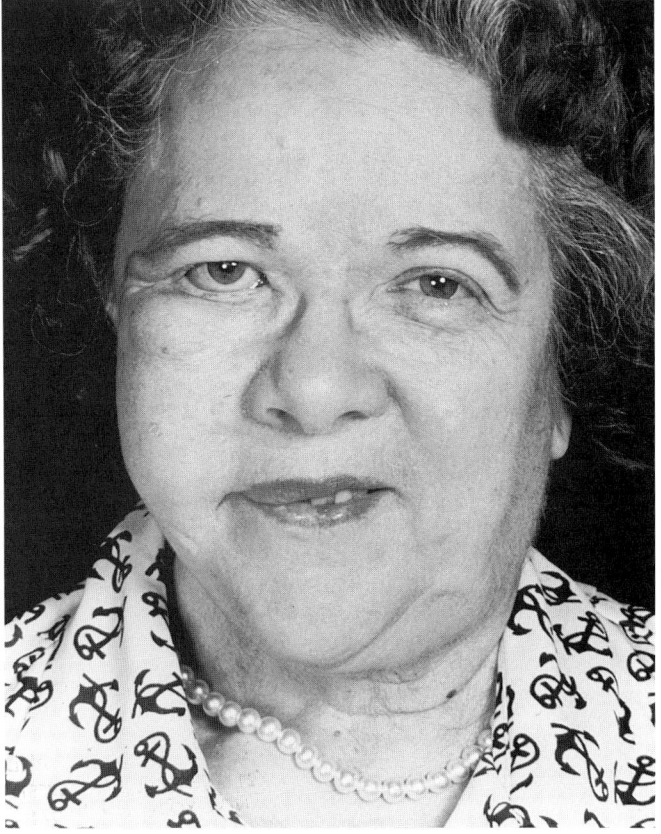

Fig. 8.**38d** The patient has fair return of movement of the face six years after surgery

8 Surgical Treatment

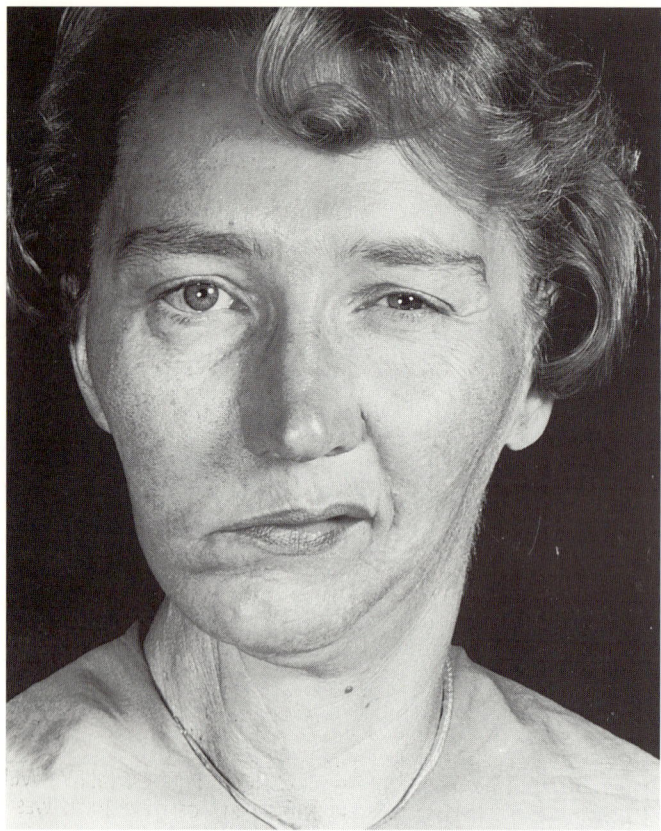

Fig. 8.39a This patient had extensive adenoid cystic carcinoma of the right parotid gland treated by radical resection

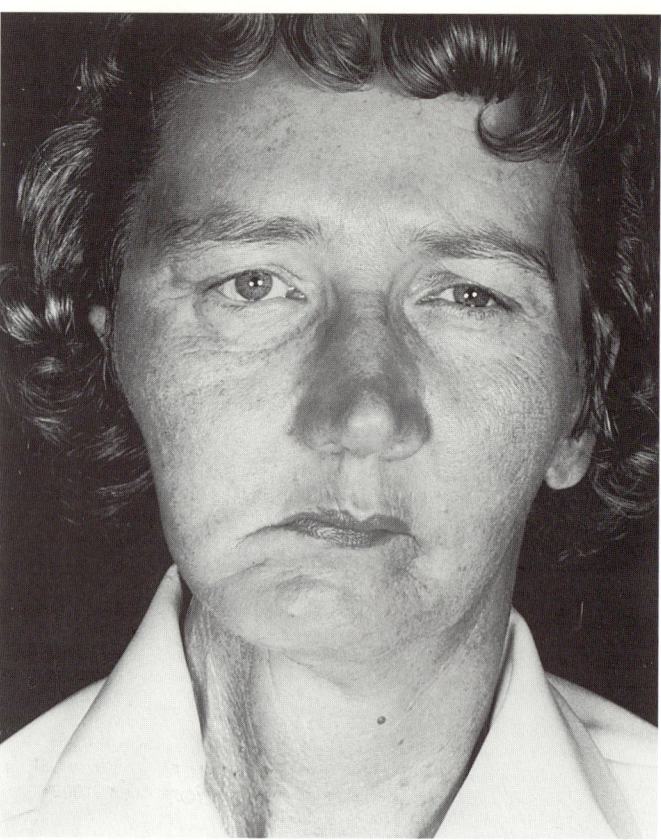

Fig. 8.39b She had local recurrence and reoperation three years later. The face was rehabilitated with a facial nerve graft

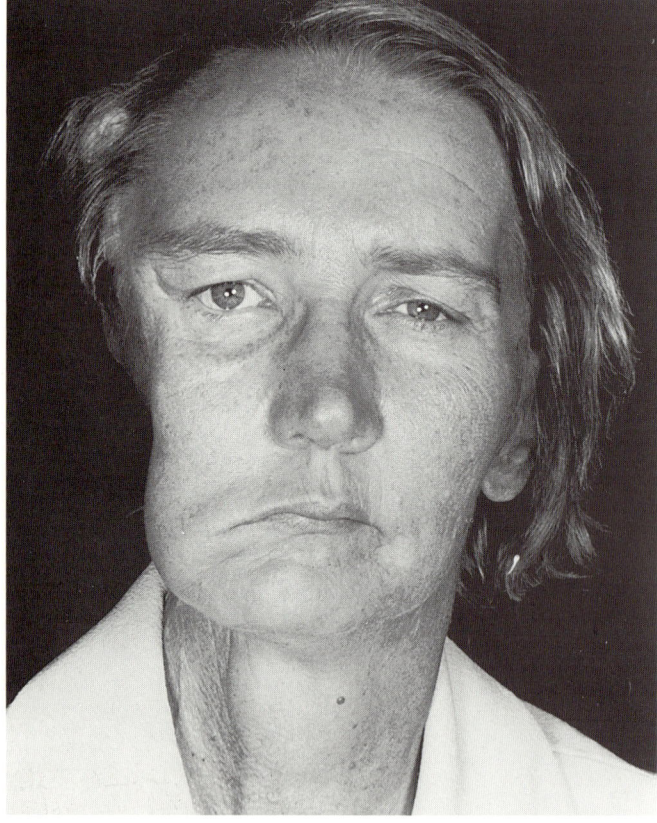

Fig. 8.39c Subsequently, she developed extensive local recurrence and underwent radical local ablation two years later

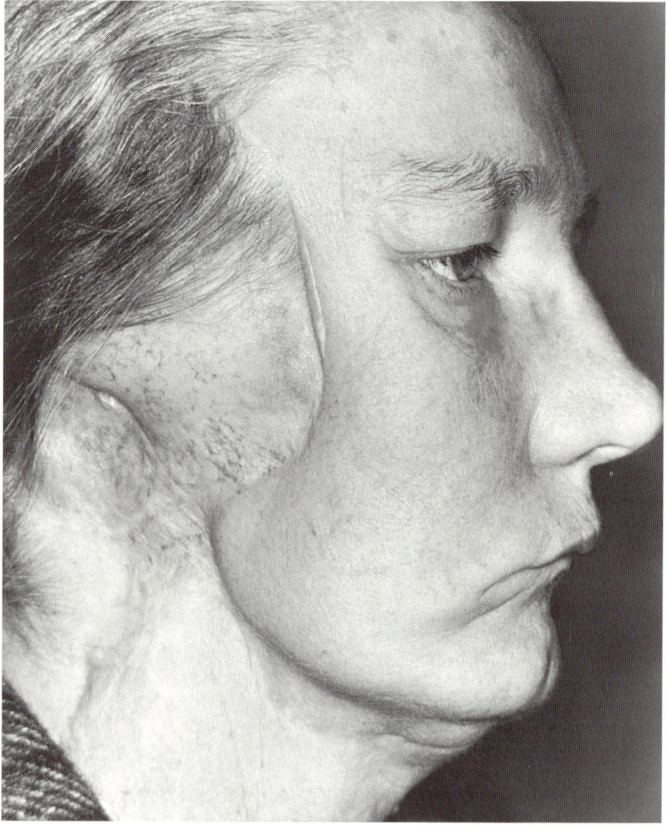

Fig. 8.39d Reconstruction of the wound was accomplished by a posterior cervical flap

Major Salivary Glands

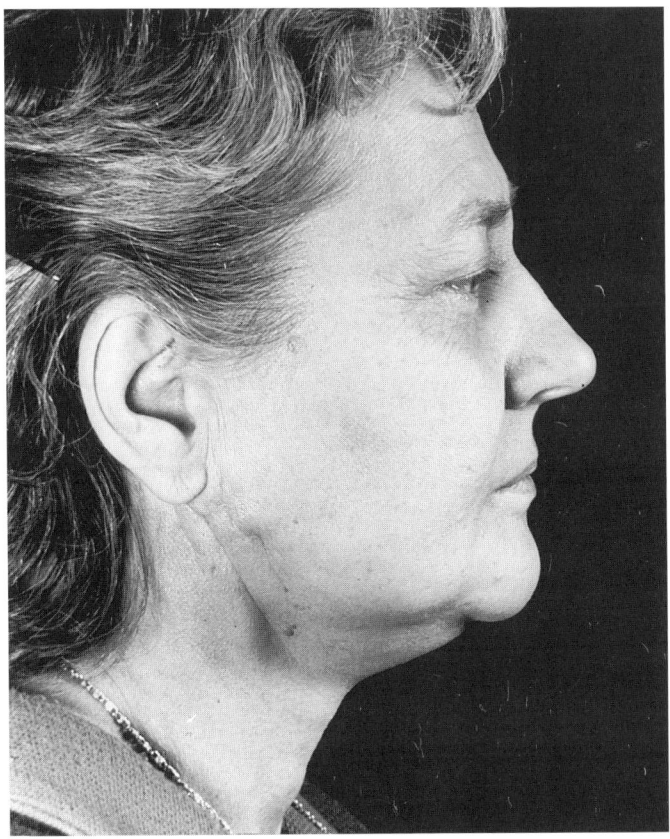

Fig. 8.**40a** This patient had extensive recurrent adenoid cystic carcinoma involving the parotid gland, upper neck, and temporal bone

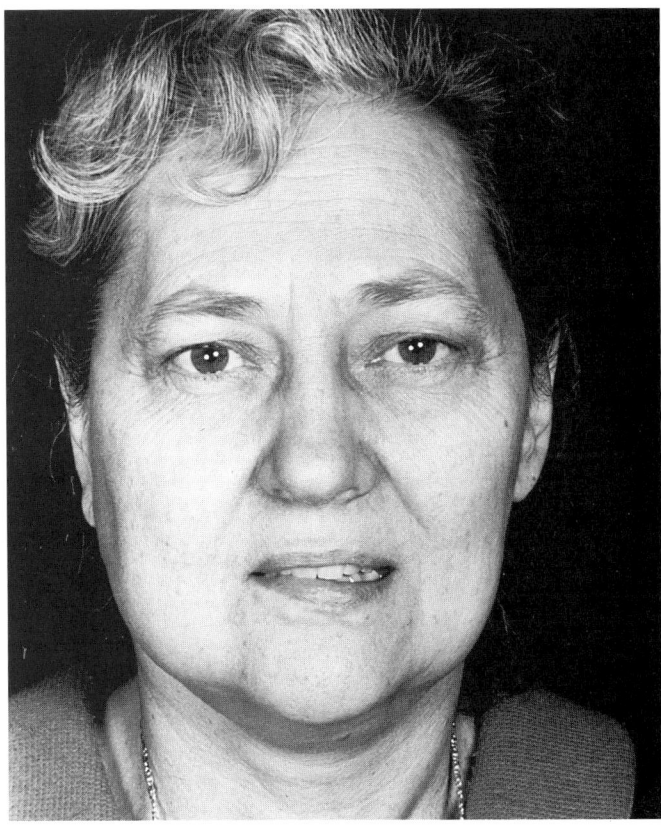

Fig. 8.**40b** The facial nerve system was partially intact preoperatively

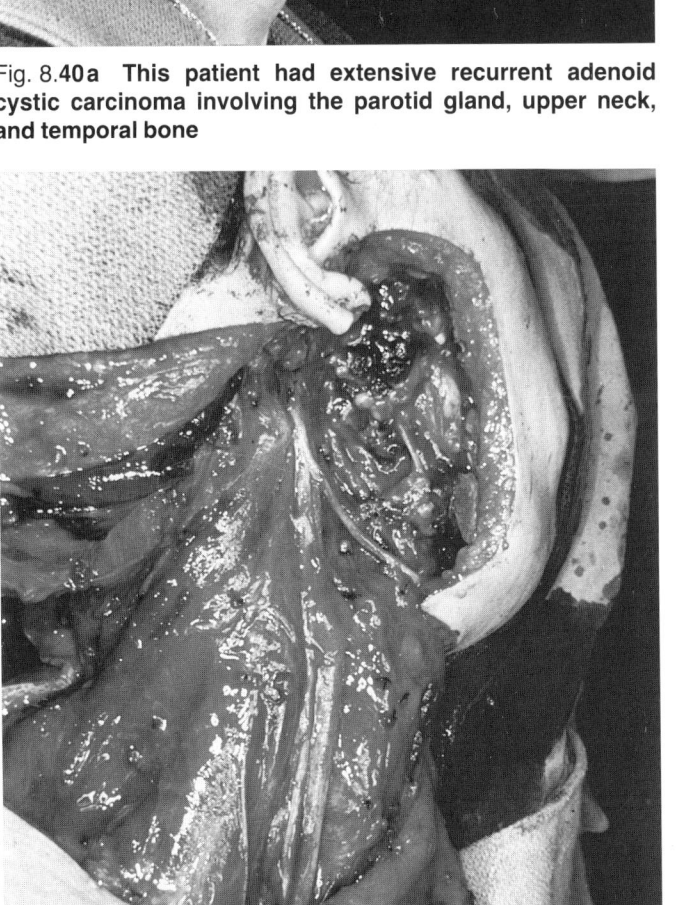

Fig. 8.**40c** It was treated by radical parotidectomy, mandibulectomy, temporal bone resection, and neck dissection

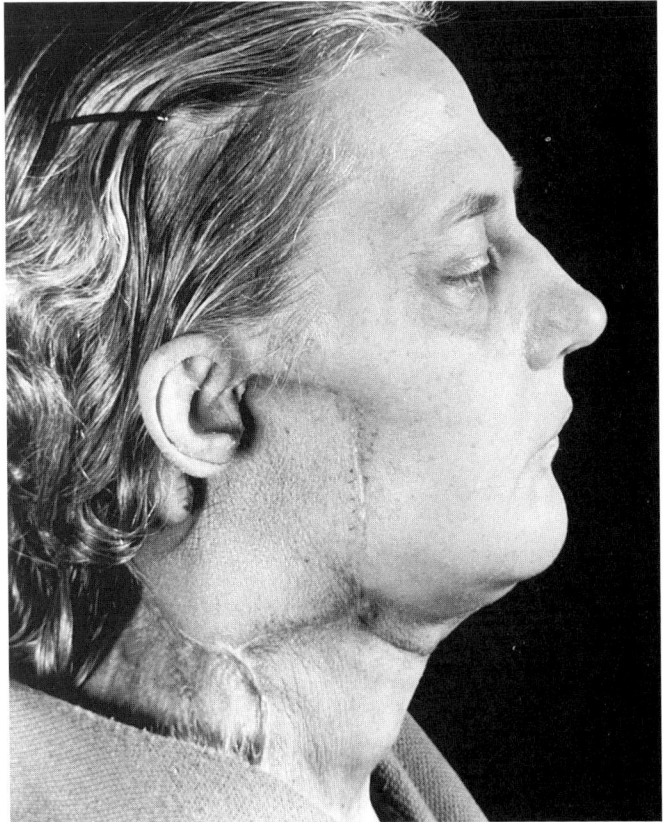

Fig. 8.**40d** The extensive wound was rehabilitated with a posterior cervical flap and skin graft. A full course of postoperative irradiation was administered to this area. These patients are highly susceptible to local recurrence and pulmonary metastasis

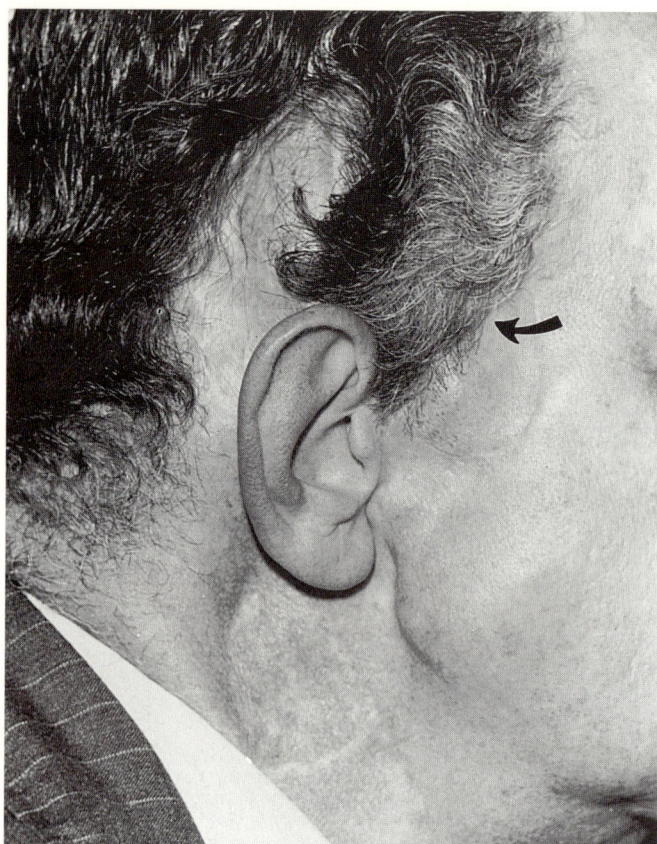

Fig. 8.41 **Radical resection of recurrent adenoid cystic carcinoma of the parotid gland, upper neck, and associated scalp and skin, rehabilitated by a facial nerve graft and posterior occipital hair-bearing flap to create a facsimile of the temple**

Major Salivary Glands 83

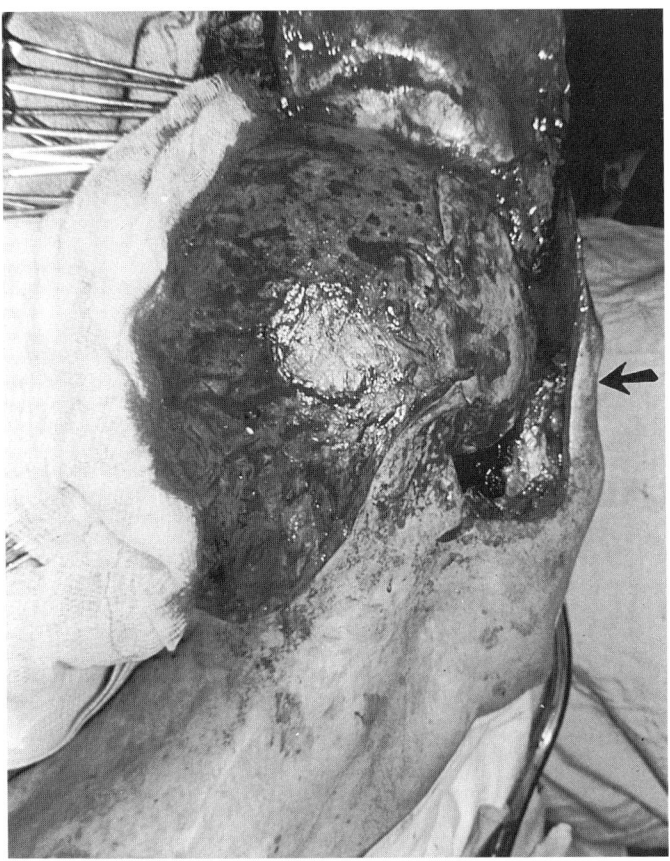

Fig. 8.42a Extensive invasion of the scalp by superior subfascial temporal extension of adenoid cystic carcinoma of the parotid. Mobilization of a large parietal flap

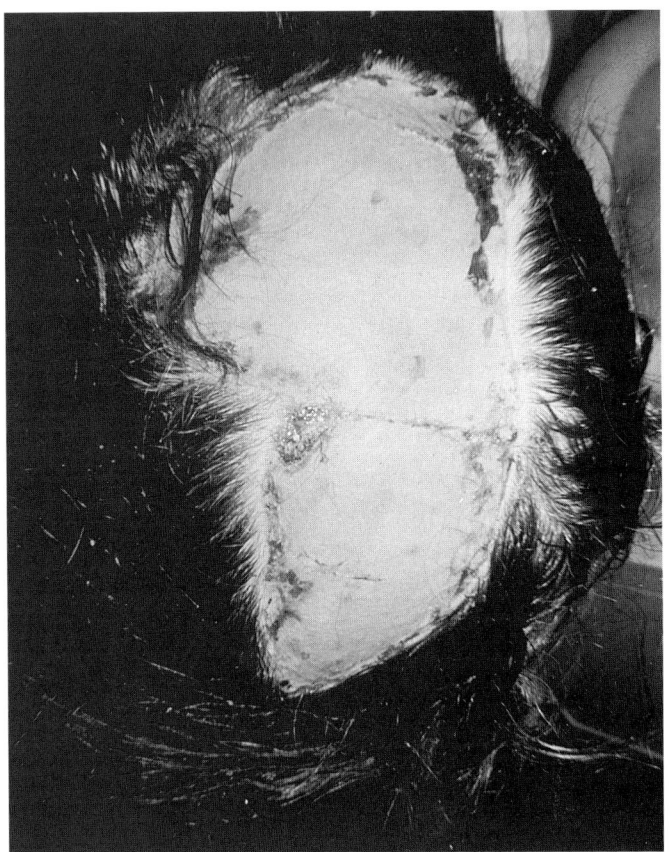

Fig. 8.42b After transfer of the flap

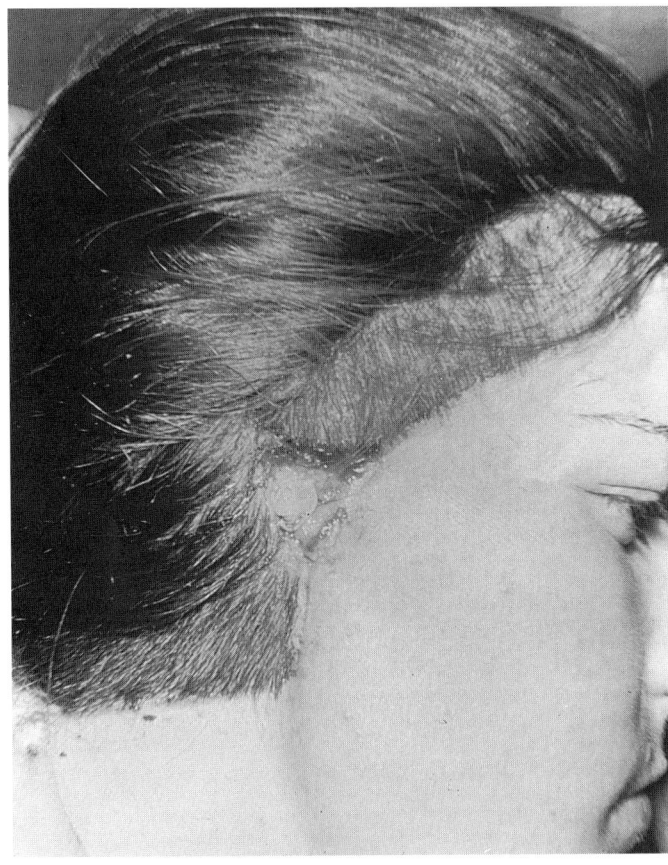

Fig. 8.42c Hairline, parotid, and auricular areas covered by new scalp flaps

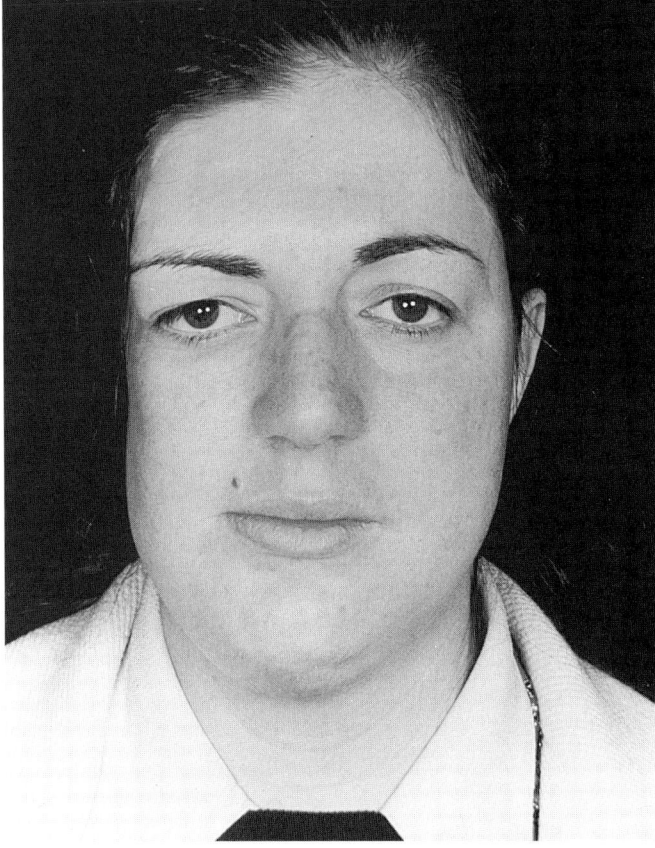

Fig. 8.42d The patient had rehabilitation of the face with a nerve graft

The Facial Nerve in Adenoid Cystic Cancer of the Parotid Gland

(Figs. 8.43–45)

One of the most difficult decisions in the treatment of adenoid cystic cancer of the parotid gland relates to the resection of the facial nerve. This problem has certainly not been solved. The original surgical trend in managing this tumor was to preserve the facial nerve at all costs. After decades of unsatisfactory results, a more radical approach entered the picture, but was not universally accepted because of the mutilating effects of facial paralysis, the capricious behavior of this tumor in some instances, in spite of any form of treatment, and the failure to document a significant improvement in prognosis as a result of this extensive surgery. Radicality made reconstruction of the surgical wound and the facial nerve system more difficult, and many surgeons were not prepared to execute these reconstructive procedures. A compromise was made by many surgeons to preserve the nerve if it was not grossly involved by the cancer. This was not at variance with the general principle of saving the vital structures that were not involved with the malignant process, even if there was critical proximity.

Irradiation had been rejected as the prime method of treatment of this tumor because of its failure to cure, but it was later discovered that it did have an effect in reducing the volume of the cancer in almost every case. Irradiation has therefore come back into the therapeutic picture as a palliative tool and as an adjunct to surgery in high-risk cases and gross subtotal resections. It has proved to effect an extension of life for patients with minor salivary gland tumors, but for patients with major salivary gland tumors, this effect is only marginal. Thus, there is ample reason for the dilemma of when to cut the facial nerve to persist, with convictions and emotions being expressed without factual proof about what is best for the patient and most effective against the disease. This worrisome situation is not completely resolved by our study, but suggests that when there is a chance for cure by technically removing all of the adenoid cystic cancer from the body, it is rational to use the most effective operation that can be developed for that purpose. The presence of the normally functioning facial nerve prevents that in certain instances. The question then arises as to how big a price one wishes to pay to possibly accomplish this objective. All patients, all surgeons, and all family groups resist this mutilation, yet it could be a lifesaving decision in certain instances. The psychological urge to preserve the integrity of the body is normal, and even if overwhelming proof is finally presented that it is better for prognosis to resect the nerve, there will still be resistance to this proposition in certain instances. It is no wonder that there is disagreement at this stage of our understanding.

There is no reason to think that resection of this nerve in high-risk cases will cause a spectacular improvement in prognosis. This type of surgery would have to be selectively applied to the cases in which it has the best chance of providing detectable improvement. Yet our data suggest that even some advanced cases were improved and others were cured. Perhaps the most rewarding cases would include T1 and T2 tumors that approximated the facial nerve, were centrally positioned in the gland, and were amenable to complete excision with a high degree of marginal security. Not all of this information could be absolutely accurately established preoperatively, which introduces an indeterminate variable. It must also be admitted that this is precisely the type of case that might be cured with an operation that preserves the facial nerve. This dilemma will not be solved by a double-blind experiment because of human factors, but it is possible to do retrograde studies that may be suggestive. The basic question is whether the price of an elective facial paralysis is too high or too unreal. Although CT scanning would be helpful in selection preoperatively, there would be cases in which a judgmental decision would be necessary during the operation.

No one will deny the gravity of elective facial paralysis. There is no doubt that it irrevocably changes the quality of life of each patient in a unique and unmeasurable way. On the other hand, this condition today can be ameliorated by three basic reconstructive procedures and a variety of minor selective fine-tuning procedures. The basic rehabilitative techniques are ipsilateral facial-nerve grafting, regional masticatory muscle transposition, and hypoglossal crossover. Free muscle transfer with microsurgical techniques is rarely indicated in this particular situation. The quality of the clinical result and the patient's adaptation to its effects vary in each instance. It is therefore reasonable to state that facial paralysis can be improved in almost every instance, but that the face will never be completely normal. These factors must be weighed against a possible improvement of prognosis. The final question is whether this type of risk-taking is justifiable for the patient and for the doctor.

It can be categorically stated that if the facial nerve were not in the parotid gland, a radical parotidectomy would be routinely done for this malignancy. No one advocates partial resection of a salivary gland for adenoid cystic carcinoma except in parotids, and that is done only to preserve the facial nerve. Of course this is risky with a malignant tumor that has an affinity for nerve tissue, and presents the surgeon with restraints as well as stimulants.

The fundamental purpose of the operation is to remove all of the cancer from the patient's body within justifiable perimeters. A high incidence of systemic spread will defeat all efforts, regardless of the nature of the primary operation. A high incidence of local recurrence can augment the incidence of systemic spread, so it is reasonable to do an adequate primary operation, to have free surgical margins, and to have accountability for possible nerve involvement. Compliance with these demands requires a selection of cases that favors all of these factors, namely, early cases which are not architecturally disadvantaged and which have a normally functioning facial nerve. This certainly does not exclude the possibility of cure by a lesser operation in these cases, but the theoretical and real advantages of a more inclusive procedure should not be denied.

Many authors have made significant contributions to the discussion of this problem; some support radical surgery, others conservative surgery, irradiation, or various combinations of these modalities, but no single method of management for all cases has prevailed. This is not the result of confusion, but of different experiences with a variable, unpredictable tumor, combined with the opinions and experience of surgeons. These opinions are ultimately measured by the patients, by the quality of their lives and the number saved. Our experience with this tumor is not at variance with these data and these attitudes in many instances.

Of 108 patients seen with adenoid cystic carcinoma of the parotid gland between 1945 and 1988, those who had only diagnostic procedures, who had systemic metastases, and who were lost to follow-up within five years were eliminated, leaving 75 charts available for in-depth study.

These patients were divided into four surgical groups: group 1, cases involving lateral lobectomy (8 patients); group 2, total parotidectomy with preservation of the facial nerve system (16 patients); group 3, radical total parotidectomy with cutting of facial nerve (32 patients); and group 4, radical parotidectomy or augmented radical parotidectomy for those patients with preoperative facial paralysis (19 patients). A subgroup included within group 3 consisted of 14 patients who had recurrent tumor and were reoperated on for palliative purposes. None of the patients in groups 1, 2 and 3 had preoperative facial paralysis. The patients who had undergone these four types of surgical procedures were then staged according to tumor size from T1 to T4. In groups 2 and 3, TX was used for those who had indeterminate initial staging. Chi-squared testing was employed to determine whether the clinical outcome was related to the type of surgery performed. There are obviously statistical limitations to this type of analysis, but it presents a picture which has specific implications.

Group 1 had only 8 patients with tumors in a favorable position relative to the facial nerve. They were T1 and T2 lesions and were treated by conservation surgery of the facial nerve and by lateral lobectomy. This group had the highest 15-year and 20-year survival rates. It also had the lowest incidence of metastasis; however, it had a higher incidence of local recurrence than groups 3 and 4, in which the facial nerve was resected.

Group 2 had 16 patients with T1 and T2 lesions that were treated by total parotidectomy with preservation of the facial-nerve system. These tumors were closer to the facial nerve and somewhat larger than the tumors in group 1. This procedure was basically a lateral lobectomy plus piecemeal resection of the isthmus and deep lobe of the parotid. This group fared as well as groups 1 and 3 up to five years and then had a significant drop in survival over the next ten years. Fifty percent had metastases and slightly over 60% had local recurrence.

Group 3 contained 32 patients with a somewhat more advanced tumor and with a normally functioning facial nerve. These patients were treated by radical parotidectomy, including cutting of the facial nerve system. Ultimately, 50% had metastases, but only 12% had local recurrence. Their 15-year survival rate approximated that of group 1. The figures in this group for the control of local recurrence and for survival are statistically significant. A subgroup of 14 patients with recurrent turmor was operated on for palliation and the results also support the concept of radical parotidectomy.

Group 4 contained 19 patients, all of whom had preoperative regional facial paresis or total paralysis. The prognostic gravity of this situation is obvious. These patients were treated by radical parotidectomy or augmented radical parotidectomy. This group had the highest incidence of metastasis, but only a 10% incidence of local recurrence. At 15 years after surgery, 12% of these patients were living. These data also support the effectiveness of radical surgery in the control of local recurrence, even in these advanced cases.

Statistical Conclusions

Staging. Staging was a most significant factor in planing treatment and establishing prognosis. The rate of metastasis for each stage was in arithmetical progression, from 33.5% for T1 primary lesions to 100% for T4 primary lesions.

Margins. The status of surgical margins was the next most important factor in attaining a cure. Of the patients with clear surgical margins, 59.6% were disease-free, whereas only 11.6% of those with violated margins were disease-free. This was statistically significant.

Histopathology. Our data support the conclusion that the tubular and cribriform types of adenoid cystic carcinoma are less aggressive and have a better survival rate than the small-cell, undifferentiated adenoid cystic carcinomas.

Metastasis. Curability was unlikely after regional or systemic metastases. Systemic metastases in group-3 individuals, who had radical parotidectomy, was significantly less frequent than in group-2 patients, who had conservation surgery. The lower number of metastases in group 3 may also be coupled with the fact that this group also had fewer local recurrences.

Local recurrence. This was less frequent in T1 lesions and also when the margins of the surgical specimen were not violated. The rate of local recurrence in total parotidectomy with preservation of the facial nerve in group 2 was statistically significant. At ten years after surgery, 46% with multiple recurrences were alive, whereas 70.4% of those without local recurrences were alive.

Comparison of group 2 with group 3. Group 3 contained more advanced disease and underwent radical parotidectomy with sacrifice of the facial nerve. Group 2 had somewhat less advanced disease and underwent total parotidectomy with preservation of the facial nerve. Those cases with radical parotidectomy showed better local control than the piecemeal resections with preservation of the facial nerve. They also had a better survival rate.

Local control. This factor was enhanced in group 4, in which all patients had preoperative facial paralysis, had a radical parotidectomy, and received postoperative irradiation. The ten-year survival rate in this group was 36%.

Irradiation. Although all types of adenoid cystic carcinoma are affected by irradiation to a favorable degree, it was only marginally successful in treatment of tumor of the parotid gland. Data on tumors of the minor salivary glands indicate that irradiation is more successful in these cases. It delayed and reduced local recurrence, although it did not ultimately improve the survival rate. The longest period of time in which an individual remained free of clinical disease following irradiation was eight years. The specific role of irradiation in the treatment of adenoid cystic carcinoma requires further evaluation.

Facial paralysis is a tragic situation that has influenced the treatment of all tumors in the parotid gland. The patient, the surgeon, and the family react with considerable distress when confronted not only with the burden of cancer, but also with the consequences of a mutilating operation and the knowledge that the condition is life-threatening. Until the 1960s, patients accepted the possibility of a facial paralysis with adenoid cystic cancer of the parotid gland with the rationale that, if the choice was to be made between living with paralysis or dying of cancer, the paralysis would be endured. Cosmetic considerations, self-image, life-style, and the stigma of deformity have become powerful factors in the decision-making process of treatment. In some instances, they are more decisive than the cancer itself in establishing the options. They are not necessarily the wisest with respect to life-saving, but are significant factors in many instances, and represent a social change in medical service.

Fortunately, there are many ways to rehabilitate the paralyzed face today. It is important that the patient understands that his or her face will never be normal again, that the rehabilitative procedures only mitigate the effects of the paralysis, but if one technique does not give an optimal result, there are also ancillary procedures that can be applied. These techniques were not routinely applied 40 years ago, indeed, some were unknown.

Rehabilitative Techniques

There are a variety of different surgical techniques used to rehabilitate the paralyzed face. The most effective technique is ipsilateral facial-nerve grafting. The best time to do this repair is at the operation that initiates the paralysis. It is not always realistic to incorporate it into the ablative procedure, but when it is possible, the patient's capacity for movement in the face begins to return in approximately six months, and continues to improve over the next two years. The possibility that some degree and type of movement will return under these circumstances is 90–95%. It is, of course, never perfect, requires concentration and constant practice on the part of the patient, who can be assisted professionally by biofeedback orientation. If this type of rehabilitation is not suitable for the patient for psychological or technical reasons, the next best rehabilitative operation is the transfer of the masseter muscle or the temporal muscle. The masseter muscle is within the original surgical field and can be transferred to the upper and lower lips and cheek in a short period of time. It is necessary to overcorrect the lift on the face and lips, as some sagging always occurs postoperatively. If this muscle is not available for transfer, then the temporal muscle may be transferred. In contrast to facial nerve grafting, which is specific axonal replacement, this transfer of masticatory muscles supplies fifth-nerve axonal buds to the middle one-third of the face through the distal recipient facial nerve segments, and also supplies intrinsic masticatory movement. This combination of fifth-nerve neural elements begins to function within two to three months and continues to improve for two years. If none of these procedures are possible, one may be forced to apply static elevation with autogenous fascial strips or Marlex strips or crossover techniques.

Special attention must be directed to the eye, as it needs special protection from exposure and drying. This is accomplished by tarsorrhaphy, Fatio-spring or gold-weight implantation in the upper lid, cartilage implantation in the lower lid, external taping, and artificial ocular lubrication. The immobilization and sagging of the face that was not corrected at the primary operation can be improved at a later date. An assessment of the possible use of the techniques mentioned above is made along with the other, more involved procedures of cross-face grafting and free microvascular muscle grafting.

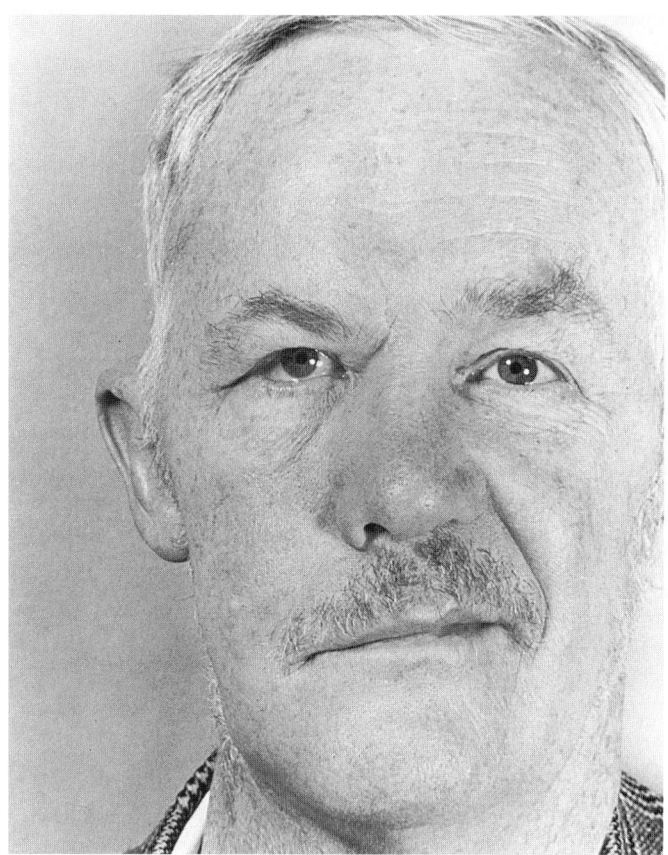

Fig. 8.**43b** He underwent radical parotidectomy and facial nerve graft

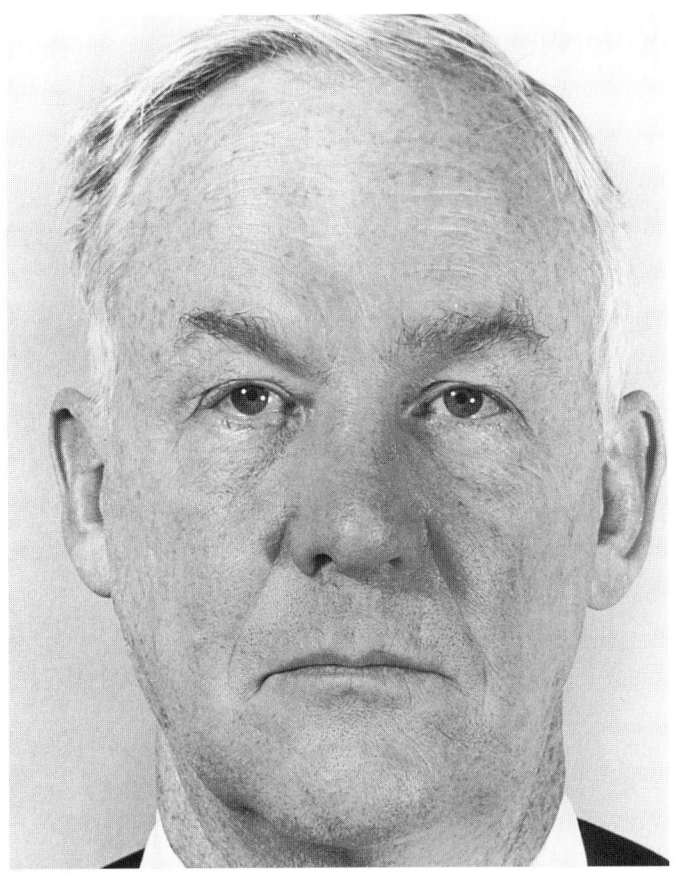

Fig. 8.**43a** **This patient had extensive, recurrent adenoid cystic carcinoma of the right parotid gland with normal facial movement**

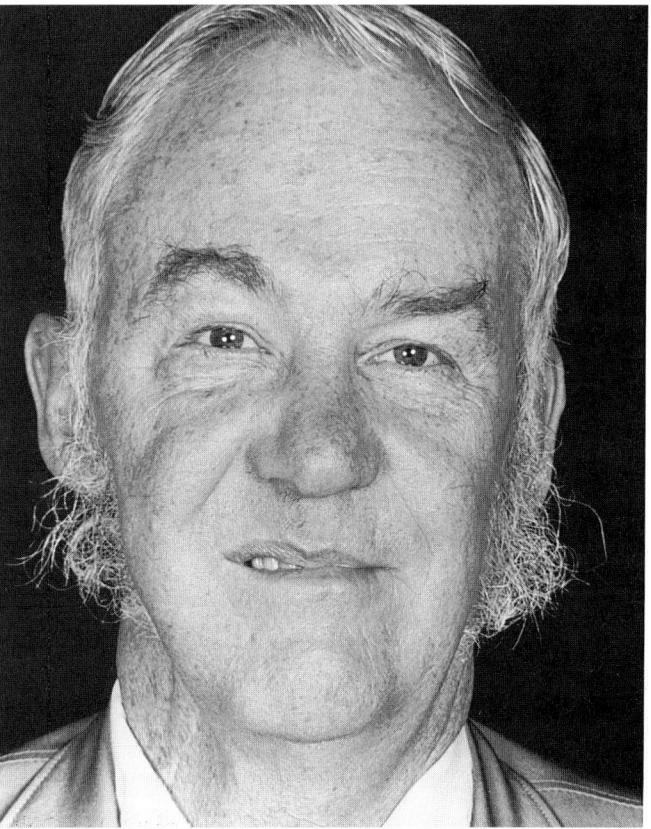

Fig. 8.**43c** The patient three years after surgery with excellent return of movement of the graft. He also had postoperative radiotherapy

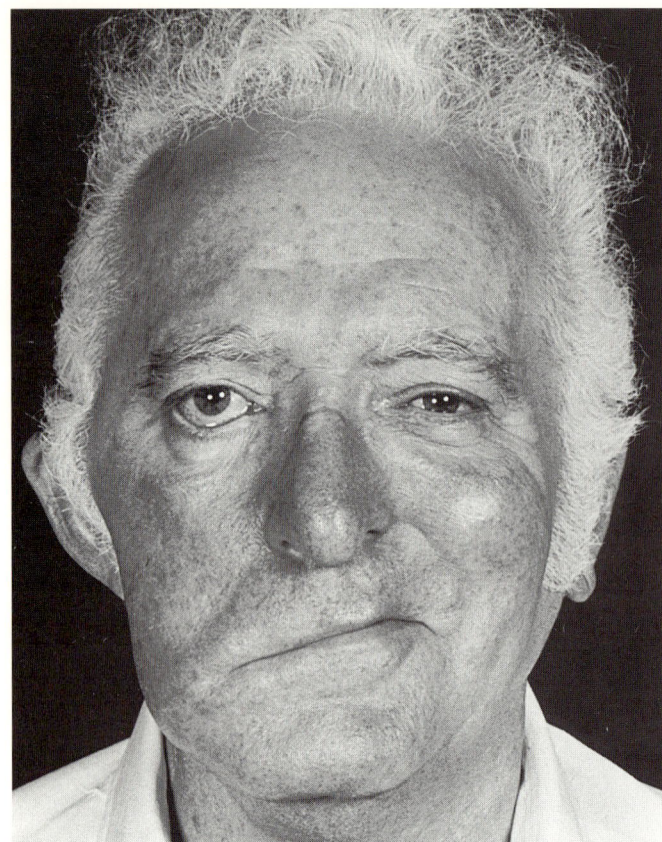
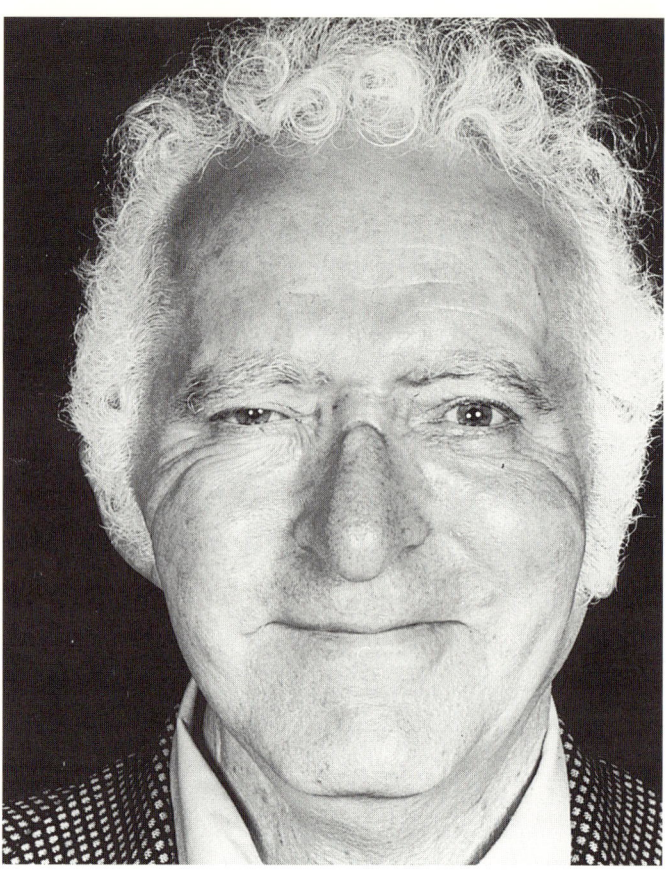

Fig. 8.44a **This patient had radical resection of the right parotid gland for adenoid cystic carcinoma.** The face was rehabilitated immediately with a facial nerve graft. The face was normal preoperatively

Fig. 8.44b There is excellent return of movement of the face. This patient lived free of disease for over 15 years

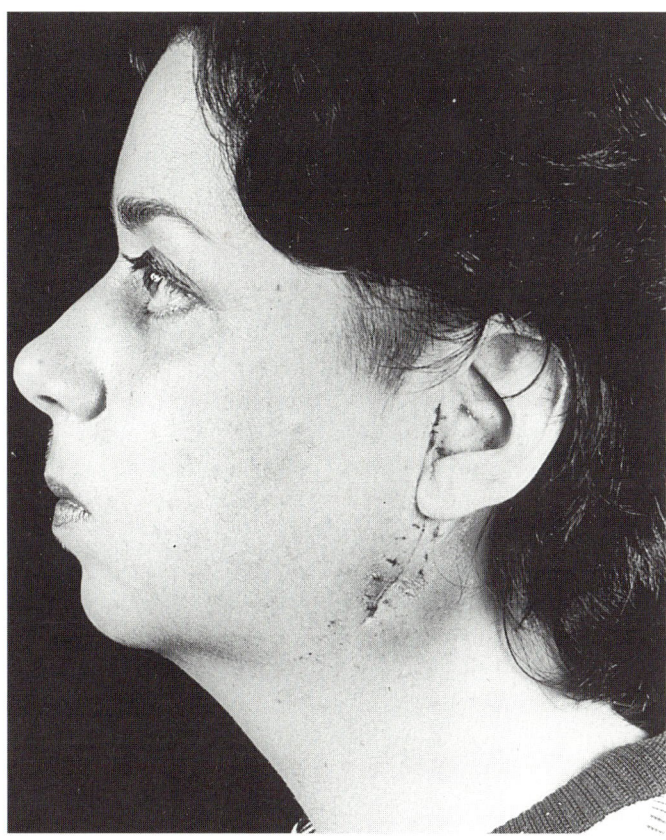

Fig. 8.45a **This patient had extensive adenoid cystic carcinoma of the left parotid gland and an open biopsy.** A fine-needle aspiration biopsy or lateral lobectomy is preferred

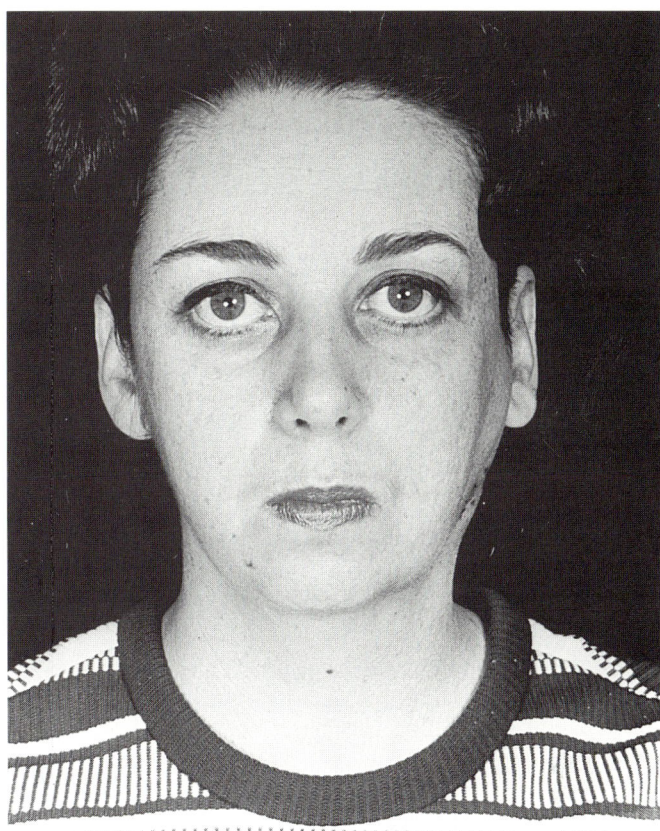

Fig. 8.45b Facial movement is normal

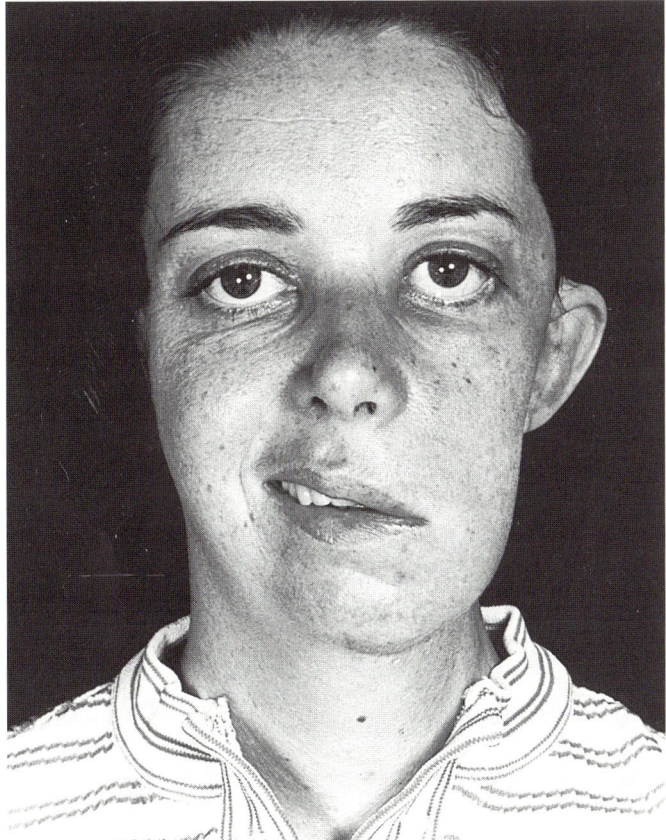

Fig. 8.45c A radical parotidectomy and upper neck dissection was done with immediate facial nerve grafting

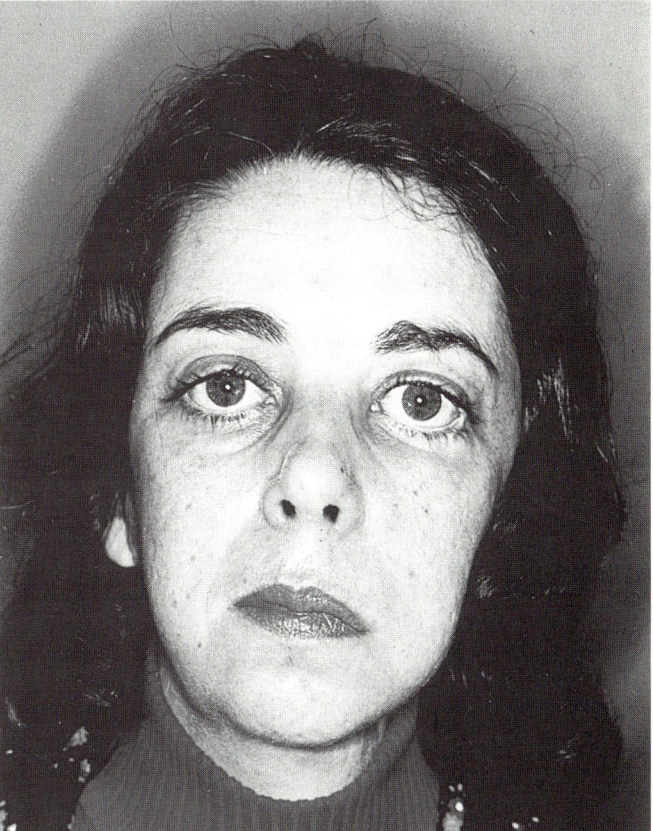

Fig. 8.45d The patient had good return of movement to the face three years after surgery, but ultimately developed metastases to the lungs

Submandibular Gland

(Figs. 8.46–55)

Approximately 35% of the cancers in the submandibular gland are adenoid cystic cancers. The presence of tumor in this gland is more serious than in the parotid gland, even though it is surgically more accessible for ablation. The paucity of lymph vessels and lymph follicles in this gland reduces the incidence of spread within the gland via lymph channels, but apparently enhances the possibility of hematogenous spread. Cervical metastases are more common from this gland, possibly because of the position of the gland in the upper neck and also its surgical anatomy. It is paradoxical, however, that the frequency of cervical metastases is greater in the gland that has a less extensive internal lymph system.

This gland is loosely snuggled against the floor of the mouth in a high position of the lateral neck underneath the horizontal ramus of the mandible. It is surrounded by a capsule of areolar tissue, muscles, mucous membrane, skin, and bone. There are three nerves in this vicinity: the hypoglossal nerve, the sublingual nerve, and the mandibular branch of the facial nerve. The alveolar nerve is also close by, but is protected in the alveolar canal of the mandible. As the tumor expands into the mandible and bone, the alveolar nerve becomes susceptible to invasion. One dramatic case of adenoid cystic carcinoma of this gland kept under observation for 25 years exhibited relentless pernicious growth into the neck, mandible, skin, tongue, and floor of the mouth, with extension to the base of the skull. Gross pulmonary metastases appeared along with local recurrence one year after the major ablation of the primary cancer. The histology of this tumor was a cribriform type and illustrates the extreme chronicity that some of these neoplasms may present. The tumor is capriciously unpredictable in some instances, and the end result in this case dispels any rationality to be found in incorporating this chronicity as part of the therapeutic program, except in a very small percentage of the cases.

The fact that this gland has less volume than the parotid gland and is more accessible for bimanual examination should permit and earlier discovery. As the vast majority of swellings in this gland are due to inflammation and calculi, the diagnostic process must eliminate these conditions first. Once the **diagnosis** of neoplasia is suspected, further investigation is initiated with imaging and fine-needle aspiration biopsy. This type of biopsy may reveal an unequivocal diagnosis of adenoid cystic carcinoma or it may not. An absolute diagnosis of cancer is sufficient before proceeding with an ablative procedure, even though the specific cell type may not be discovered preoperatively. Under these circumstances, a closer diagnosis of the tumor's histological type can be made by fast frozen-section technique if this is deemed necessary during the operation. Open biopsy is rarely necessary today. A basic problem arises, however, when this tumor is resected by a submandibular-gland removal only, with the hope that the microscopy will be benign, or when the surgeon is surprised to receive a diagnosis of malignancy from frozen-section technique, or from the permanent sections several days later. This situation is addressed directly with the patient after the tumor and the gland have been more thoroughly studied to determine violation or adequacy. It is indeed rare for a procedure that has amounted to an excisional glandular biopsy to cure a cancer, and indeed, no one recommends this as a philosophy or technique. It is not inconceivable that it might cure the cancer, but it is not realistic as an adequate therapeutic process. These patients usually require reoperation of the primary site and regional tissues.

The **surgical treatment** of adenoid cystic carcinoma in this location when there has been an open biopsy, or if it is a reoperation, depends upon the size of the original tumor and its spread beyond the gland. If it is contained within the gland, a resection of the gland, the mylohyoid and digastric muscles, and the floor of the mouth would hopefully be adequate. If it is a recurrence or gross spillage or spread beyond the gland, then a composite resection of the gland, the floor of the mouth, a section of the tongue, part of the parotid, the sublingual gland, associated muscles is necessary along with a conservation neck dissection. If it adheres to the mandible or the periosteum, then a

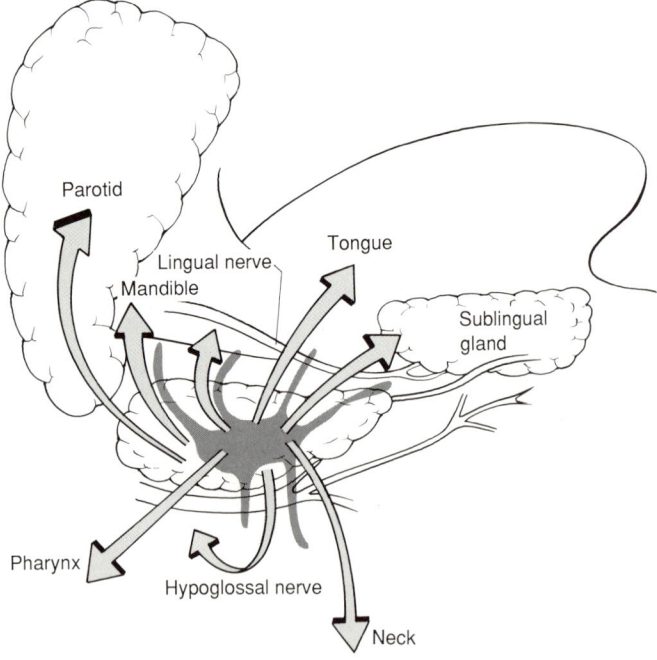

Fig. 8.46 **Primary adenoid cystic carcinoma in the submandibular gland.** Arrows indicate areas most frequently involved by direct extension

partial mandibulectomy should be included. A mandibular swing will provide access to the base of the skull. This is certainly the most adequate process to attempt to gain local control. Some surgeons and some patients may resist this type of surgery, and it is always possible for the operating surgeon to modify his or her technique, if he or she so chooses. Many of these patients will succumb to distant metastases after 10 or 15 years without a local recurrence, but this type of operation has the best chance of gaining local control during that interval of time.

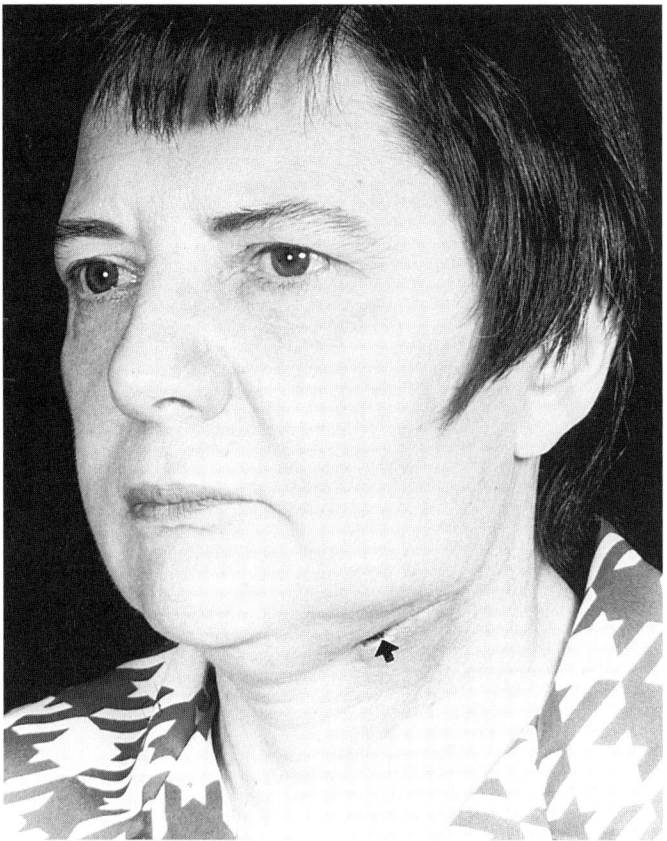

Fig. 8.47 **This patient had an open incisional biopsy for adenoid cystic carcinoma of the submandibular gland (arrow).** Preferably, a removal of the submandibular gland is carried out with frozen-section biopsy or fine-needle aspiration biopsy preoperatively

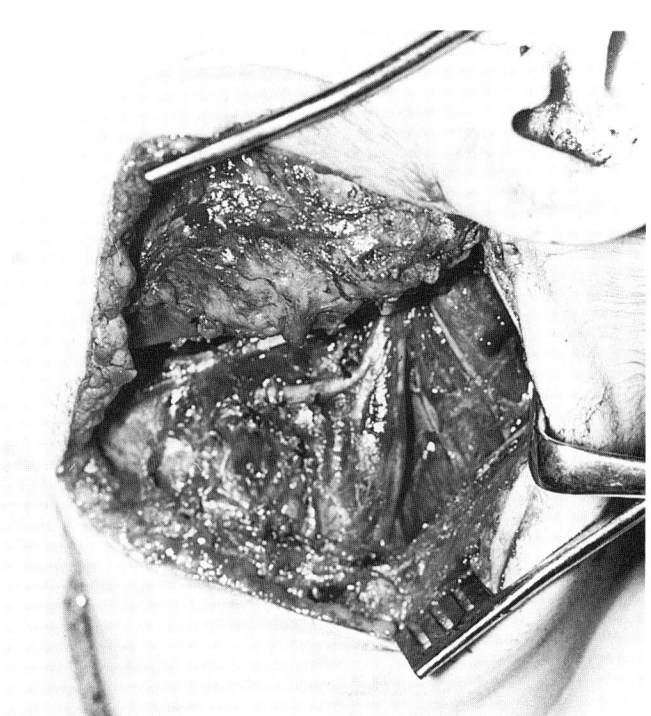

Fig. 8.48a **Surgical removal of the submandibular gland, periglandular structures, and the abutting portion of the parotid.** This is a minimal procedure for a small, localized adenoid cystic carcinoma in this region

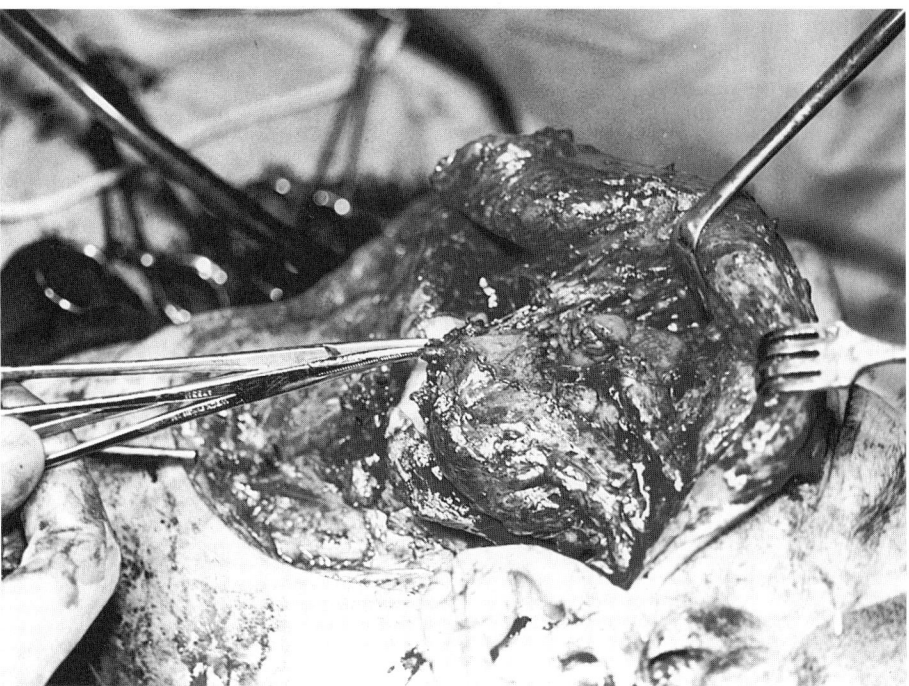

Fig. 8.48b A more extensive resection of the submandibular gland with extension up into the parotid

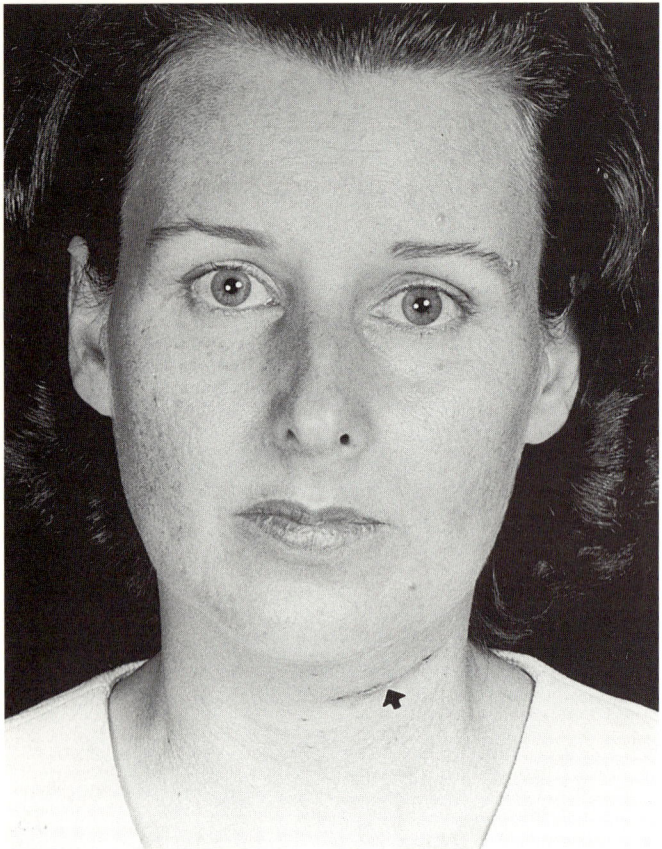

Fig. 8.49a **This patient had a removal of the submandibular gland (arrow),** and the diagnosis of adenoid cystic carcinoma was made from permanent sections. The patient desired maximum optimal reoperation

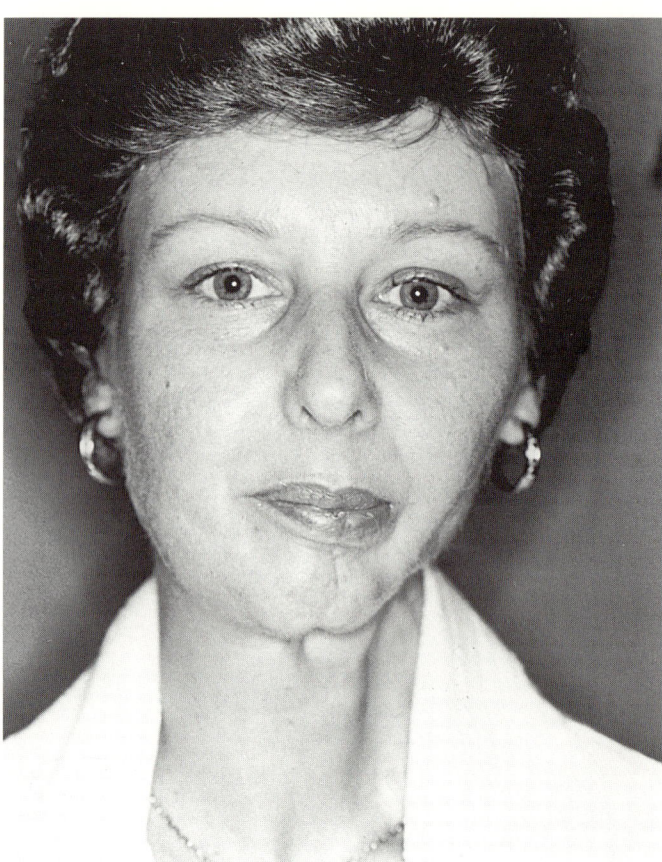

Fig. 8.49b This shows the appearance of maximum resection two years later, including the horizontal ramus of the mandible, the floor of the mouth, conservation neck dissection, the abutting portion of the parotid, and special attention to the lingual, alveolar, hypoglossal, and mandibular divisions of the facial nerve. This dissection was also carried superiorly toward the base of the skull. This is a maximum procedure for local control of this disease

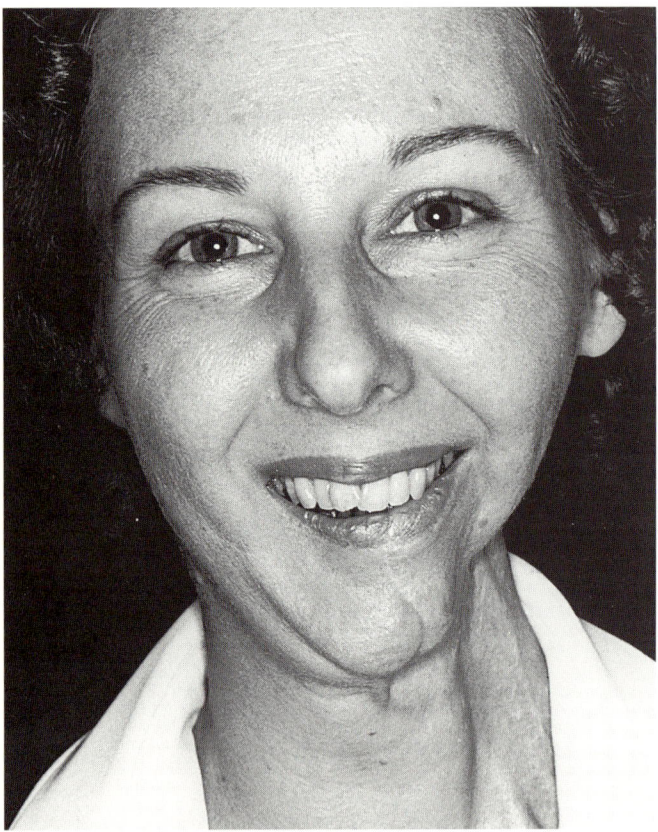

Fig. 8.49c This is the patient 5 years after surgery; she did not elect to have any reconstructive surgery

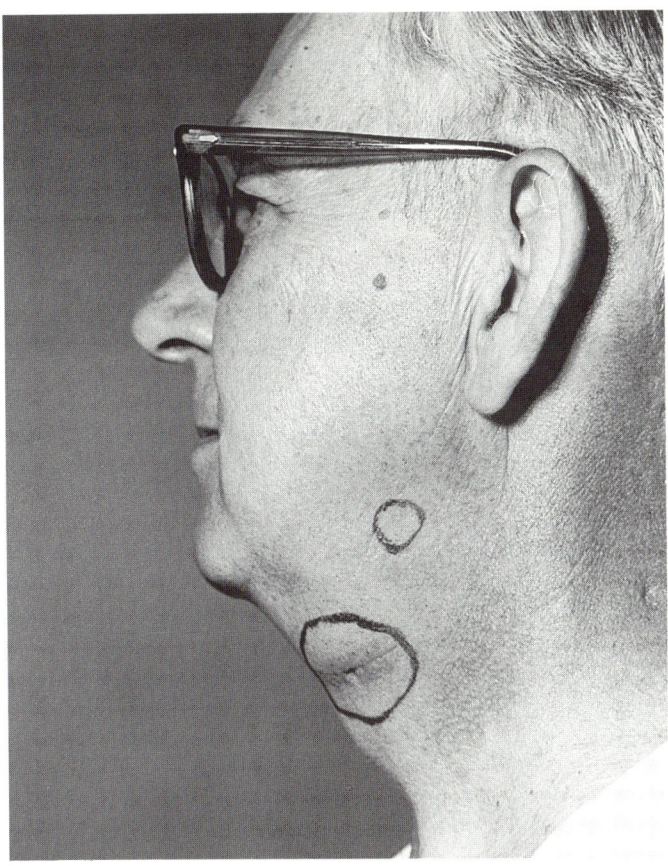

Fig. 8.50a **This patient had an open biopsy of a metastatic lymph node in the mid-anterior neck, which was adenoid cystic carcinoma.** A small primary was discovered at physical examination in the submandibular gland

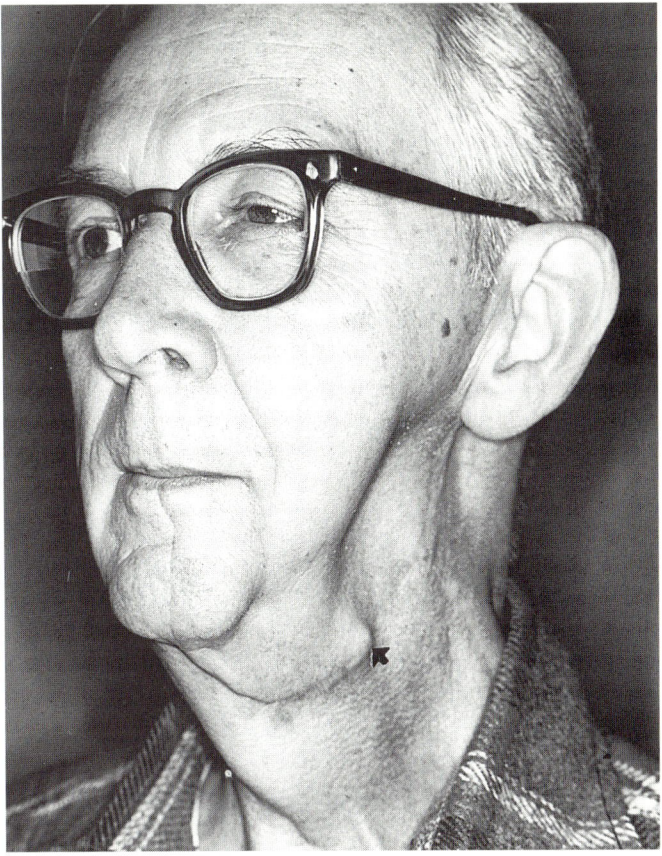

Fig. 8.50b He underwent a maximum surgical procedure for local control similar to the previous case. Arrow points to hyoid bone

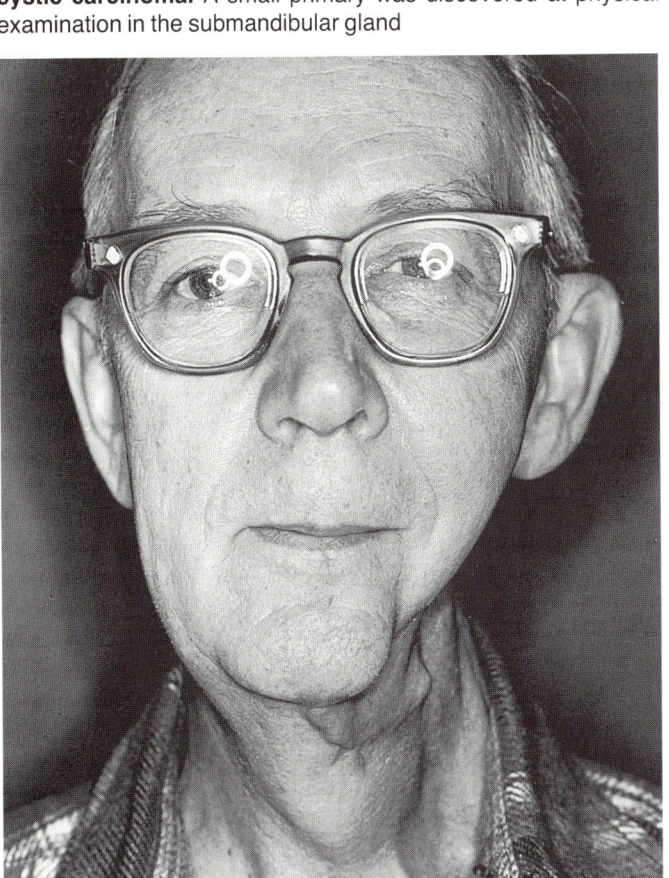

Fig. 8.50c This patient is free of disease 4 years after surgery, has adapted well to his defect, and requests no rehabilitative surgery

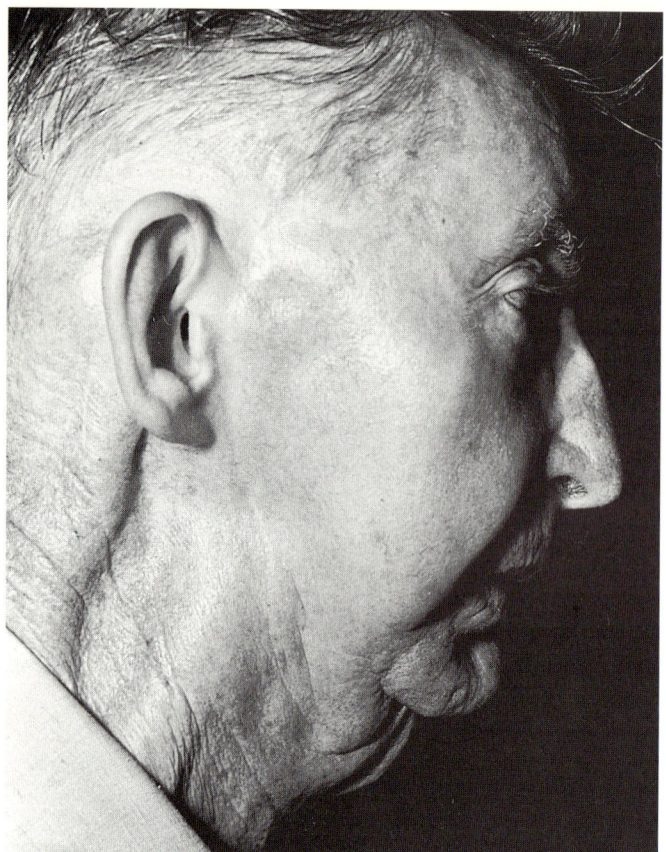

Fig. 8.51a This patient had resection of the submandibular area, the neck, and the parotid gland for recurrent adenoid cystic carcinoma of the submandibular gland

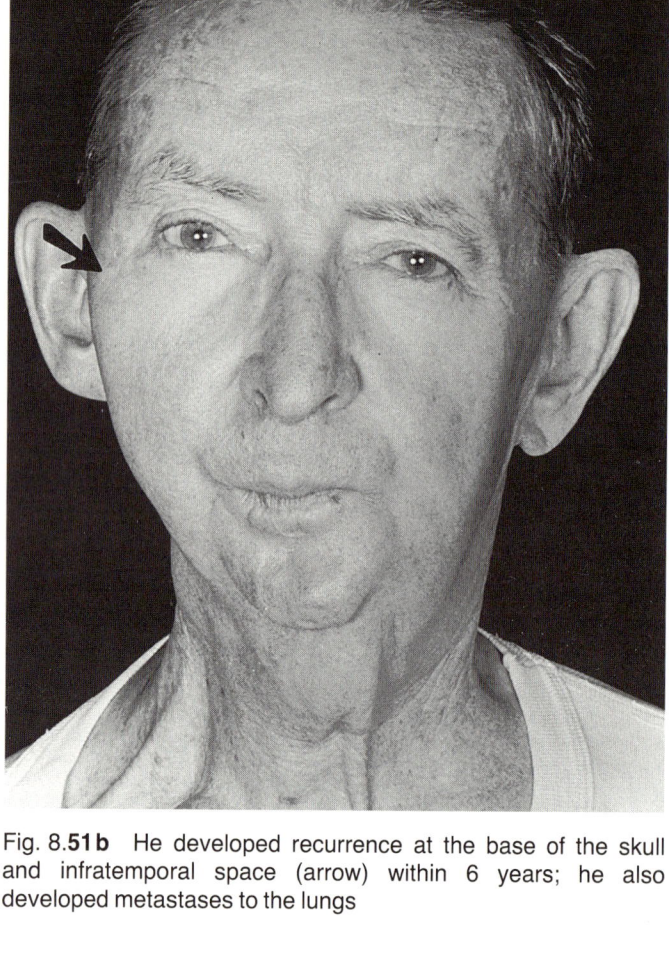

Fig. 8.51b He developed recurrence at the base of the skull and infratemporal space (arrow) within 6 years; he also developed metastases to the lungs

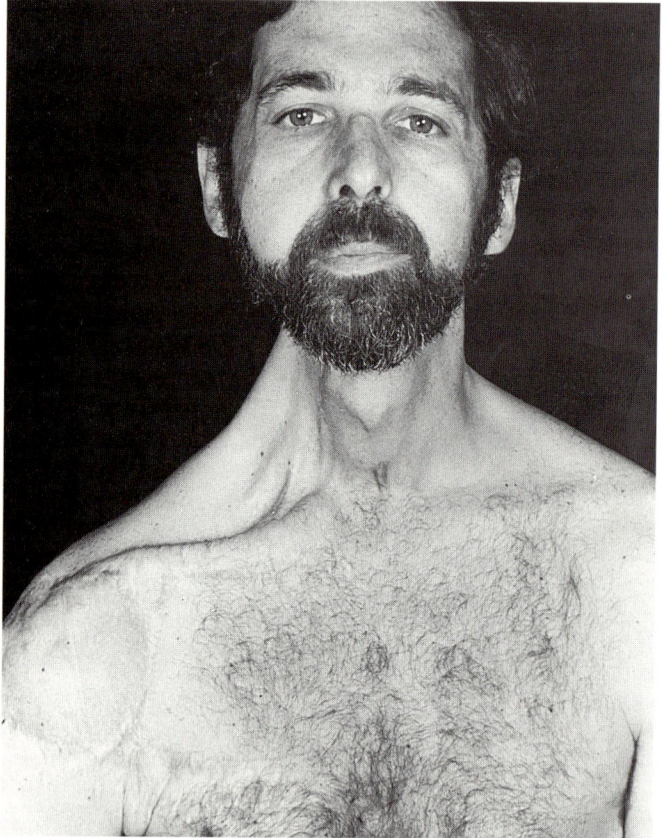

Fig. 8.52 This patient had a similar type of biological process, with radical resection of the mandible, neck, floor of the mouth, parotid gland, part of the pterygoids, and palate. The intraoral and palatal defects were corrected by a deltopectoral flap in two stages. He grew a beard to camouflage the surgical defect. He subsequently developed spread to the base of the skull and the lungs

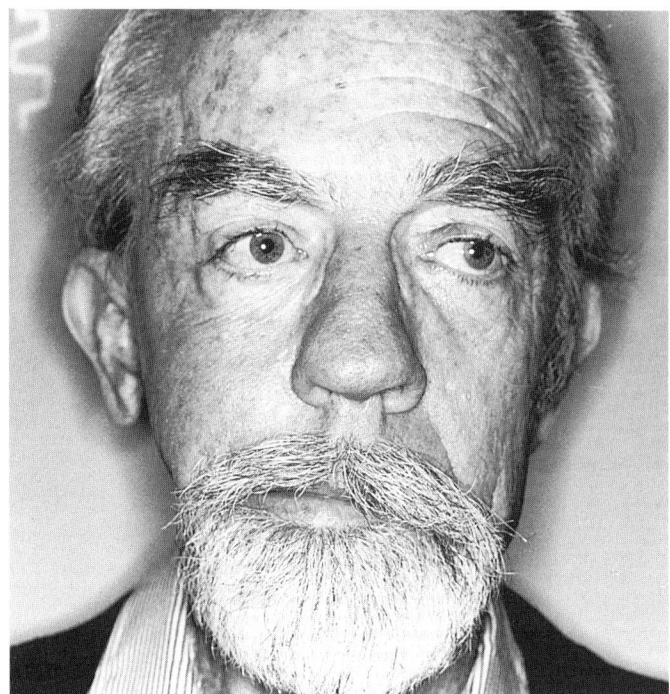

Fig. 8.53a **This patient had multiple local recurrences of adenoid cystic carcinoma of the submandibular gland** over a period of 12 years. He had surgical treatment similar to the patient in Figure 8.52 plus radiotherapy

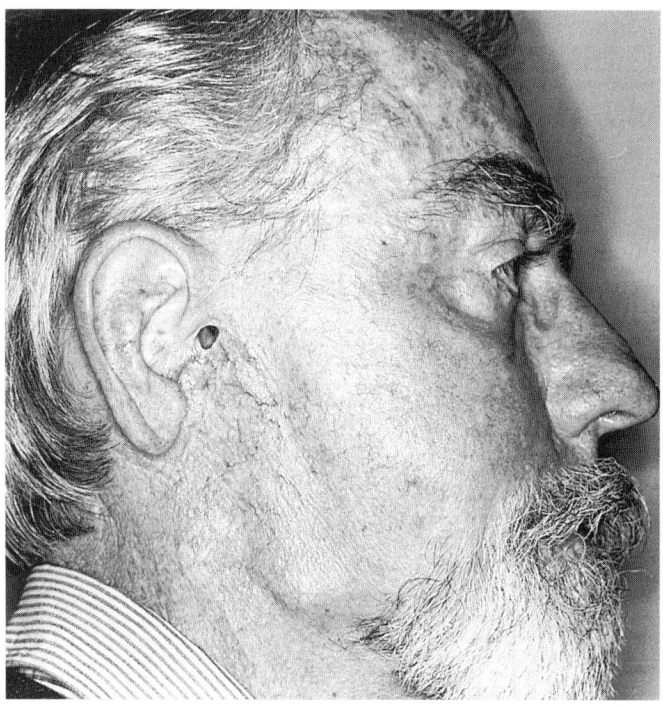

Fig. 8.53b Nine years after this definitive surgery, he manifested metastases to the lungs

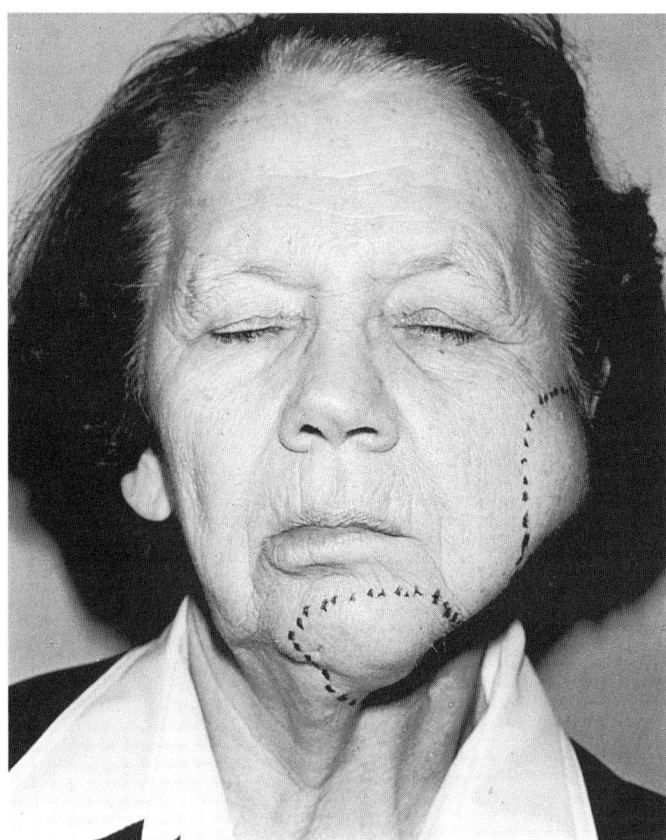

Fig. 8.54a **Massive recurrence of adenoid cystic carcinoma in the parotid-gland and mentum regions from a resected, submandibular primary tumor**

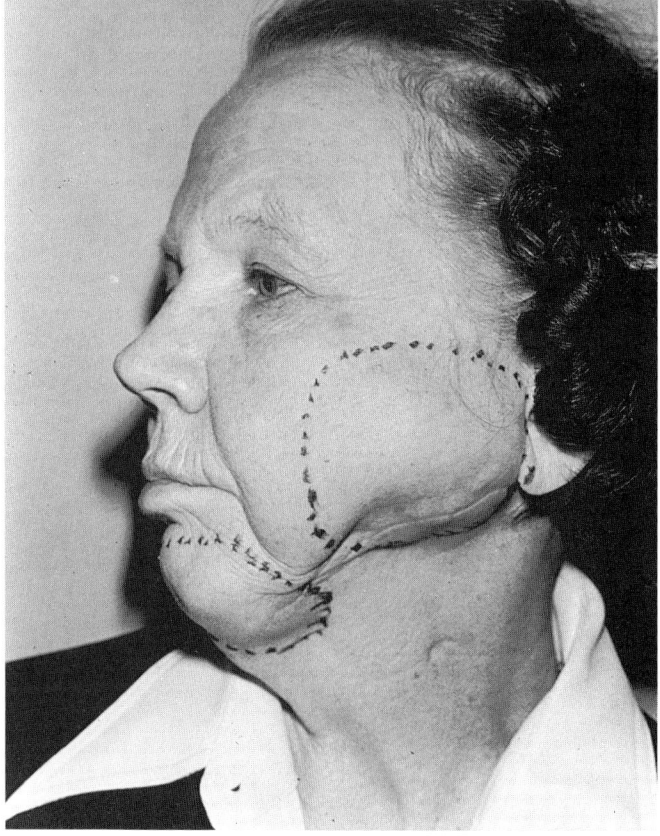

Fig. 8.54b The facial nerve remains intact

8 Surgical Treatment

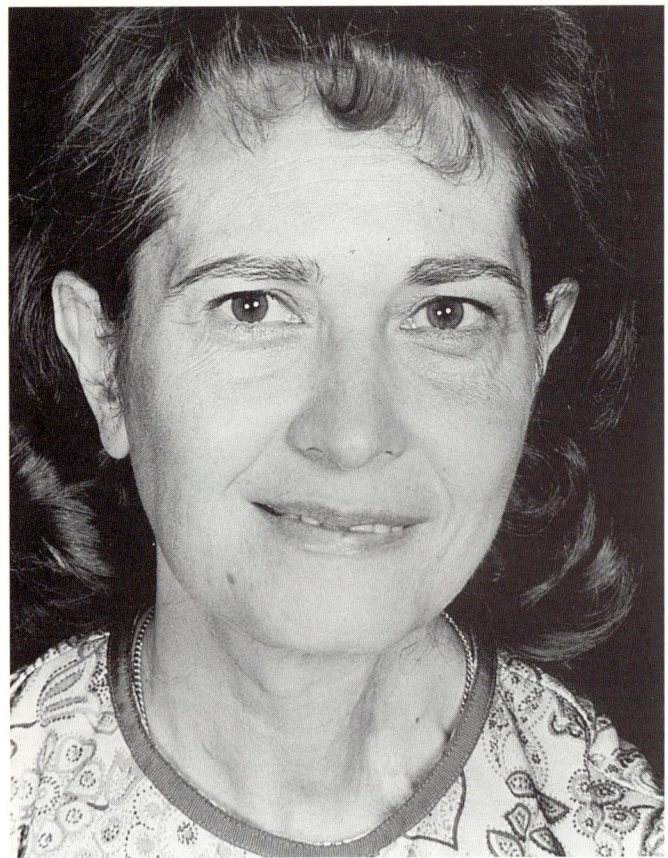

Fig. 8.55 a This patient, shown two years after surgery, had **local recurrence of adenoid cystic carcinoma in the submandibular area on the left side**

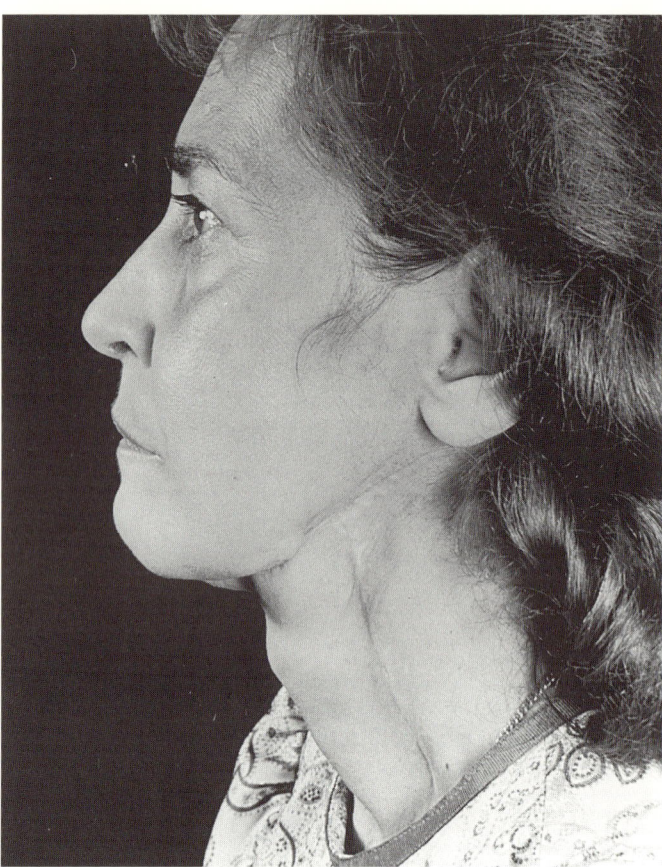

Fig. 8.55 b It was treated by wide local resection, neck dissection, and parotidectomy

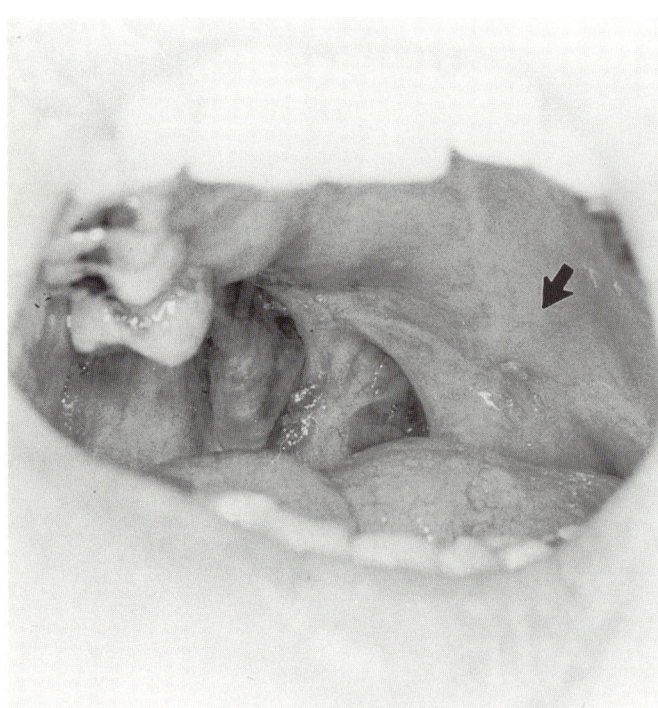

Fig. 8.55 c Four years after the first recurrence, extension into the mesopharynx and palate (arrow)

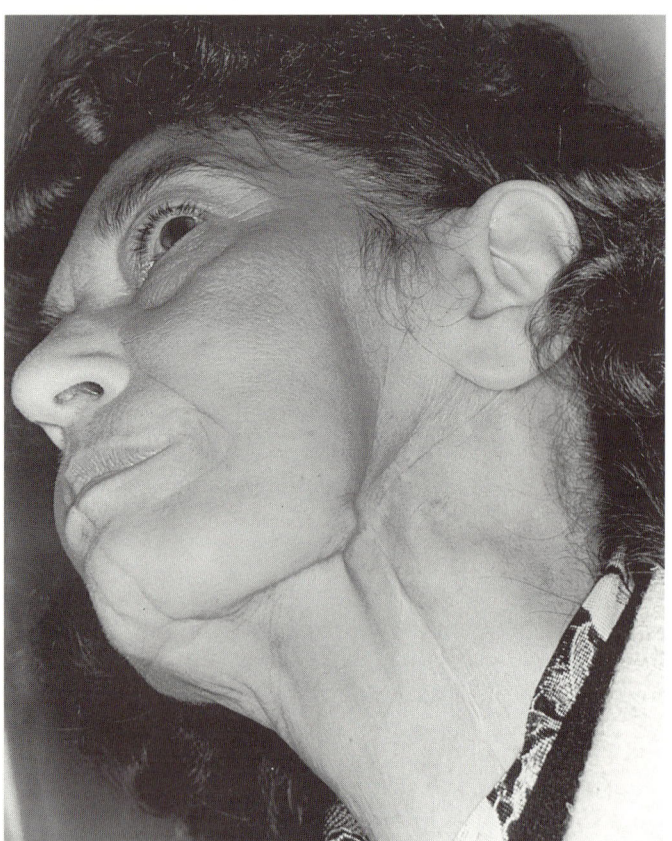

Fig. 8.55 d This is the appearance four years after reoperation of the palate and base of the skull. The patient also received postoperative radiotherapy. This patient lived with her disease for over 17 years, and is presently free of disease

Sublingual Gland

(Fig. 8.56)

The incidence of malignancy and the incidence of adenoid cystic carcinoma in this gland are 65% and 50%, respectively. It is indeed fortunate that the occurrence of neoplasia in this gland is uncommon because of the probabilities it presents in treatment and prognosis.

This gland is situated in the anterior floor of the mouth between the mylohyoid muscle and mucous membrane, with the tongue on one side and the mandible on the other. It is situated very close to the lingual extension of the submandibular gland, its duct, the lingual nerve, and associated vasculature. A tumor in this gland presents first in the floor of the mouth. In its incipiency, it is asymptomatic and inconspicuous, but could possibly be recognized by a dentist or by the patient. In this case, there is a chance for early diagnosis. Unfortunately, many of these tumors are not recognized until much later in the disease process.

The volume of the sublingual gland is much less than that of the other major salivary glands, and the adenoid cystic cancer spreads beyond its capsule into the surrounding tissue in a shorter period of time. Because of the compactness of this region, it quickly comes into contact with the lingual nerve, the mylohyoid muscle, the tongue, and the periosteum of the mandible.

Diagnosis is made first by analysis of the history, by physical examination, and then by CT scan and MRI. An incisional biopsy can be carried out in most cases. This gives the patient and the doctor an opportunity to discuss the aspects of treatment in more detail. This protraction can be circumvented by doing a frozen section with the patient under general anesthesia and, if positive, proceeding with an ablative procedure. This is one area in which it is difficult for the patient to comprehend the full extent of an adequate resection for a relatively small lesion that has not caused any symptoms. A few days for the patient to absorb this information, and to get another opinion, will help clarify some of the issues.

In some instances, the decision on adequate **surgical treatment** for an early adenoid cystic carcinoma in this region is problematic. The basic objective, again, is to remove all of the cancer cells, and the best first step is to analyze the capsule of the primary tumor, which was removed for biopsy, for microinvasion or macroinvasion. If this investigation is negative, which is quite unlikely, one should still attempt to develop a soft tissue cuff about the gland. The mucous membrane, the lingual nerve, the mylohyoid muscle, a sliver of the tongue, and the periosteum of the mandible should be sufficient for additional mi-

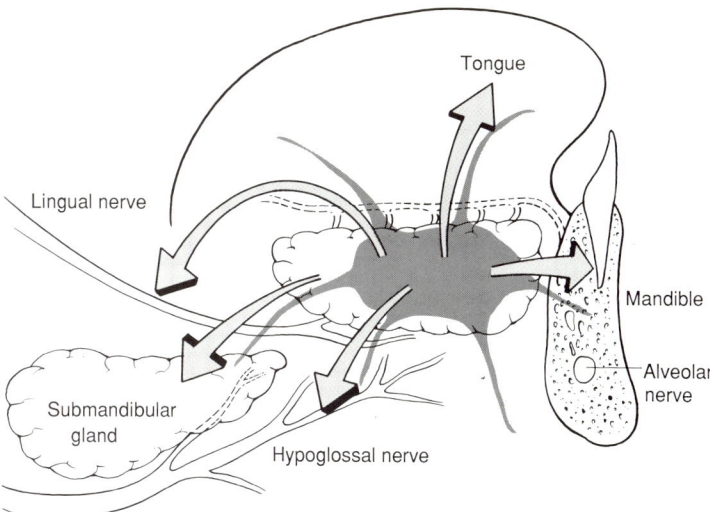

Fig. 8.56 **Primary adenoid cystic carcinoma of the sublingual gland.** Arrows indicate areas most frequently involved by direct extension

croscopic documentation and biologic security. The wound is repaired with a skin graft. Many doctors and patients are reluctant to undergo this type of intraoral crippling, yet inadequate operation at this site creates a more severe type of crippling, and results in repetitive operations for local recurrences, and ultimate death.

The surgical treatment of the more advanced and chronic recurrent adenoid cystic carcinoma at this site may require a resection of the floor of the mouth, a section of the tongue, the adjacent mandible, supra-omohyoid structures, the lingual and hypoglossal nerves. This serious functional and aesthetic deficit requires augmentation with skin, muscle, and bone replacement. The precise technique of rehabilitation is the operator's choice; it can be attempted in a single stage with a composite microvascular flap transposition, with regional myocutaneous flap transfer, or with sequentially staged techniques. The gravity of the problem is very serious in some cases. One patient in this series underwent six operations for local recurrence, had a full course of irradiation and chemotherapy, was severely handicapped physiologically, suffered a poor physical appearance, and ultimately died of pulmonary metastases.

Ear Canal

(Figs. 8.57–68)

There are not enough cases of adenoid cystic carcinoma of the ear canal to create a statistical analysis, and the majority of the cases reviewed here have been published before by Conley and Dingman (1974), and by Perzin, Gullane, and Conley (1982); an unpublished study of a group of cases of adenoid cystic carcinomas, of which 20 occurred in the ear canal, was done by Baker, Conley, and Joss in 1982. Thus, the reports obviously overlap considerably; however, 20 cases with a minimum follow-up of ten years qualified for careful study and analysis. This material is not being presented as a definitive position on this tumor, but presents an extensive, 40-year personal experience, from which certain deductions are possible, in the hope that it will encourage introspection and, ultimately, improvement of the management of these problems.

Benign and malignant tumors of the ear canal are extremely rare. One might have to examine over 30 000 patients in an ear clinic to see one case of adenoid cystic cancer in the canal. Consequently, it is encountered very rarely in the pathology department. Perzin reports that 395 000 specimens at the Columbia Presbyterian Medical Center revealed only 16 adenoid cystic carcinomas of the ear canal. Because of the paucity of cases, the patient, the surgeon, the pathologist, and the medical profession tend not to be aware of this possibility during a routine examination. This certainly reduces the probability of this tumor being diagnosed at an early stage of development; however, as the neoplasm develops in the deep layers of the skin in the ear canal adjacent to the conchal cartilage, it will produce definite signs and symptoms when it has attained an obstructive volume. The interval for this development may extend over two to five years before a diagnosis is made.

In the early stages, there are no signs or symptoms. This characteristic of adenoid cystic carcinoma at all locations causes an automatic delay in **diagnosis** because the patient has no complaints and a routine examination at this stage is not usually productive. This may be the case for several years. Eventually, the patient has a feeling of discomfort in the ear, or the examining doctor may notice a lump or constriction in the ear canal. The patient is indeed fortunate if an incisional biopsy is done at that time. CT scanning shows narrowing of the canal at this stage, which is not impressive, and bone destruction would not be suspected. It requires quite a bit of conviction and courage for a surgeon to advise this patient to have an open biopsy in the early stages of this disease.

The specific signs of a mass or nodule, a "cyst" or "pimple," with specific narrowing of the external canal at one point or circumferential swelling, is a sign of advanced disease. In the beginning, these signs are limited to the canal itself, but as the tumor enlarges, pain, otitis externa, otitis media, drainage, ulceration, bleeding, invasion of the parotid gland, swelling about the ear, and facial paralysis come into the clinical picture one after the other. At this stage, CT scanning shows a soft tissue mass with regional swelling and possibly shows bone destruction. In the majority of instances, these signs and symptoms point to an infection in the ear canal and this is, understandably, treated first. If the swelling does not resolve, an incisional biopsy or forceps biopsy is taken.

Establishing the diagnosis microscopically may be very easy, as the histologic pattern is similar to the other adenoid cystic carcinomas of the aerodigestive system, but there are also subtleties that can and do mislead an inexperienced pathologist. The majority of pathologists are inexperienced in diagnosing this tumor because of the paucity of cases and the lack of training. Many pathologists may see only a few of these tumors in a lifetime. In addition to this handicap, there has been a confusion of terms and nomenclature in the evolution of the classification of all tumors in the ear canal.

The general term ceruminoma, which was often a misleading term, has been abandoned for a histologic description that identifies the lesion as a benign type of adenoma of the ceruminous glands or a carcinoma of the ceruminous glands. The distinction between a ceruminous adenoma and sweat gland adenoma is not always easy. The distinction between the malignant ceruminomatous tumors is also complicated, including adenoid cystic carcinoma, ceruminous gland adenocarcinomas, mucoepidermoid carcinomas, and some benign adenomas. Neoplasms in the eccrine sweat glands add an additional challenge to the differentiations in certain instances. Adenoid cystic carcinoma may arise from the eccrine or the ceruminous glands, but usually has the characteristic histopathologic picture. The use of the term cylindroma for any of these tumors may correctly imply an adenoid cystic carcinoma, but may also be confusing if it refers to a benign sweat gland adenoma. Cylindroma is no longer advocated as a synonym for adenoid cystic carcinoma. In addition to these hazards of misdiagnosis within this family of tumors of skin appendages in the ear canal, the pathologist must occasionally differentiate between basal cell epithelioma and squamous cell cancer, which are much more common epithelial tumors in this area than the skin appendage tumors.

The biologic behavior of adenoid cystic carcinoma of the ear canal is in many ways similar to other adenoid cystic carcinomas of the aerodigestive system, particularly those of the minor salivary glands. In the cases studied, the development of signs and symptoms was always delayed, therefore, the diagnosis was delayed, patients were rarely cured after the first operation, and they were never cured after multiple recurrences set in. None of these tumors metastasized to the cervical area.

The ear canal is primarily a tubular conduit for sound waves to the tympanic membrane. There is a conjoint segment of cartilage and bone which maintains its lumen. It is the cartilaginous segment that contains ceruminous glands, sweat glands, and hair follicles in the deep part of the subcutaneous tissue between the skin and the conchal cartilage. These structures are absent in the bony canal, where a thin layer of skin is stretched over the periosteum of the tympanic bone. Adenoid cystic carcinoma arises primarily in the ceruminous glands, but has also been reported in the eccrine glands, both of which are found in the membranous portion of the ear canal. These skin appendages are microscopic in size, and any neoplasm growing from them would, in a short period of time, be in the fascial and subcutaneous tissue spaces. The most proximal barrier is the extension of the conchal cartilage. This space is richly populated with terminal nerve endings from the cervical, glossopharyngeal, vagal, trigeminal, and facial branches, and this helps to explain why 30% of these patients complained of pain. It is extremely significant that, in 70% of these cases, perineural involvement was found upon histologic examination of their specimens. These facts point to the significance of nerve involvement in cases of local recurrence and to a very poor prognosis.

Special attention must also be directed to the parotid gland, cartilage, and bone because of their proximity to the ear canal and their potential for involvement. The parotid gland was involved in 40% of the cases. In one instance, it was not possible to determine whether the tumor had originated in the parotid gland and involved the ear canal by extension or not. This emphasizes the fact that the parotid gland adjacent to the canal should be included in the operation as a routine measure. The cartilage was involved by tumor in 50% of the cases and should also be routinely excised at the initial operation. The tympanic bone or mastoid bone was involved in 40% of the cases, which indicates advanced disease and the necessity for considering some type of bone resection in the initial operation, both as a therapeutic measure and also for documentation. Two cases (10%) had extensive involvement of the mastoid bone. Ten percent of these patients had preoperative facial paralysis.

Local recurrence occurred in 70% of the cases, extending over a period of 2 to 20 years. This group underwent multiple, repetitive local operations, irradiation, and chemotherapy; the patients died primarily of uncontrolled local disease after a protracted morbidity. Three patients in this group had metastases to the lung along with local recurrence, and two had metastases to the brain with local recurrence.

It is doubtful that, at this time and with the facilities available to us, this disease can be dealt with in its early stages because of its paucity of signs and symptoms, the physicians' frequent failure to discover gross abnormalities, the unproductive scientific scanning tests, and the patients' reluctance to undergo an invasive biopsy to diagnose the cause of minimal symptoms. Pain in the ear is the earliest warning in most instances, and although it is such a ubiquitous and common complaint, it is rarely associated with the possibility of adenoid cystic carcinoma, even though it may represent the earliest lead in this direction.

The minimum **surgical treatment** for this tumor is a resection of the membranous and bony ear canal, with a cuff of cartilage and tympanic bone and the cortex of the mastoid bone. The parotid gland and postauricular lymph node should be included. This would include T1 and T2 tumors, each operation being tailored to the tumor's position, its size, and the tissue involvement. Because of the silent progression of extensions of this tumor along fascial planes, soft tissues planes, vascular channels, and lymph channels, it is important to have a cuff of normal tissue around it. It is appropriate to include this tissue in the operative technique, when it can be done without causing serious handicap or deformity.

Obviously, this tumor has a high propensity for local recurrence, and the vast majority of initial operations are inadequate as far as the total removal of the neoplasm is concerned. These tumors are always much larger biologically than all the clinical deductions and scientific tests might indicate. The philosophy of cutting as close as you can to the edges of the neoplasm has no place in the management of this tumor. Of the patients in this series, 14 had previously had some type of treatment which had failed, and 16 ultimately had surgical excisions that included all of the previous boundaries or more. Half of these tumors were originally misdiagnosed by the pathologist, and often the surgeon was misled by what had been identified as a "low-grade tumor."

It is almost impossible to cure an adenoid cystic carcinoma of the ear that is chronically recurrent over a period of years, but this in itself does not invalidate attempts at adequate removal. When the tumors are larger and have extended beyond the ear canal, all operations could be considered palliative. The balance of technique, philosophy, and humanistic factors in grappling with these problems is not found in sentences dictating a surgical policy, but in the art of medicine and the involvement of the highest ethics. Some of the more extensive procedures include the ear, mastoid, temporal bone, parotid gland, mandible, and upper neck. These extensive wounds are rehabilitated immediately with a superiorly based trapezius myocutaneous flap from the nape of the neck. This gives skin coverage, bulk, and nourishment to the area. It does not restore function, however. Hearing is lost, there is temporary vertigo after the operation, and there is facial paralysis; however, these deficits are welcome substitutes for the cancer. The facial paralysis should be rehabilitated immediately by hypoglossal crossover, masseter muscle rotation, or facial-nerve graft. Morbidity can extend over 2 to 20 years, which highlights the importance of an adequate first operation with free margins.

If the final report from the pathology department reveals violation of the surgical margins by tumor, the surgeon should consider reoperation of that area. Some surgeons and many patients will avoid this issue by choosing the alternative of close clinical observation or postoperative irradiation. These usually fail within one to eight years, and further, extensive surgery is then required. This position is justifiable if the patient has led a normal life without serious mutilation during this period of time, or if the patient had rejected additional surgery, however, it usually defeats the purpose of saving life.

All of the cases in this study have received or will receive postoperative radiotherapy, with the exception of early lesions that have safe margins as established by the india-ink technique. It has therefore become an integral part of the therapeutic program at some stage of treatment. All adenoid cystic carcinomas will respond to irradiation to some degree. The disappointment is that they may only partially respond, or even if they completely disappear, that they will ultimately recur. The interval before recurrence may extend over years, and in this sense, radiotherapy is an effective palliative agent. Because the data at the present time is inadequate, it cannot yet be stated that it is curative when combined with surgery for the treatment of possible residual microscopic tumor, but that is the hope for and the intent of its application.

The number of cases of this tumor is too small for a comprehensive statistical analysis, but it is significant enough to warn of its serious nature, the difficulty of its early diagnosis, a reluctance to do an adequate operation initially, the high incidence of local recurrence, and the protracted morbidity, extending in some instances over 10 and 20 years. Of these 20 patients, who have been observed for a minimum of ten years, 14 are dead of the disease, 2 are living with tumor, and 2 are allegedly cured; 1 patient was lost in follow-up, and 1 died of other causes, free of disease at 8 years after initial surgery. An approximate 80% mortality rate illustrates the gravity of the problem and the need for improvement.

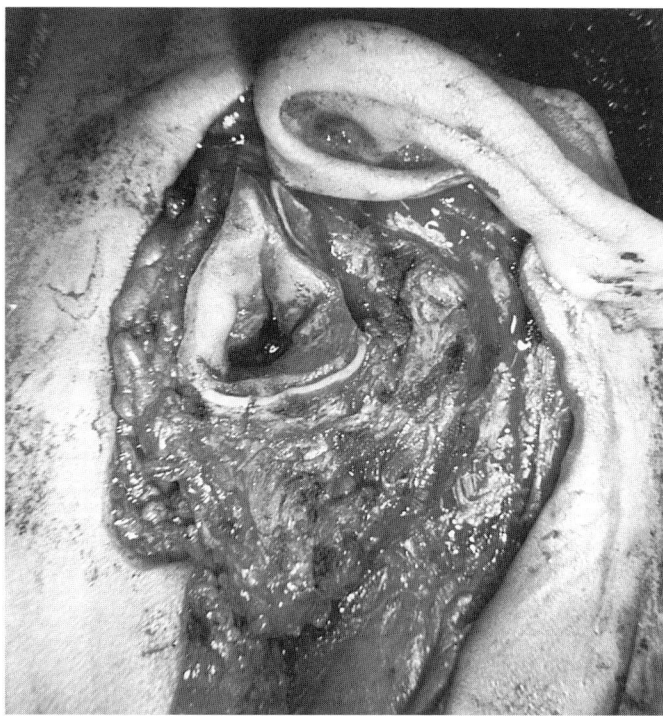

Fig. 8.57a **Classical approach for adenoid cystic carcinoma of the ear canal,** including the entire membranous and cartilagenous canal, with portion of the concha and tragus, total conservative parotidectomy, and conservation uper neck dissection

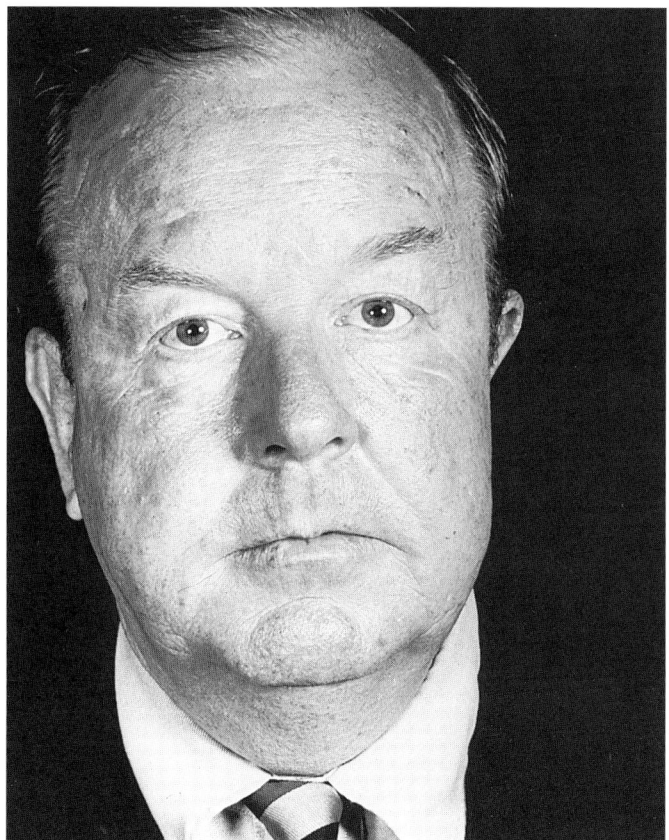

Fig. 8.57b The patient three years after surgery with normal facial movement

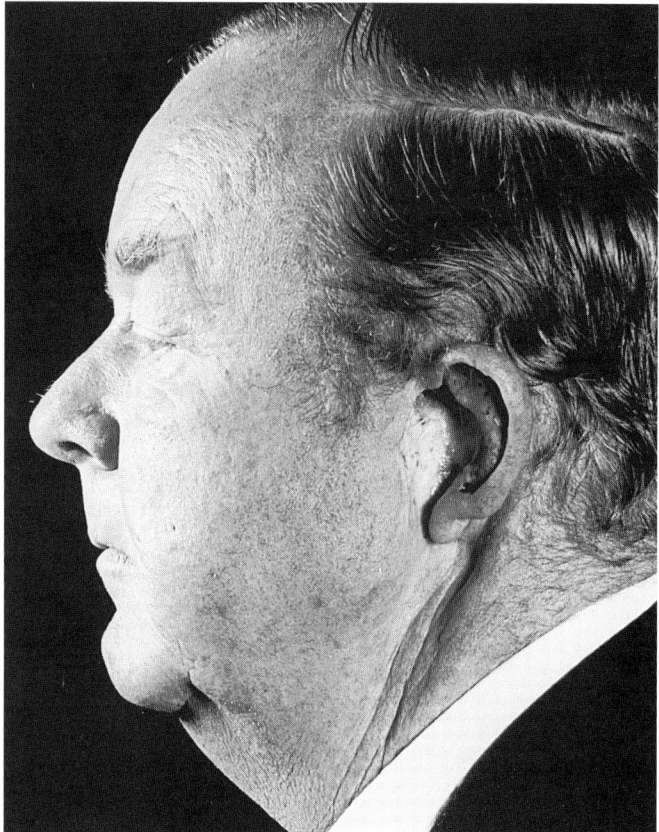

Fig. 8.57c Lateral view showing skin-graft dressing in the ear canal

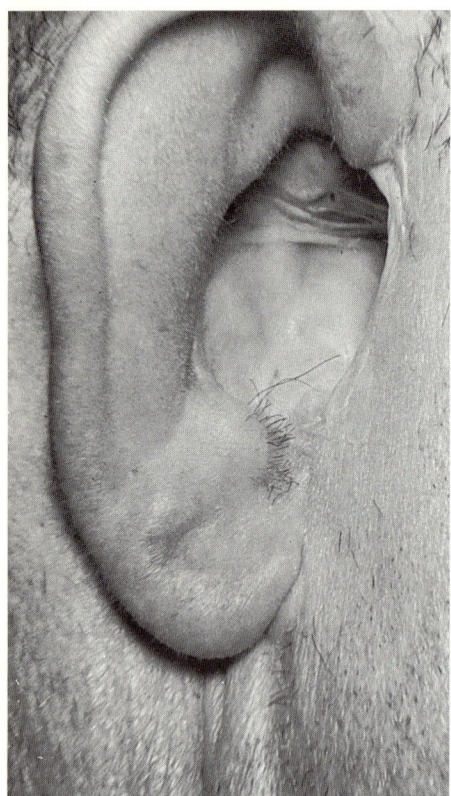

Fig. 8.**58a Skin-graft dressing in the ear canal, concha, and mastoid area**

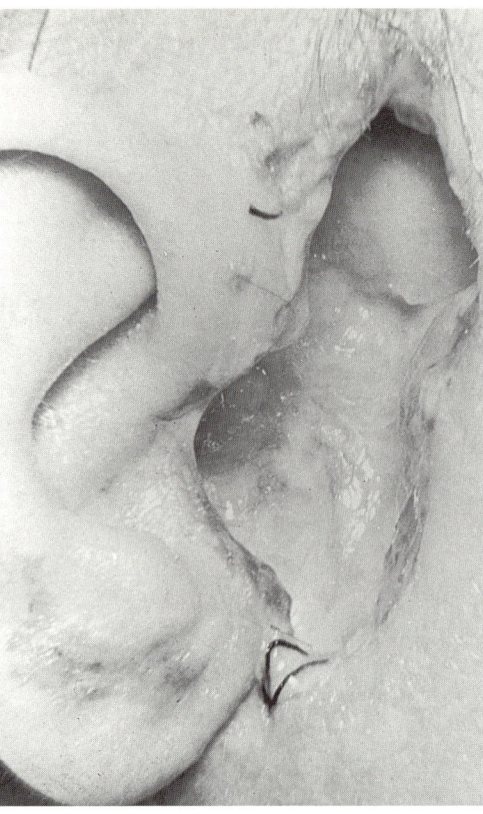

Fig. 8.**58b** More extensive resection of skin, extending toward infratemporal area, with partial mastoidectomy and skin-graft dressing

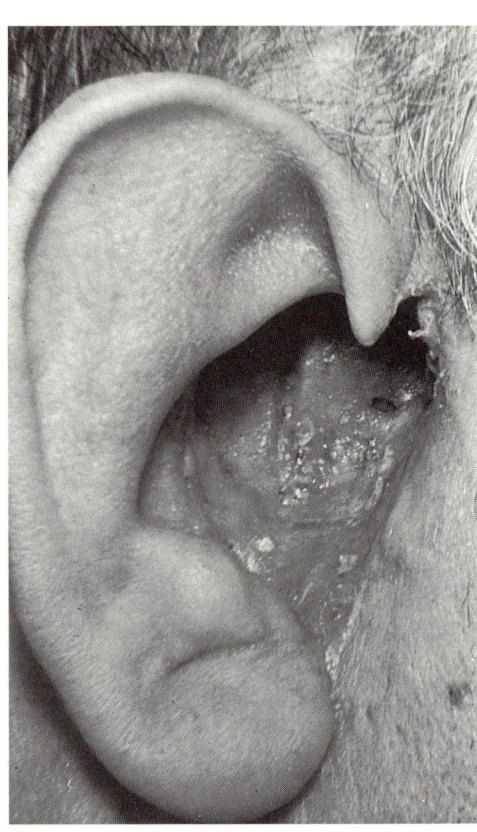

Fig. 8.**58c** Wider excision, including ear canal, parotid, concha, and partial temporal bone, and the skin-graft dressing

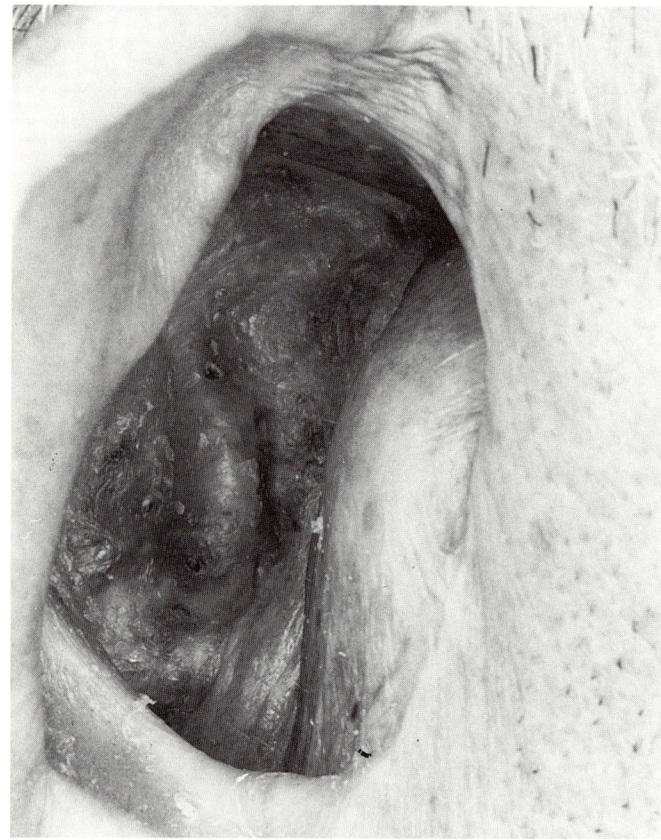

Fig. 8.**58d** More extensive dissection showing deep penetration into the temporal bone region and also over the head of the mandible with skin-graft dressing

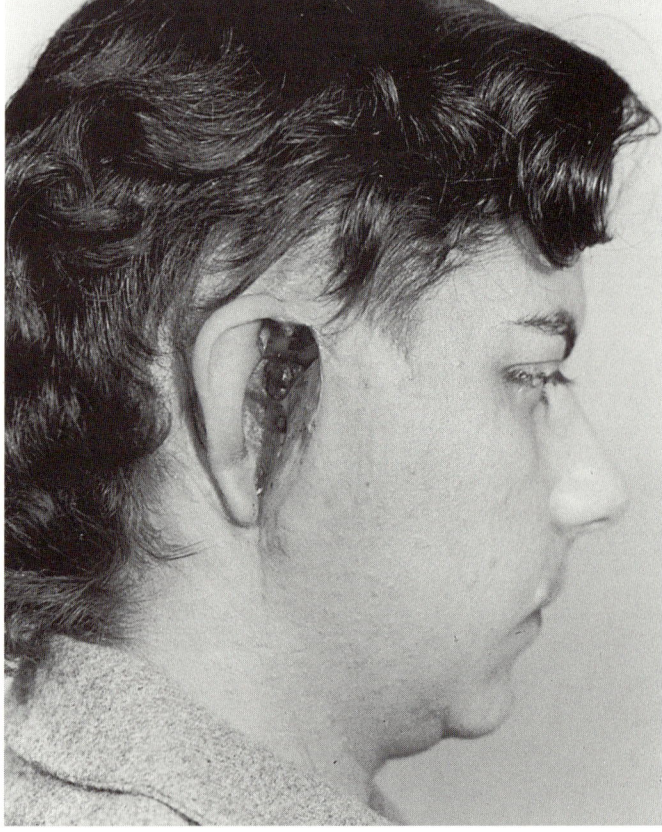

Fig. 8.**58e** A more extensive resection of skin, cartilage, bone, parotid, and neck. These cases, which have been rehabilitated with a free skin graft, require some cleaning of the cavity from time to time. The cavity may connect to the eustachian tube. Skin graft is a direct and simple way of rehabilitation. These skin grafts will tolerate 6000 rads (60 Gy) postoperatively in most instances

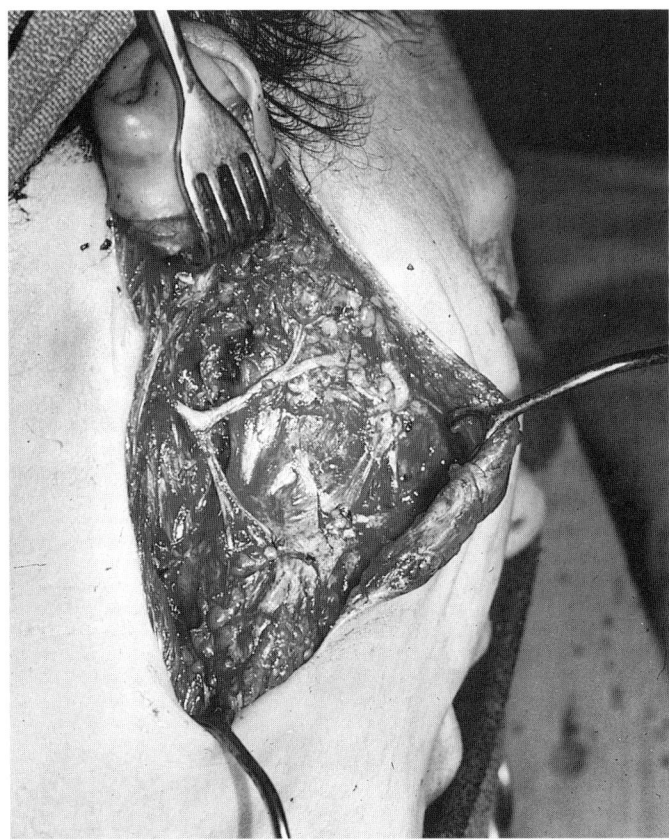

Fig. 8.**59 Adenoid cystic cancer of the ear canal with early invasion of the parotid gland.** Resection of the ear canal, mastoidectomy, and total parotidectomy with preservation of the nerve

8 Surgical Treatment

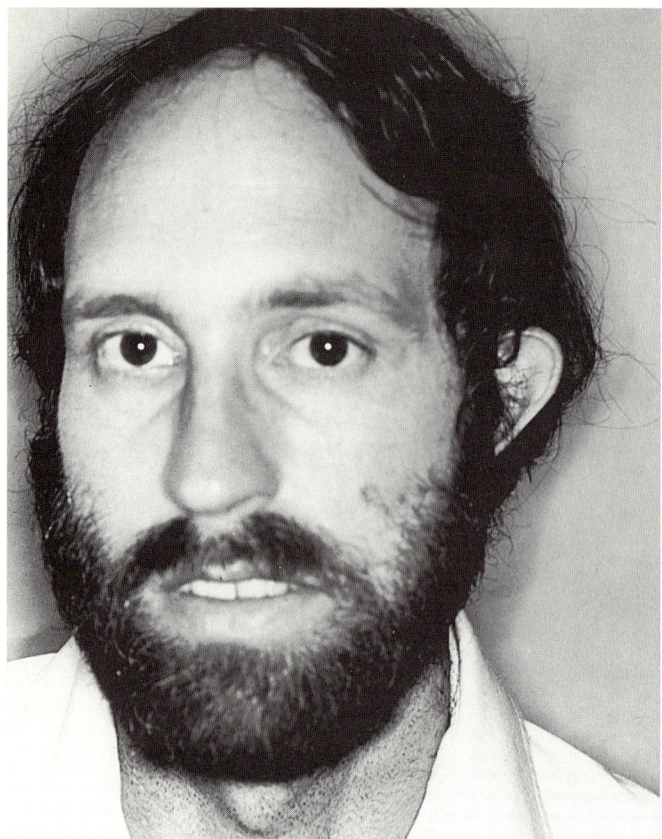

Fig. 8.**60a** **This patient has early adenoid cystic carcinoma of the left ear canal;** his face is normal

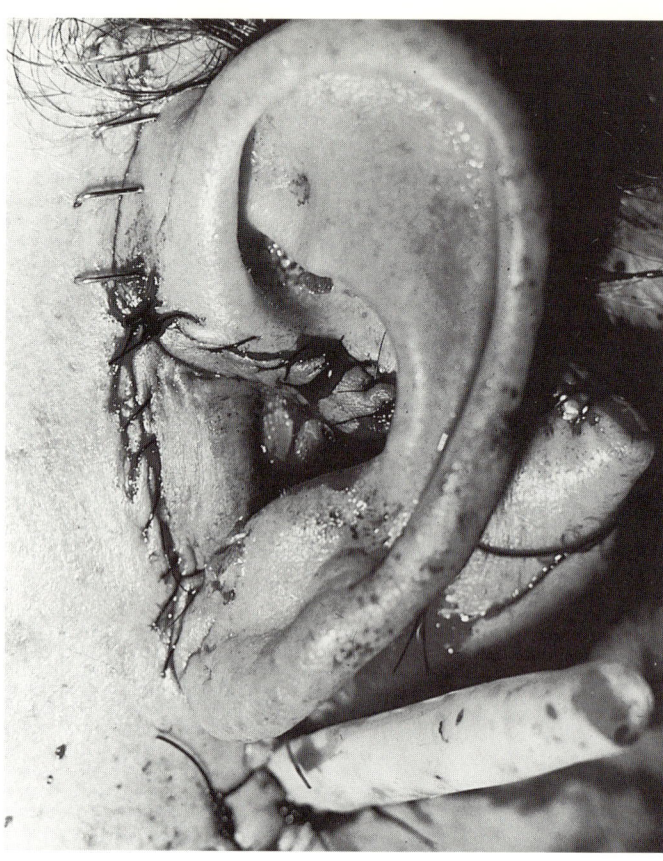

Fig. 8.**60b** A classical resection of the ear canal, a mastoidectomy, and a parotidectomy was carried out and the area was rehabilitated with a small posterior cervical flap and free skin graft

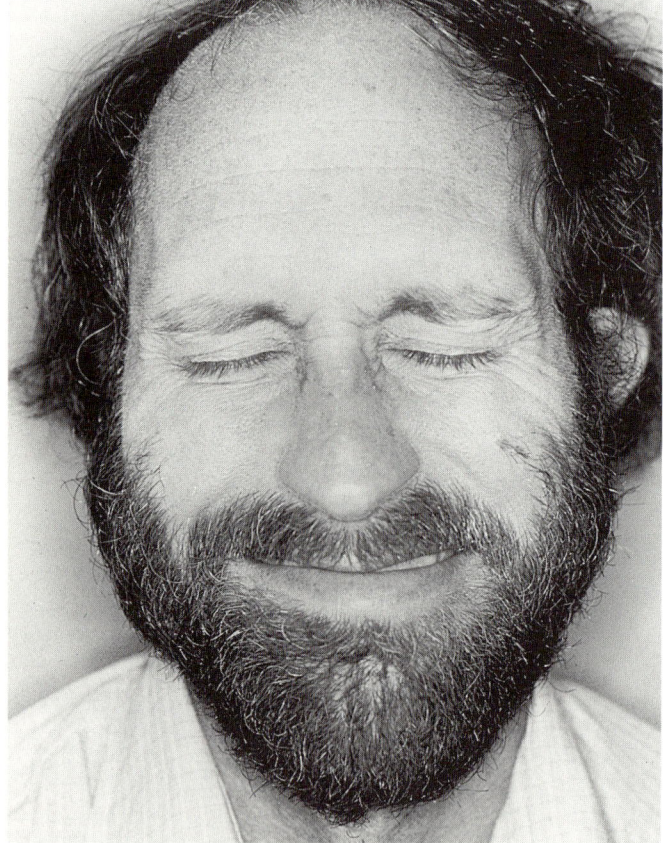

Fig. 8.**60c** The patient has normal facial movement and has been free of disease for 12 years since surgery

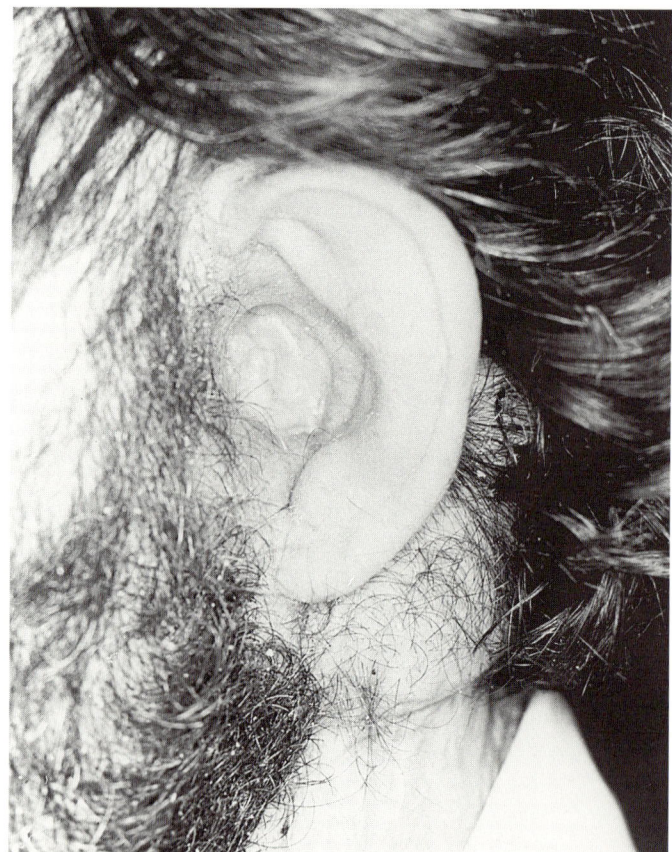

Fig. 8.**60d** Lateral view showing skin graft and flap

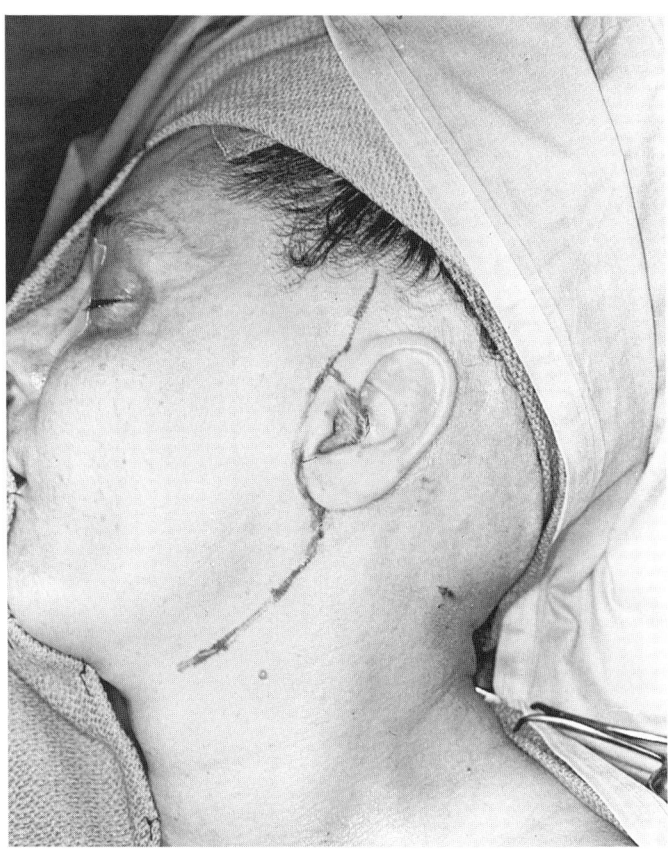

Fig. 8.**61a** **Skin incisions for adenoid cystic carcinoma of the ear canal** with resection of the ear canal, mastoid bone, parotid gland, and upper neck

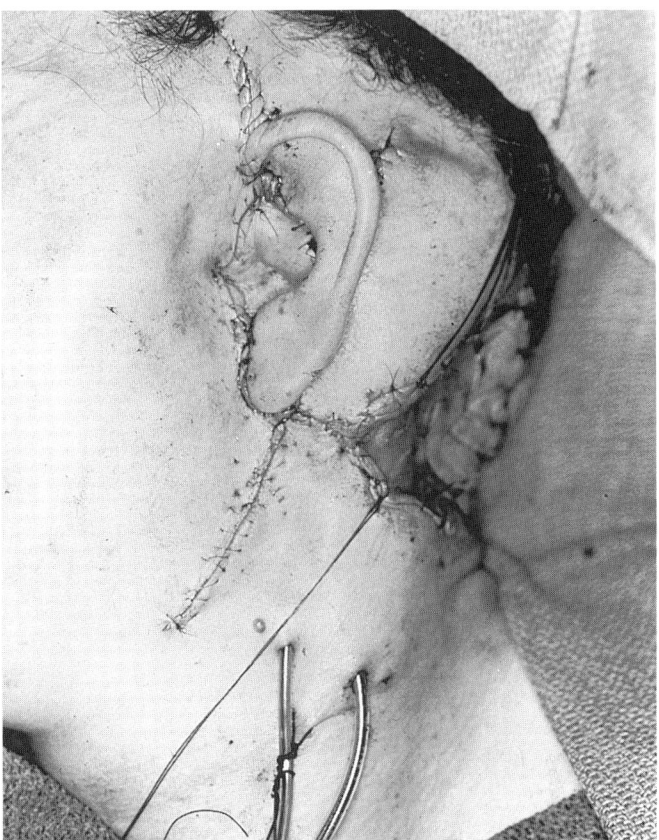

Fig. 8.**61b** This cavity is rehabilitated with a postauricular flap and skin graft. The facial nerve remains intact

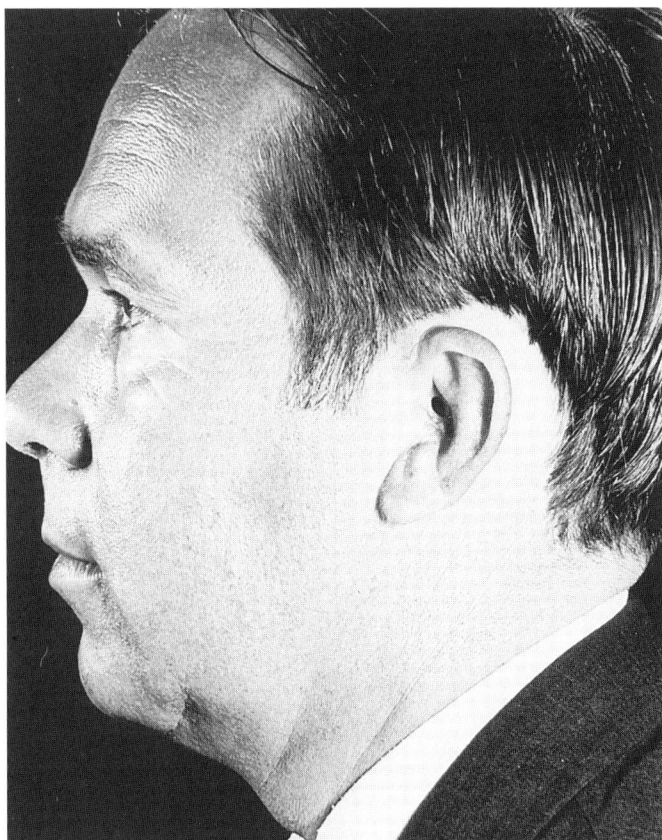

Fig. 8.**62a** **Recurrent and more advanced adenoid cystic carcinoma of the ear canal**

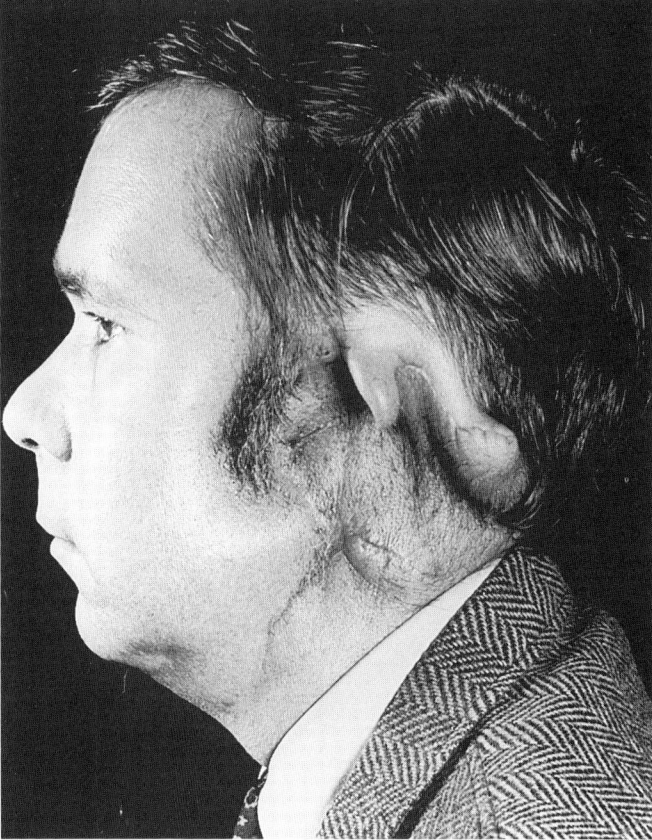

Fig. 8.**62b** Resection included a major part of auricle, the parotid gland, the mandible, and the temporal bone. Rehabilitation of this wound with a larger, superiorly based posterior cervical flap

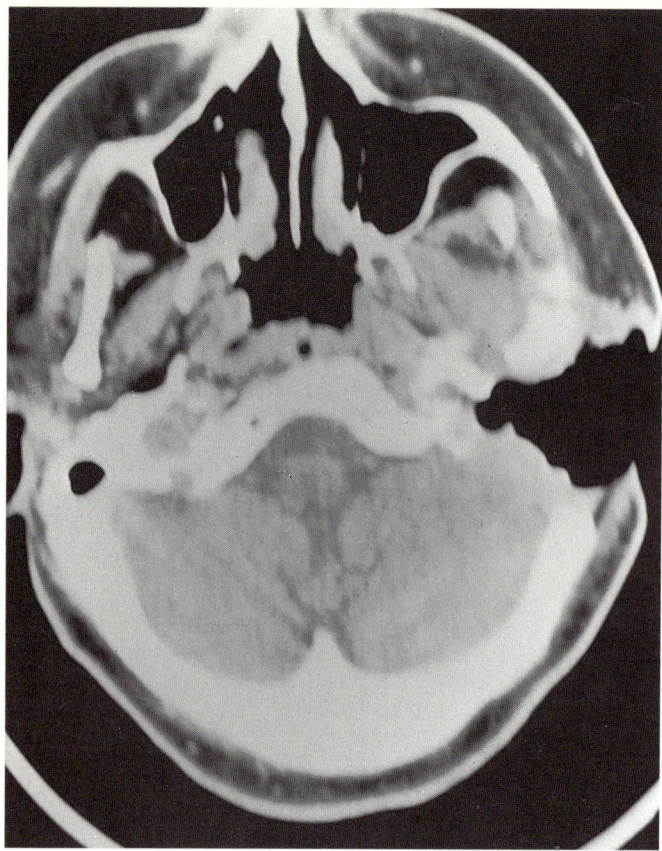

Fig. 8.**63** **X-ray documentation of resection of the adjacent bone in the mastoid, middle ear, and petrous pyramid**

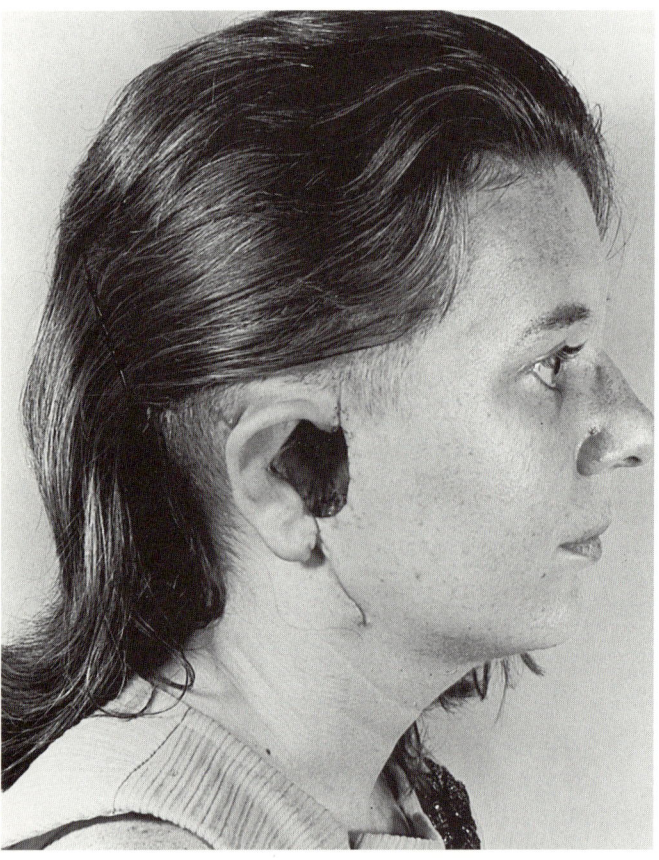

Fig. 8.**64a** **This patient had partial temporal-bone resection along with more extensive resection of conchal cartilage, the ear canal, and the parotid gland, with preservation of the facial nerve.** This cavity was dressed with a skin graft

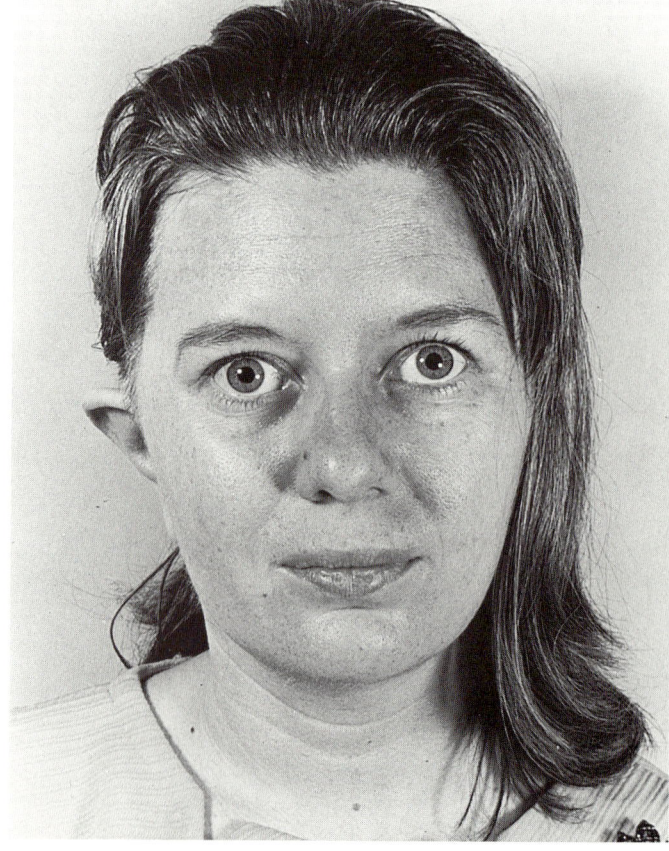

Fig. 8.**64b** Her face is essentially normal

Ear Canal

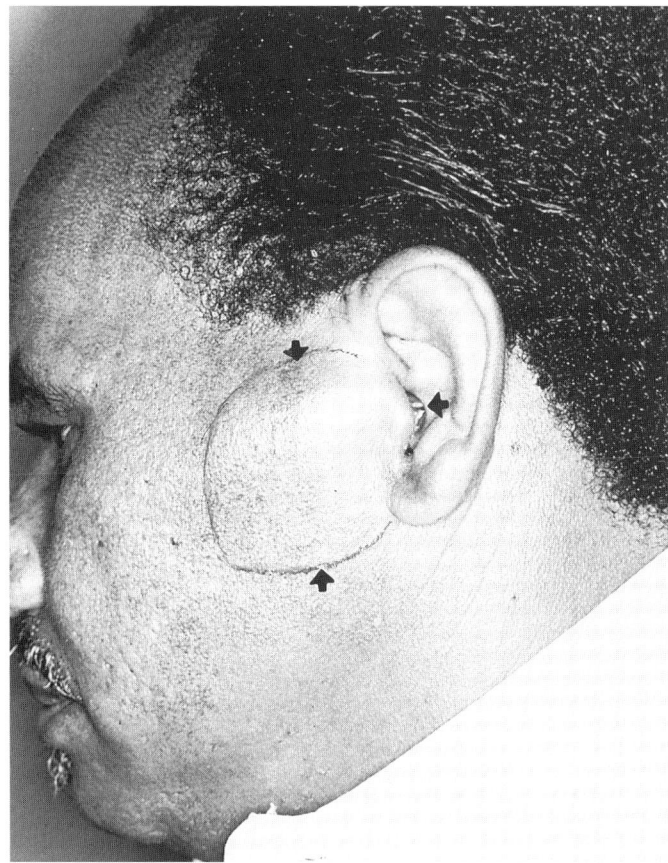

Fig. 8.65a **This patient's tumor demonstrates the close relation of adenoid cystic carcinoma of the ear canal to the parotid gland (arrows)**

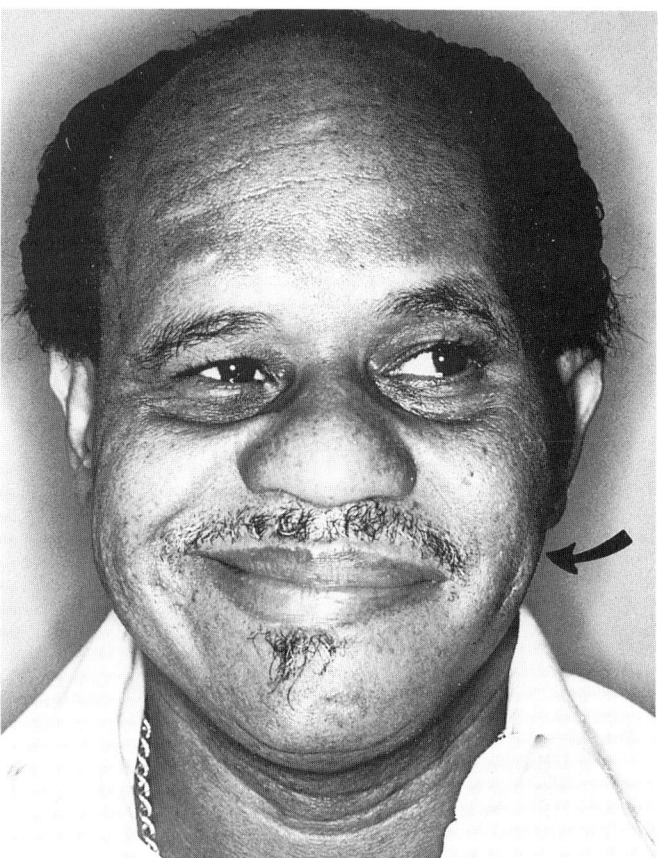

Fig. 8.65b He was treated with radical parotidectomy, modified temporal bone resection, and rehabilitation of the facial nerve with hypoglossal crossover. He has excellent movement of the face three years after surgery (arrow)

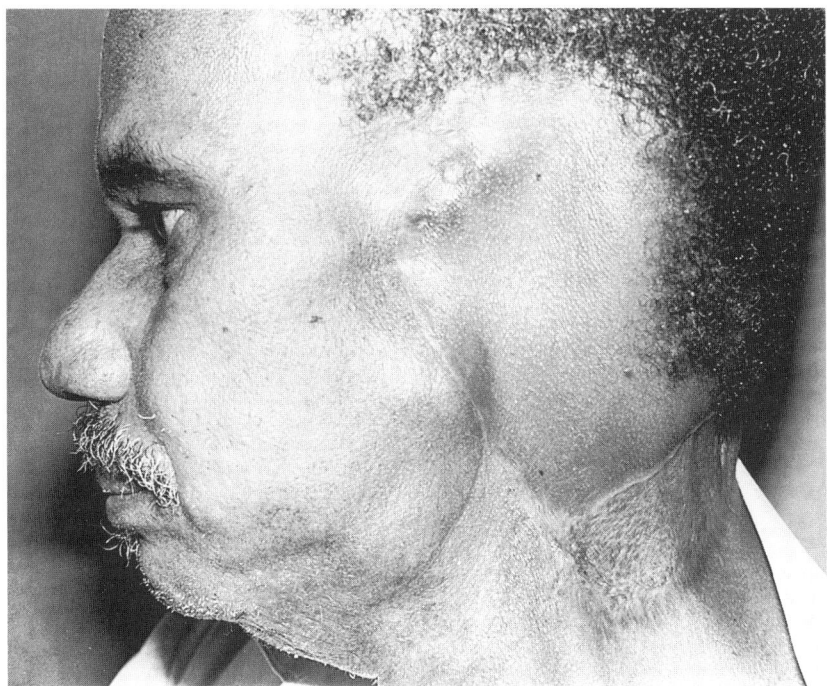

Fig. 8.65c The patient developed local recurrence, even though he had postoperative radiotherapy, and had local resection of the ear and skin and rehabilitation with a posterior cervical flap. The patient ultimately developed pulmonary metastases

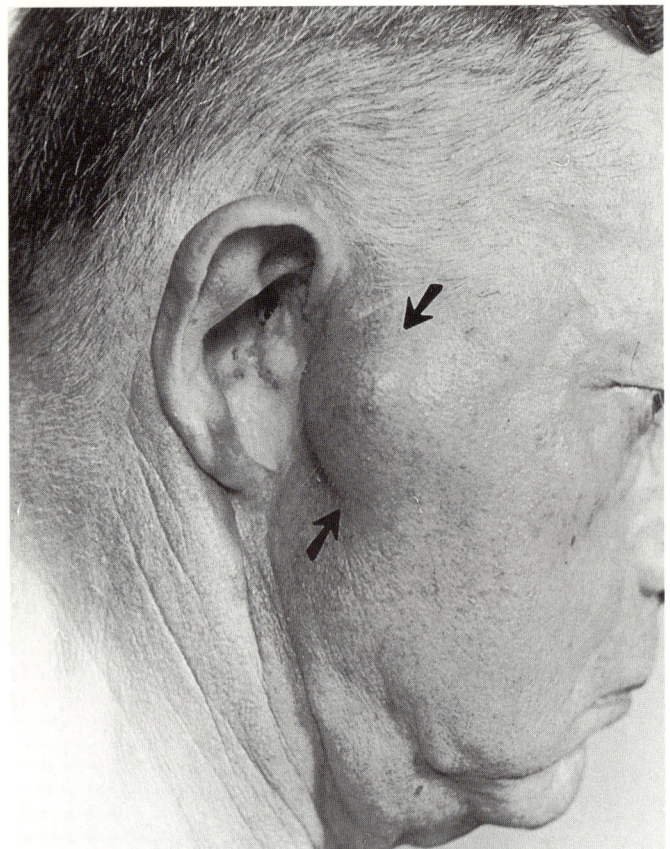

Fig. 8.66 **This patient had recurrence in the parotid gland (arrow) following previous resection** of adenoid cystic carcinoma in the ear canal six years before. This emphasizes the necessity of including the parotid gland in the primary resection

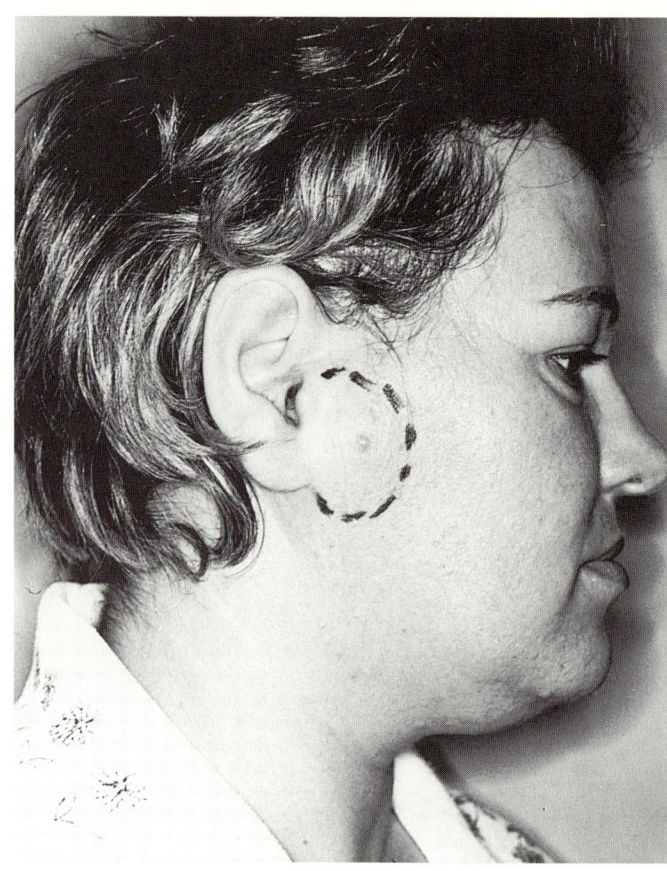

Fig. 8.67a Advanced involvement of the ear canal by adenoid cystic carcinoma with extension to the parotid gland

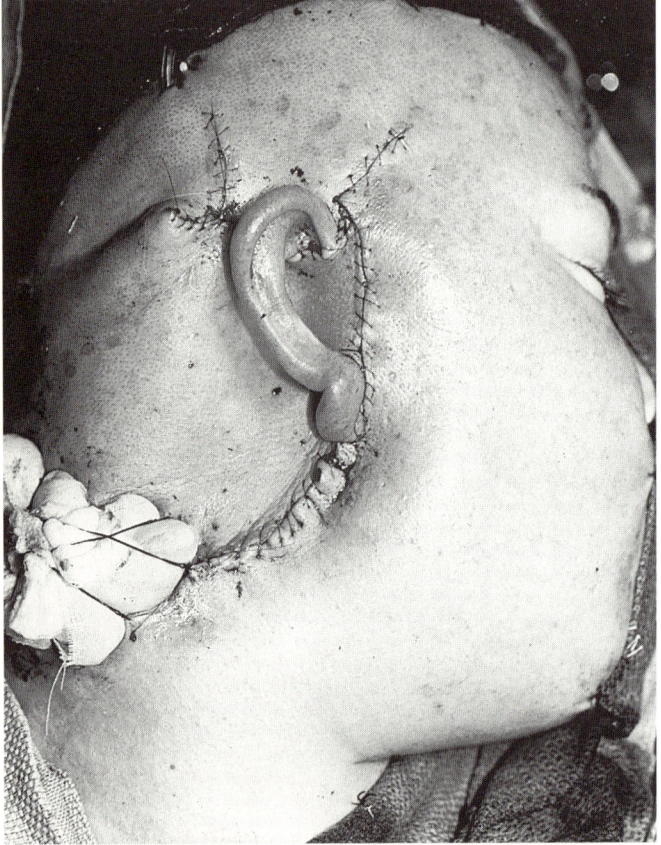

Fig. 8.67b This patient underwent radical resection of the ear canal, partial temporal bone, associated skin, and the parotid gland. The wound was rehabilitated with a posterior cervical flap and skin graft

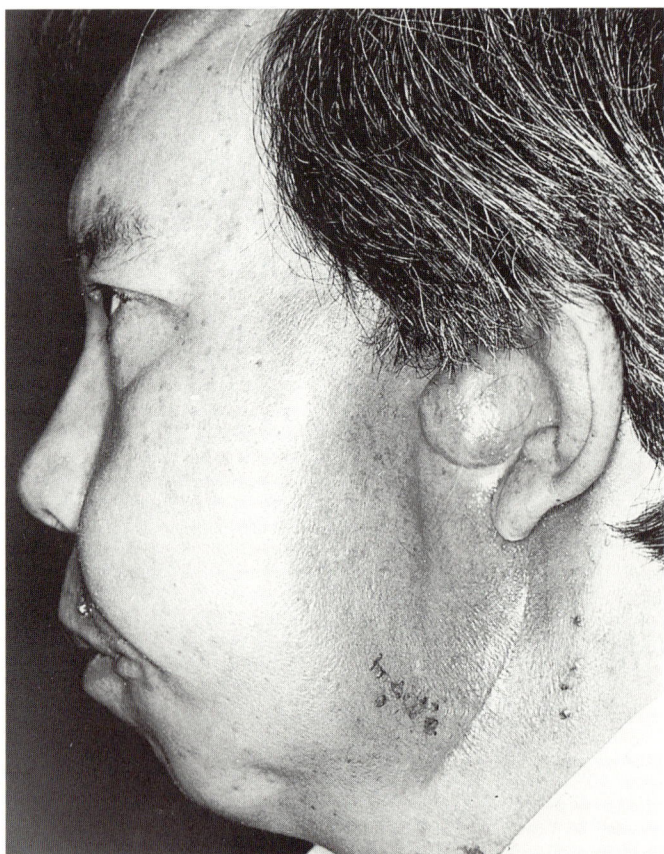

Fig. 8.68 **This patient exhibits erythema from postoperative irradiation applied to the area of the primary carcinoma and its regional environment.** This patient has been living free of disease for 11 years since surgery. Postoperative irradiation is an essential part of the management of the majority of adenoid cystic carcinomas in this area

9
Management of Persistent Tumor

As the majority of these cases are not cured by any method of treatment, it is appropriate to be prepared for a protracted morbidity that requires treatment and management as the dying process runs its course. This program of palliation must deal with local recurrence, regional metastasis, and systemic spread. Taken together, these occurrences ultimately appear in 70–80% of the cases.

Local Recurrence
(Figs. 9.**1–3**)

Local recurrence occurs in approximately 74% of the cases. This alarming figure emphasizes the fact that the majority of operations are inadequate, either as a result of initial planning, or as a result of unresectability. Neither of these answers seems justified in view of the fact that only a small percentage of patients with local recurrence can be salved by reoperation or any other form of treatment. The clinician cannot be blamed for this unfortunate predicament in every instance, however, as 73% of the cases involve tumors beyond T1 when they are first seen. The challenge is basically the ominous one of advanced disease. The best solution to this problem is earlier diagnosis, but this is unrealistic when treating a disease that does not produce early symptoms and, in many cases, is not discoverable because it is submucosal and anatomically concealed from discovery.

Local recurrence was developed in 74% of these cases at the site of the patient's primary operation; 37% were discovered within five years. This statistic would indicate that gross tumor was present in the wound at the termination of the first operation. Local recurrence was experienced by 22% of the patients 5–10 years after surgery, and 10% had local recurrence 10–15 years after surgery. In 4%, the local recurrence appeared 15–20 years after surgery and in 1%, 20 years and later. This chronicity and persistence of local recurrence is a hallmark of this tumor and challenges the clinician with the protracted problems of extended morbidity and retreatment. These problems are further compounded by a wide range of recurrence, with an incidence of 56% for the submandibular gland tumors and 87% for the sublingual gland tumors.

A review of the tumors in the salivary gland systems showed that some regions and systems are more susceptible to recurrent tumor. Minor salivary gland tumors had a 79% incidence of recurrence, with 37% appearing in less than 5 years, 23% occurred 5–10 years after surgery, 12% in 10–15 years, 6% in 15–20 years, and 1% over 20 years later. This emphasizes the extended period of chronicity of this disease in minor salivary glands with a gradual tapering-off after 15 years, but is also a reminder that in 1% of the cases a recurrence may not become apparent until after 20 years.

The parotid gland tumors had a 71% incidence of recurrence, with 40% appearing within 5 years after surgery, 21% between 5 and 10 years, and 10% between 10 and 15 years. There were no recurrences after 15 years.

The submandibular gland tumors had a 56% incidence of recurrence, which was the lowest; 32%

occurred within 5 years after surgery, 16% between 5 and 10 years, and 8% between 10 and 15 years. There were no recurrences after 15 years.

The sublingual gland tumors had the highest recurrence rate: 87%. Fifty percent recurred within 5 years after surgery, 31% in 5–10 years, and 6% in 10–15 years. There were no recurrences after 15 years.

The majority of recurrences occur in the soft tissues adjacent to the primary tumor. In the parotid gland, it may occur in any parenchymal tissue that might remain, but in all other glands, it is assumed that all of the parenchymal salivary-gland tissue was removed at the primary operation. This elimination of the primary regional tissue with its zones of fascial spaces, and the embedment of neoplastic tissue in the surrounding mesenchymal structures with new spaces and new planes, puts this area at risk for unchallenged, random growth of the tumor in these new tissues. This means that the neoplasm is no longer contained in the salivary gland system, but has actually invaded the substance of the body.

All of these data point to incurability in the vast majority of cases. This does not, however, mean that the patient will be immediately incapacitated or suffer pain, or experience severe deterioration in quality of life. It does mean that he or she has most likely entered the dying phase and that he or she may still have good quality of life for up to 15 additional years. Some of these primary recurrences can be controlled by reoperation or irradiation, or both, for a period of 10 to 15 years. During this interval, the patient usually develops systemic spread from the recurrent primary focus and dies of it. Some of these patients, who have had only irradiation for the recurrence, are controlled for 3 to 14 years, do not develop an additional recurrence, but die of distant metastases. It is also possible that the local recurrence be controlled by reexcision for a period of ten years, and then controlled again for ten years, and then again for ten years, and that, after 30 years, the patient develops pulmonary metastases and has it controlled by lobectomy. One such case is in this series, and this most unusual patient died at the age of 90, having had no recurrence after the lobectomy for five years, no evidence of adenoid cystic carcinoma at the primary buccal site or in the lungs, and no irradiation during this entire interval. No one could believe that he had been cured of this cancer during that 41-year period. He lived a normal life with his cancer for four decades, with the exception of the morbidity associated with three operations at the primary site and one operation for systemic disease. On the other hand, this is a most unusual and fortuitous situation that proves the extreme chronicity of this disease, its so-called "benign behavior," and how little we really know about its fundamental biological factors. In addition to this, it emphasizes the justification for the adequate and effective treatment of local recurrences, when it is realistic.

Local Recurrence

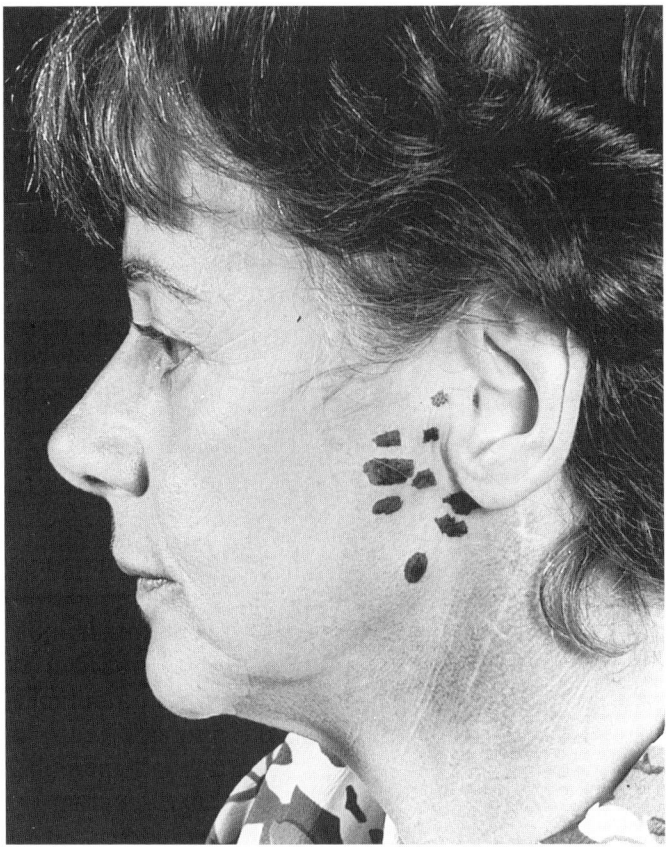

Fig. 9.**1 Multiple and disseminated recurrent adenoid cystic carcinoma throughout the parotid gland** with an interval of three years. This is most likely associated with spillage

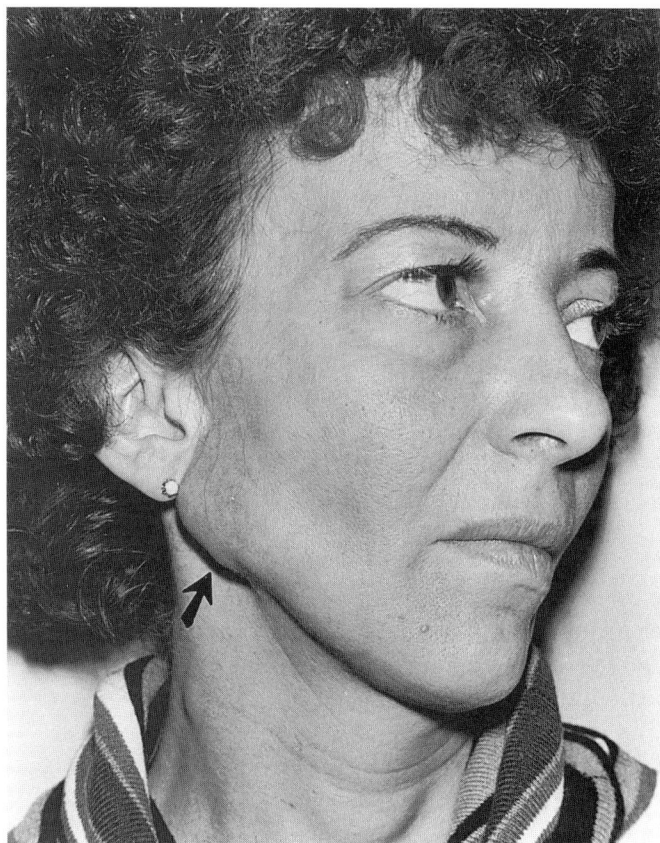

Fig. 9.**2 Large recurrence of adenoid cystic carcinoma over the mandible four years after surgery**

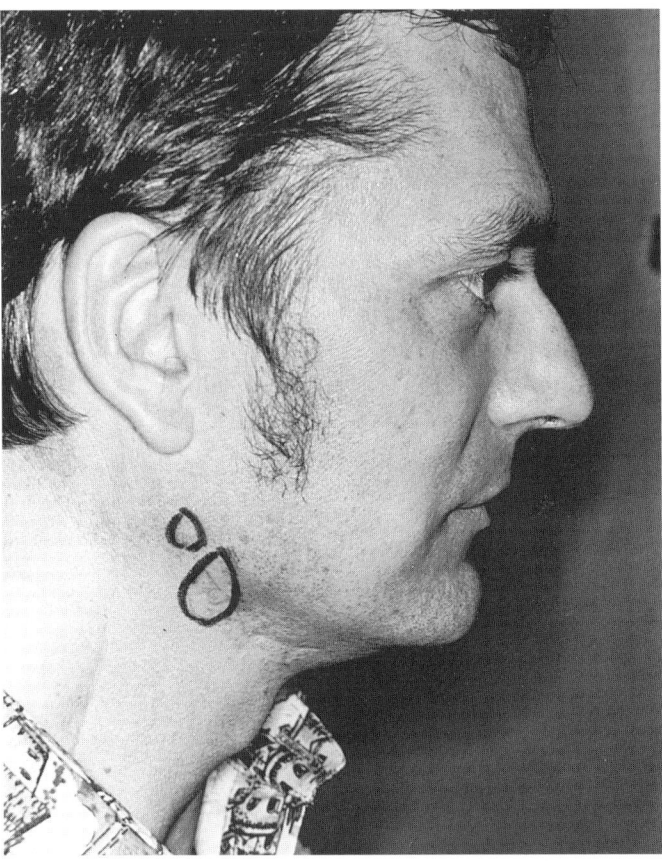

Fig. 9.**3 Multiple, localized recurrence of adenoid cystic carcinoma in the area of the tail of the parotid gland, adjacent to the submandibular gland, after three years**

Regional Metastasis

Adenoid cystic carcinoma does not commonly metastasize to regional lymph nodes. In this series, 5% had regional metastases at the initial examination, 3% developed metastases within the first five years after treatment, 2% in 5 to 10 years, 1% in 10 to 15 years, and 1% in 15 to 25 years. The total incidence of metastasis to regional lymph nodes was 12%. The low number of lymph-node metastases is indeed an unusual cancer behavior pattern, as the disease recurs locally for over two decades. The high incidence of local recurrence over a long period of time gives the tumor favorable opportunities to invade regional afferent lymph vessels and to spread to regional lymph nodes, but this is infrequent. The fact that it prefers to invade the venous system and spread systemically is an ominous characteristic of its biologic behavior. In some instances, extensions of the primary cancer invade regional lymph nodes and simulate metastases, thus making primary embolic metastases difficult to identify. The incidence of metastasis with the basaloid type was higher than with the tubular and cribriform types. It is therefore appropriate not to include elective neck dissection in the primary therapeutic program, unless it facilitates the primary operation and has a minimal surgical deficit.

Systemic Metastasis

In this series, 2% of the patients had pulmonary metastases at their initial visit. Fifty percent of the patients ultimately had a variety or combination of systemic metastases, with 27% ultimately going to the lungs; in 12% of the cases, the pulmonary metastasis appeared in less than five years. In another 14%, it appeared in 5 to 35 years, indicating that there was a persistent risk for pulmonary metastasis as the disease continued over decades. The question is whether chronicity of the disease, repetitive operations for recurrences, or a special affinity for venous invasion enhanced this occurrence of pulmonary metastasis.

The brain was the next most common metastatic repository for adenoid cystic carcinoma. Only 1% of the patients had it at the initial examination, but 5% had it within five years. An additional 7% developed it in 5 to 15 years. The proximity of adenoid cystic cancer of the sinuses in particular, and also of the ear canal and the palate, unquestionably puts the brain at risk for direct extension and regional metastasis. Unsuccessful surgery at these sites followed by local recurrence further increases this risk.

Six of the adenoid cystic carcinomas metastasized to bone. Only 0.5% were present at the initial examination, 3% were manifest within the first five years and 1% occurred more than 15 years after surgery.

Metastases to other organs of the body occurred in 4% of the cases, but according to these data, this cancer does not have a tendency toward wide dissemination. It has a predilection for the lungs, the brain and bone, and although only 3% of the patients had systemic metastases at the initial examination, 20% had it within five years and another 14% had it within ten years. Only 10% developed it more than ten years after surgery. These data indicate a significant risk (30%) of systemic metastases within the first ten years after treatment; however, these data are primarily applicable to tumors of the major salivary glands. Curiously, in minor salivary glands, the incidence of systemic metastasis is greatest between 15 and 20 years after initial treatment and continues beyond 20 years, which gives the biological behavior of this neoplasm a prolonged danger and increased lethality. In the major salivary glands, metastasis alone is past its crescendo in ten years; local recurrence then becomes the dominant factor. After ten years, there is still the pernicious continuation of local recurrence, alone or combined with systemic metastases, which becomes a hallmark of this disease and a serious addition to the ever-diminishing prognosis extending up to and beyond 20 years.

10
Risk Factors

Morbidity and Mutilation

One of the difficult decisions patients must make in dealing with certain advanced adenoid cystic carcinomas is the amount of mutilation they are willing to accept. Indeed, this also becomes a problem for their operating surgeons, who must advise, and then carry out the act of surgery with its consequences. It must be appreciated that the definition of surgical mutilation in life-threatening disease processes cannot be an arbitrary decision and must contain some rational parameters. Fortunately, significant and negative alteration in appearance and function can be quite accurately assessed preoperatively today. There are, of course, biological imponderables that are unpredictable. All patients are anxious about every cancer operation, and most patients depend on their surgeon's advice on the treatment with the best consequences possible. All of this takes place before the fact and may prove to be disappointing postoperatively.

Some of the factors that require consideration are: 1) the size and duration of the cancer, 2) its histologic classification, 3) its anatomical site, 4) the general plan of treatment, 5) its rationale and consequences, and 6) its effect on the patient. These six proposals pertain to the quality of life, the chance of survival, the degree of the alteration of appearance, and the patient's intrinsic right to be involved in this aspect of his or her destiny.

The *size and duration* of the tumor are directly involved with the prognosis. The longer the tumor has been present and the greater its volumetric proportions are, the higher is the danger, in all aspects.

Large adenoid cystic carcinomas that have been present for years have the gravest prognoses. They also require the most extensive operations and adequate postoperative radiotherapy. This obviously presents serious considerations in planning and management. There are no easy or simple answers to some of these decisions.

The *histologic classification* of the tumor may add considerable gravity to the outlook, particularly if it presents microscopically as a compact, small-cell, undifferentiated variety of adenoid cystic carcinoma. The tubular and the cribriform types have a more favorable prognosis. Many of the histologic patterns are mixed, in which case the preponderant pattern is usually selected as the histologic type.

The *site* of the neoplasm is significant both in prognosis and in treatment. Those tumors arising in minor salivary glands have a much more serious prognosis than those arising in the major salivary glands. The minor salivary gland tumors are contained in the submucosal tissues af the mucous-membrane patterns of the oral cavity, nasal cavity, and pharynx. This often presents a more serious problem than the presence of this tumor in the parotid gland and the submandibular gland, which have a large mass of tissue to contain the tumor and are in more accessible positions for surgical ablation. The adenoid cystic cancer in the minor salivary glands in the nasal cavity may threaten the orbit, the brain, and the base of the skull. In the oral cavity, they can threaten the mandible and maxilla, and in the pharynx, affect swallowing, breathing, and speaking.

The *general plan of treatment* must include a program of adequate surgery for cure, surgical excision and postoperative irradiation, irradiation for cure, irradiation for palliation, massive palliative surgery and irradiation, or no treatment at all. In the majority of cases the first two options are usually the most desirable and the most frequently selected. There are special cases, however, to which the other forms of management are suited.

The *rationale and consequences* of the treatment are more difficult to assess because of training, personal bias, some confusion in the statistics, and because the success of a bolder program is an "outside chance." All of this must be mixed with a realistic estimation of the actual chance for cure and the severity of the postoperative alterations and their consequences, or with the decision to emphasize temporary palliation over a possible cure. Certainly, these pervasive negative aspects and possibilities are reinforced in cases of T3 and T4 tumors, where the local recurrence rate is at least 50%, and the systemic metastasis rate is at least 50%.

The *effect* of these analyses and the philosophizing on the part of the surgeon are wittingly and unwittingly transmitted to the patients. They then not only have the burden of their cancer, but the responsibility of deciding which treatment they would prefer. Fortunately, it is not as agonizing a process as it seems, as a consensus develops on the basis of shared information. In this decision-making process, the patient, the doctor, the family, and indeed, even society are involved.

Consultation with the radiotherapist incorporates another opinion that may conform to the surgical program or may demand its modification. Certainly in the vast majority of cases, surgery and irradiation are used on more than one occasion as patients struggle with recurrences and metastases in a program which amounts to a strategic retreat from life. It is well-recognized that uncontrolled cancer can be the most severe mutilator of the patient's life. With this disease, it is often a question of the balance between the disease process, the quality of life, and the possibilities of therapeutic help. Many of these decisions cannot be made in advance and must be made on an individual basis.

Rehabilitation

The majority of T1 and T2 adenoid cystic carcinomas do not require specific rehabilitative procedures. On the other hand, the majority of the advanced cases and recurrent cases of adenoid cystic carcinoma require some type of rehabilitation following their ablative surgery. This varies with the site and volume of the disease. There is no need for reconstruction around the sinuses or nasal cavity when the bony arch and the skin of the face remain intact. When these structures have been sacrificed along with the orbit or the palate, or both, some form of rehabilitation is essential. The simple and most direct method around the orbit and sinuses is the application of a skin graft. It is preferred in cases in which only the sinuses are removed in order to permit the wounds to heal by secondary intention. A closed nasal cavity that allows irrigation only through the nostrils is frequently inadequate for thorough cleaning, and skin grafts in many of these nasal cavities will develop an unpleasant odor. This does not happen if irrigation can be accomplished through a palatal or orbital opening. Regional and free microvascular flaps may be used to add bulk, skin, or palatal resurfacing. Some individuals desire a facial prosthesis for certain aesthetic effects, and under specific circumstances, this result may be very pleasing; however, one must be prepared for disappointment in the craftsmanship and artistry, poor fitting, the additional burden of putting this prosthesis on and taking it off, and the necessity for refabrication as it wears out. They are usually not a realistic substitute for a simple black patch.

Facial paralysis is immediately rehabilitated by autogenous nerve graft or muscle (masseter or temporalis) transfer (see chapter 7, under "The Facial Nerve in Adenoid Cystic Carcinoma of the Parotid Gland").

The major resections in the oral and pharyngeal cavities as the result of advanced or recurrent adenoid cystic carcinoma comprise the palate, buccal areas, tongue, mandible, pharyngeal structures, and various parts of each anatomical region. The best rehabilitation in these areas is direct approximation of the regional tissues if that is feasible, or free skin grafts or flap replacements. In the palate, the patient requires bulk plus resurfacing in order to swallow and speak. This is usually accomplished by a regional myocutaneous flap such as platysma, trapezius, or pectoralis major tissue. Some modifications may include the masseter muscle plus skin grafting or skin grafting and posterior palatal prosthesis.

Rehabilitation of the tongue is usually associated with mandibular and partial pharyngeal resections. The most direct, simplest, and in many respects most functional, method is the mobilization and direct approximation of the regional tissues. One of the classical technical procedures is to sew the residuum of the tongue to the buccal mucosa. If the magnitude of the ablation obviates this possibility, a myocotaneous flap is the preferred alternative. It should be stated that the security and appeal of some of the flaps have induced a tendency to overuse them, and it has been discovered that some of these flaps are too bulky, become pendulous, and interfere with physiological function. The criteria for their use have matured over the past decade. There is no limit to the imagination for reconstruction except the reality of the product itself. New mandibular segments have been successfully transferred from the iliac crest, scapula, radius, tibia, and rib by microvascular flaps, which are custom-designed to accommodate that particular deficit. These techniques are maximized by master planners and craftsmen and are certainly beyond the routine procedures carried out in the majority of hospitals where these operations are not standard procedures. These efforts, however, are under trial by many different surgeons in many institutions who will ultimately clarify the criteria for their use and improve the quality of the surgery and treatment program.

11
References

General

Ancell H. History of a remarkable case of tumours, developed on the head and face, accompanied with a similar disease on the abdomen. Med Chir Trans 1842;25:227–31.

Batsakis JG. Mucous gland tumors of the nose and paranasal sinuses. Ann Otol 1970;79:557–62.

Batsakis JG. Tumors of the major salivary glands. In: Batsakis JG. Tumors of the head and neck: clinical and pathological considerations. Baltimore: Williams and Wilkins, 1979.

Billroth T. Beobachtungen über Geschwülste der Speicheldrüsen. Virchows Arch A 1859;17:357.

Blanck C, Eneroth CM, Jacobsson F, Jakobson PA. Adenoid cystic carcinoma of the parotid gland. Acta Radiol Ther Phys Biol 1967;6:177–96.

Bosch A, Brandenburg JH, Gilchrist KW. Lymph node metastases in adenoid cystic carcinoma of the submaxillary gland. Cancer 1980;45:2872–7.

Buffoli A, Olivetti L, Micheletti E, Facchetti F, Moretti R. Degree of malignancy of maxillary sinus cylindromas in relation to histologic characteristics. Tumori 1982;68:127–31.

Byers RM, Berkeley RG, Luna M, Jesse RH. Combined therapeutic approach to malignant lacrimal gland tumors. Am J Ophthalmol 1975;79:53.

Chilla R, Schrot R, Eysholdt, Droese M. Adenoid cystic carcinoma of the head and neck: controllable and uncontrollable factors in the therapy and prognosis. ORL J Otorhinolaryngol Relat Spec 1980;42:346–67.

Chilla R, Schrot R, Eysholdt, Droese M. Über die therapeutische Beeinflussbarkeit adenoidzystischer Karzinome im Parotisbereich. HNO 1981;29:118–23.

Chommette G, Auriol M, Tranbalol P, Vaillant JM. Adenoid cystic carcinoma of the minor salivary glands: analysis of 86 cases, clinico-pathological and ultrastructural studies. Virchows Arch A 1982;395:289–301.

Conley J, Dingman D. Adenoid cystic carcinoma in the head and neck (cylindroma). Arch Otolaryngol 1974;100:81–90.

Conley J, Hamaker RC. Prognosis of malignant tumors of the parotid gland with facial paralysis. Arch Otolaryngol 1975;101:39–41.

Conley J. Salivary glands and the facial nerve. Stuttgart: Thieme, 1975.

Cooper DL. Cylindroma: report of an unusually extensive case. JAMA 1946;132:575.

Crain RC, Helwig EB. Dermal cylindroma (dermal eccrine cylindroma). Am J Clin Pathol 1961;35:504.

Cummings CW. Adenoid cystic carcinoma (cylindroma) of the parotid gland. Ann Otol Rhinol Laryngol 1977;86:280–92.

Donovan DT, Conley J. Adenoid cystic carcinoma of the subglottic region. Ann Otol Rhinol Laryngol 1983;92:491–5.

Eby LS, Johnson DS, Baker HW. Adenoid cystic carcinoma of the head and neck. Cancer 1972;29:1160–8.

Edgerton MT, Snyder GB. Combined intracranial-extracranial approach and use of the two stage split flap technic for reconstruction with craniofacial malignancies. Am J Surg 1965;110:595.

Elisa LT. Statistical methods for survival data analysis. Belmont, CA: Lifetime Learning, 1980.

Eneroth CM. Facial nerve paralysis. A criterion of malignancy in parotid tumors. Arch Otolaryngol 1972;95:300–4.

Eneroth CM, Hjertman G, Moberger G. Adenoid cystic carcinoma of the palate. Acta Otolaryngol 1968;66:248–60.

Evans, CD. Turban tumor. Br J Dermatol 1945;66:434.

Font RL, Gamel JW. Epithelial tumors of the lacrimal gland: An analysis of 265 cases. In: FA Jakobiec, ed. Ocular and adnexal tumors. Birmingham: Aesculapius, 1978;787–805.

Font RL, Gamel JW. Adenoid cystic carcinoma of the lacrimal gland. A clinicopathologic study of 79 cases. In: DH Nicholson, ed. Ocular pathology update. New York: Masson, 1980:227–83.

Foote FW Jr, Frazell EL. Tumors of the major salivary glands. In: Atlas of Tumor pathology. 1954.

Fu KK, Leibel SA, Levine ML, Friedlander LM, Boles R, Phillips TL. Carcinoma of the major and minor salivary glands: analysis of treatment, results and sites and causes of failures. Cancer 1977;40:2882.

Gabarro P, Baker SL. An enormous epithelioma adenoides cysticum of the scalp with a pathological report. Br J Surg 1945;33:188.

Guillamondegui OM, Byers RM, Luna MA, Chiminazzo H Jr, Jesse RH, Fletcher GH. Aggressive surgery in treatment for parotid cancer: The role of adjunctive postoperative radiotherapy. AJR 1975;123:49.

Hageman MEJ, Becker AE. Intracranial invasion of a ceruminous gland tumor. Arch Otolaryngol 1974;100:395.

Henderson JW, Neault RW. En bloc removal of intrinsic neoplasms of the lacrimal gland. Trans Am Ophthalmol Soc 1976;74:133.

Horree WA. Adenoid cystic carcinoma of the maxilla. Arch Otolaryngol 1974;100:469–72.

Jones IS. Surgical considerations in the management of lacrimal gland tumors. Clin Plast Surg 1978;5:561.

Koopot R, Reyes C, Pifarré R. Multiple pulmonary metastases from adenoid cystic carcinoma of ceruminous glands of external auditory canal. J Thorac Cardiovasc Surg 1973;65:909.

Leafstedt SW, Gaeta JF, Sako K, et al. Adenoid cystic carcinoma of major and minor salivary glands. Am J Surg 1971;122:765–62.

Luger A. Das Cylindrom der Haut und seine maligne Degeneration. Arch Dermatol Syphilol 1949;188:155.

Murray JE, Matson DD, Habal MB, Geelhoed GW. Regional cranio-orbital resection for recurrent tumors with delayed reconstruction. Surg Gynecol Obstet 1972;134:437.

Olofsson J, Van Nostrand AWP. Adenoid cystic carcinoma of the larynx: a report of four cases and a review of the literature. Cancer 1977;40:1307–13.

Perzin KH, Gullane P, Clairmont AC. Adenoid cystic carcinoma in the salivary glands: a correlation of histologic features and clinical course. Cancer 1978;42:265–82.

Perzin KH, Gullane P, Gonley J. Adenoid cystic carcinoma involving the external auditory canal: a clinicopathological study of 16 cases. Cancer 1982;50:2873–83.

Pulec JL. Glandular tumors of the external auditory canal. Laryngoscope 1977;87:1601.

Seaver PR Jr, Kuehn PG. Adenoid cystic carcinoma of the salivary glands: a study of ninety-three cases. Am J Surg 1974;128:512–20.

Spiro RH, Huvos AG, Strong EW. Adenoid cystic carcinoma of salivary origin: a clinicopathologic study of 242 cases. Am J Surg 1974;128:512–20.

Spiro RH, Huvos AG, Strong EW. Adenoid cystic carcinoma: factors influencing survival. Am J Surg 1979;138:579–83.

Szanto PA, Luna MA, Tortoledo ME, White RA. Histologic grading of adenoid cystic carcinoma of the salivary glands. Cancer 1984;154:1062–9.

Turner HA, Carter H, Neptune WB. Pulmonary metastases from ceruminous adenocarcinoma (cylindroma) of external auditory canal. Cancer 1971;28:775.

Weinstein GS, Conley J. Adenoid cystic carcinoma of the parotid gland: a review of surgical management with reference to the facial nerve. Ann Otol Rhinol Laryngol 1989;98:845–7.

Whiffen JD. Dermal cylindroma. Plast Reconstr Surg 1963;31:70.

Adenoid Cystic Carcinoma at Aberrant Sites

Abrao FS et al. Adenoid cystic carcinoma of Bartholin's gland: review of the literature and report of two cases. J Surg Oncol 1985;30:132–7.

Akamatsu T, Honda T, Nakayama J, Nakamura Y, Katsuyama T. Primary adenoid cystic carcinoma of the esophagus. Acta Pathol Jpn 1986;36:1707–17.

Amichetti M, Aldovini D. Primary adenoic cystic carcinoma of the Bartholin's gland: a clinical, histological and immunocytochemical study of a case. Eur J Surg Oncol 1988;14:335–9.

Anthony PP, James PD. Adenoid cystic carcinoma of the breast: prevalence, diagnostic criteria, and histogenesis. J Clin Pathol 1975;28:647–55.

Chapman GW, Benda J, Lifshitz S. Adenoid cystic carcinoma of the vulva with lung metastases. J Reprod Med 1985;30:217–20.

Copeland LJ et al. Adenoid cystic carcinoma of Bartholin gland. Obstet Gynecol 1986;67:115–120.

Ferry JA, Scully RE. Adenoid cystic carcinoma and adenoid basal carcinoma of the uterine cervix. Am J Surg Pathol 1988;12:134–44.

Fowler WC et al. Adenoid cystic carcinoma of the cervix. Obstet Gynecol 1978;52:337–42.

Freedman AM, Woods JE. Total scalp excision and auricular resurfacing for dermal cylindroma (turban tumor). Ann Plast Surg 1989;22:50–7.

Friedman BA, Oberman HA. Adenoid cystic carcinoma of the breast. Am J Clin Pathol 1970;54:1–14.

Gallagher CG, Stark R, Teskey J, Kryger M. Atypical manifestations of pulmonary adenoid cystic carcinoma. Br J Dis Chest 1986;80:396–9.

Gamel JW, Font RL. Adenoid cystic carcinoma of the lacrimal gland: the clinical significance of a basaloid pattern. Hum Pathol 1982;13:219–25.

Gilmour AM, Bell TJ. Adenoid cystic carcinoma of the prostate. Br J Urol 1986;58:105–96.

Gordon HW et al. Adenoid cystic (cylindromatous) carcinoma of the uterine cervix: report of two cases. Am J Clin Pathol 1972;58:51–7.

Grillo HC. Tracheal surgery. Scan J Thorac Cardiovasc Surg 1983;17:67–73.

Harris M. Pseudoadenoid cystic carcinoma of the breast. Arch Pathol Lab Med 1977;101:307–9.

Henderson JW. Orbital tumors. Philadelphia: WB Saunders, 1973:430–7.

Henderson JW. Past, present, and future surgical management of malignant epithelial neoplasms of the lacrimal gland. Br J Ophthalmol 1986;70:727–31.

Henderson JW. Adenoid cystic carcinoma of the lacrimal gland: is there a cure? Trans Am Ophthalmol Soc 1987;85:312–9.

Huber RM, Haubinger K, Niebel J, Kohler P, Held E. Adenoid cystic carcinoma masquerading as asthma: resection by laser. Eur J Respir Dis 1986;69:195–8.

Johns ME, Batsakis JG. Adenoid cystic carcinoma of the lacrimal gland. J Laryngol Otol 1975;89:641–4.

Jones IS. Surgical considerations in the management of lacrimal gland tumors. Clin Plast Surg 1978;5:561–9.

Josephson JS, Wenig BL. Dermal cylindroma. Arch Otolaryngol Head Neck Surg 1987;113:1000–3.

Koller M, Ram Z, Findler G, Lipshitz M. Brain metastasis: a rare manifestation of adenoid cystic carcinoma of the breast. Surg Neurol 1986;26:470–2.

Lang PG, Metcalf JS, Maize JC. Recurrent adenoid cystic carcinoma of the skin managed by microscopically controlled surgery (Mohs' surgery). J Dermatol Surg Oncol 1986;12:395–8.

Lawrence JB, Mazur MT. Adenoid cystic carcinoma: a comparative pathologic study of tumors in salivary gland, breast, lung, and cervix. Hum Pathol 1982;13:916–24.

Lee DA, Campbell RJ, Waller RR, Ilstrup DM. A clinicopathologic study of primary adenoid cystic carcinoma of the lacrimal gland. Ophthalmology 1985;92:128–34.

Lerner AG, Molnar JJ, Adam GG. Adenoid cystic carcinoma of the breast. Am J Surg 1974;127:585–7.

Munsch C, Westaby S, Sturridge M. Urgent treatment for nonresectable asphyxiating tracheal cylindroma. Ann Thorac Surg 1987;43:663–4.

Musa AG, Hughes RP, Coleman SA. Adenoid cystic carcinoma of the cervix: a report of 17 cases. Gynecol Oncol 1985;22:167–73.

Nerad JA, Folberg R. Multiple cylindromas: the "turban tumor." Arch Ophthalmol 1987;105:1137.

Nomori H, Kaseda S, Kobayashi K, Ishahara T, Yanai N, Torikata C. Adenoid cystic carcinoma of the trachea and mainstem bronchus. J Thorac Cardiovasc Surg 1988;96:271–7.

Pearson FG, Todd TRJ, Cooper JD. Experience with primary neoplasms of the trachea and carina. J Thorac Cardiovasc Surg 1984;88:511–8.

Petursson SR. Adenoid cystic carcinoma of the esophagus. Cancer 1986;57:1464–7.

Pourzand A, Freant L, Levin R, Peabody J. Absolon K. Primary adenoid cystic carcinoma of the esophagus. J Thorac Cardiovasc Surg 1975;69:785–9.

Prempree T, Villasanta U, Tang C. Management of adenoid cystic carcinoma of the uterine cervix (cylindroma). Cancer 1980;46:1631–5.

Ro JY, Silva EG, Gallagher HS. Adenoid cystic carcinoma of the breast. Hum Pathol 1987;18:1276–81.

Saeb JA, Graham JH. Primary cutaneous adenoid cystic carcinoma. J Am Acad Dermatol 1987;17:113–8.

Shong-San C, Walters MN. Adenoid cystic carcinoma of prostate: report of a case. Pathology 1984;16:337–8.

Sumpio BE, Jennings TA, Sullivan PD, Merino MJ. Adenoid cystic carcinoma of the breast. Ann Surg 1987;205:295–301.

Tavassoli FA, Norris HJ. Mammary adenoid cystic carcinoma with sebaceous differentiation. Arch Pathol Lab Med 1986;110:1045–53.

Thomas RHM, Lowe DG, Munro DD. Primary adenoid cystic carcinoma of the skin. Clin Exp Dermatol 1987;12:378–80.

Verani RR, Van Der Bel-Kahn J. Mammary adenoid cystic carcinoma with unusual features. Am J Clin Pathol 1973;59:653–8.

Vernon HJ, Olsen EA, Vollmer RT. Autosomal dominant multiple cylindromas associated with solitary lung cylindroma. J Am Acad Dermatol 1988;19:397–400.

Weitzner S, Chaney GC, Bass HL. Adenoid cystic carcinoma of the breast. Am Surg 1970;36:571–4.

Wobbes T, Wagener DJT, Schillings PHM. Adenoid cystic carcinoma of the oesophagus: report of a case not responding to combination chemotherapy. Clin Oncol 1984;10:261–6.

Young RH, Clement PB. Adenomyoepithelioma of the breast. Am J Clin Pathol 1988;89:308–14.

Chemotherapy

Budd GT, Groppe CW. Adenoid cystic carcinoma of the salivary gland: sustained complete response to chemotherapy. Cancer 1983;51:589–90.

Dreyfuss AI et al. Cyclophosphamide, doxorubicin, and cisplatin combination chemotherapy for advanced carcinomas of salivary gland origin. Cancer 1987;60:2869–72.

Johnson RO, Lange RD, Kisken WA, Curreri AR. Infusion of 5-fluorouracil in cylindroma treatment. Arch Otolaryngol 1964;79:625–7.

Kaplan MJ, Johns ME, Cantrell RW. Chemotherapy for salivary gland cancer. Otolaryngol Head Neck Surg 1986;95:165–70.

Petursson SR. Adenoid cystic carcinoma of the esophagus: complete response to combination chemotherapy. Cancer 1986;57:1464–7.

Reddy SP, Marks JE. Treatment of locally advanced, high-grade, malignant tumors of major salivary glands. Laryngoscope 1988;98:450–4.

Schramm VL, Scrodes C, Myers EM. Cisplatin therapy for adenoid cystic carcinoma. Arch Otolaryngol 1981;107:739–41.

Sessions RB et al. Intra-arterial cisplatin treatment of adenoid cystic carcinoma. Arch Otolaryngol 1982;108:221–4.

Skibba JL, Hurley JD, Ravelo HV. Complete response of a metastatic adenoid cystic carcinoma of the parotid gland to chemotherapy. Cancer 1981;47:2543–8.

Tannock IF, Sutherland DJ. Chemotherapy for adenocystic carcinoma. Cancer 1980;46:452–4.

Triozzi PL et al. 5-Fluorouracil, cyclophosphamide, and vincristine for adenoid cystic carcinoma of the head and neck. Cancer 1987;59:887–90.

Vermeer RJ, Pinedo HM. Partial remission of advanced adenoid cystic carcinoma obtained with Adriamycin. Cancer 1979;43:1604–6.

Wobbes T, Wagener DJT, Schillings PHM. Adenoid cystic carcinoma of the oesophagus: report of a case not responding to combination chemotherapy. Clin Oncol 1984;10:261–6.

Imaging

Curtin HD, Williams R, Johnson J. CT of perineural tumor extension: Pterygopalatine fossa AJNR 1984;5:731–7.

Curtin HD, Wolfe P, Snyderman N. The facial nerve between the stylomastoid foramen and the parotid: computed tomographic imaging. Radiology 1983;149:165–9.

Dodd GD et al. The dissemination of tumors of the head and neck via the cranial nerves. Radiol Clin North Am 1970;8:445–61.

Dodd GD, Jing B. Radiographic findings in adenoid cystic carcinoma of the head and neck. Ann Otol 1972;81:591–8.

Forbes GS, Sheedy PF, Waller RR. Orbital tumors evaluated by computed tomography. Radiology 1980;136:101–11.

Hesselink JR et al. Computed tomography of the paranasal sinuses and face, part 2: pathologic anatomy. J Comput Assist Tomogr 1978;2:568–76.

Hesselink JR, Weber AL. Pathways of orbital extension of extraorbital neoplasms. J Comput Assist Tomogr 1982;6:593–7.

Lee Y, Castillo M, Nauert C. Intracranial perineural metastases of adenoid cystic carcinoma of head and neck. J Comput Assist Tomogr 1985;9:219–23.

Mafee MF, Valvassori GE, Dobben GD. The role of radiology in surgery of the ear and skull base. Otolaryngol Clin N Am 15:723–53.

Mandelblatt SM et al. Parotid masses: MR imaging. Radiology 1987;163:411–4.

Osborn AG, McIff EB. Computed tomography of the nose. Head Neck Surg 1982;4:182–99.

Pagani JJ et al. Lateral wall of the olfactory fossa in determining intracranial extension of sinus carcinomas. AJR 1979;133:497–501.

Schaefer SD et al. Evaluation of NMR versus CT for parotid masses: a preliminary report. Laryngoscope 1985;95:945–50.

Som PM. Lymph nodes of the neck. Radiology 1987;165:593–600.

Som PM et al. Tumors of the parapharyngeal space and upper neck: MR imaging characteristics. Radiology 1987;164:823–9.

Som PM, Shugar JM. The significance of bone expansion associated with the diagnosis of malignant tumors of the paranasal sinuses. Radiology 1980;136:97–100.

Spencer WH. Ophthalmic pathology. Philadelphia: WB Saunders 1986:2496–515.

Spizarny DL et al. CT of adenoid cystic carcinoma of the trachea. AJR 1986;146:1129–32.

Teresi LM et al. Parotid masses: MR imaging. Radiology 1987;163:405–9.

Weber AL, Stanton AC. Malignant tumors of the paranasal sinuses: radiologic, clinical, and histopathologic evaluation of 200 cases. Head Neck Surg 1984;6:761–76.

Pathology

Azumi N, Battifora H. The cellular composition of adenoid cystic carcinoma: an immunohistologic study. Cancer 1987;60:1589–98.

Batsakis JG. Tumors of the head and neck: clinical and pathological considerations. 2nd ed. Baltimore: Williams and Wilkins, 1979:1–99.

Caselitz J, Schulze I, Seifert G. Adenoid cystic carcinoma of the salivary glands: an immunohistochemical study. J Oral Pathol 1986;15:308–18.

Chaudhry AP, Leifer C, Cutler LS, Satchidanand S, Labay GR, Yamane GM. Histogenesis of adenoid cystic carcinoma of the salivary glands: light and electronmicroscopic study. Cancer 1986;58:72–82.

Evans RW, Cruikshank AH. Epithelial tumors of the salivary glands. Philadelphia: WB Saunders, 1970.

Matsuba HM, Spector GJ, Thawley SE, Simpson JR, Mauney M, Pikul FJ. Adenoid cystic salivary gland carcinoma: a histopathologic review of treatment failure patients. Cancer 1986;57:519–24.

Nascimento AG, Amaral ALP, Prado LAF, Kligerman J, Silveira TRP. Adenoid cystic carcinoma of salivary glands: a study of 61 cases with clinicopathologic correlations. Cancer 1986;57:312–9.

Perzin KH, Gullane P, Clairmont AC. Adenoid cystic carcinoma arising in salivary glands: a correlation of histologic features and clinical course. Cancer 1978;42:265–82.

Perzin KH, Gullane P, Conley J. Adenoid cystic carcinoma involving the external auditory canal: a clinicopathologic study of 16 cases. Cancer 1982;509:2873–83.

Thackray AC, Lucus RB. Tumors of the major salivary glands. In: Atlas of tumor pathology. Washington, DC: Armed Forces Institute of Pathology, 1974. (2nd series, fascicle 10).

12
Index

A

Aberrant sites of tumor 15–20
  Bartholin's gland 15
  breast 15
  esophagus 15
  lacrimal gland 15
  prostate 15
  skin 15
  tracheobronchial tree 15
  uterine cervix 15
ACC, *see* Adenoid cystic carcinoma
Adenoid cystic carcinoma (ACC)
  aberrant sites 15–20
  age distribtuion 21, 28
  brain involvement 59
  clinical behavior 42–46
  data and statistics 21–26
  diagnosis 27–40
  extensive 80
  general features 5
  gross features 5
  imaging methods 31–40
  incidence 28
    in females 28
  incurability of 110
  local recurrence 22
  location 5, 28
    aberrant 15–20
  metastasis, to bone 112
    to brain 112
    pulmonary 112
    regional 112
    systemic 112
  mortality rate 24
  nerve involvement 29
  occult 75
  outcome at ten years 24
  overall survival rates 25

pain 29
pathology 5–14
predictables in behavior 41–42
prognosis 30
recurrent, in maxilla 58
rehabilitation 114–115
response to irradiation 100
risk factors 113–115
sex distribution 21, 28
signs and symptoms 27–28
sites, *see also* Tumor, site 5, 14, 22, 28, 113
  aberrant 15–20
staging guidelines 30–31
surgical procedures 49, 53–108
  inadequacy 22
symptoms 27–28
  pain 27, 29
therapeutic planning 49–50
tumor behavior 41–47
  predictables 41–42
tumor management 49–52
tumor sites 5, 22
  aberrant 15–20
unusual cases 42–46
Age distribution 21, 28
Alveolus tumor, surgical treatment 67–69
Apex of orbit, compromised by tumor 38
Axial CT scan 35

B

Bartholin's gland, tumor site 20
  aberrant 15
Basaloid type of tumor 22
Base of skull, recurrent tumor 40
  tumor extension 55, 94
Behavior of tumor 41–47

chronicity 46
predictables 41–42
Benign mixed tumor, pathologic features 6
Biopsy 28
  excisional 28
  fine-needle aspiration 28
  punch 28
Bleeding, ulcerated tumor 27
Bone metastases 112
Bony erosion, ethmoidal region 36
Brain, involvement 59
  metastasis 112
Breast, tumor site 5, 18–19
  aberrant 15
Buccal area tumor, split-skin graft 65
  surgical treatment 63–65

C

Cancer, adenoid cystic, *see* Adenoid cystic carcinoma
  extensive, subglottic area 72
  undifferentiated, supraglottis 72
Cells, myoepithelial 13
Ceruminoma 98
Chemotherapy 49, 51–52
  cisplatin 52
  doxorubicin 52
  5-fluorouracil 52
  tumor management 49, 51–52
Chronicity, tumor behavior 46
Cisplatin 52
Classification, histologic of tumor 113
Clinical behavior 42–46
Cribriform pattern 6
Cribriform type, tumor incidence 22
CT scanning 28, 32

CT scanning, axial 35
   ear canal tumor 98
Cylindroma 98

D

Data and statistics 21–26
Deep lobe of parotid gland, tumor site 27
Diagnosis of ACC 27–40
   ear canal tumor 98
Doxorubicin 52

E

Ear canal tumor, CT scanning 98
   diagnosis 98
   facial-nerve graft 100
   hypoglossal crossover 100
   local recurrence 99
   masseter muscle rotation 100
   pain 99
   perineural involvement 99
   postoperative radiotherapy 100
   site 5
   surgical treatment 98–108
Esophagus, tumor site 17–18
   aberrant 15
Ethmoidal region, bony erosion 36
Ethmoids, tumor site 39, 59
Excisional biopsy 28
Extensive adenoid cystic carcinoma 80
Extensive cancer, subglottic area 72

F

Facial nerve, and parotid gland tumor 84–89
Facial-nerve graft, ear canal tumor 100
   parotid gland tumor 75, 86–88
Facial paralysis 75
   parotid gland tumor 75, 84
   rehabilitation 114
Features, of ACC, general 5
   gross 5
   pathologic, benign mixed tumor 6
   monomorphic adenoma 6
Females, incidence of ACC 28
Fine-needle aspiration biopsy 28
Flap replacement, nasal cavity tumor 55
Floor of mouth tumor, surgical treatment 67–69
5-Fluorouracil 52
Frontal sinus, compromised by tumor 39
Frozen sections 12

H

Hair-bearing flap, parotid gland tumor 82
Hard palate, tumor extension 38
Histologic classification 113
Histology, of tumor 23
Histopathology, parotid gland tumor 86
Hypoglossal crossover, ear canal tumor 100

I

Imaging techniques, ACC 31–40
Inadequacy, surgical 22
Incidence, ACC 28
   local recurrence 23
   metastasis 23
      pulmonary 22
      regional 22
      systemic 22
Incurability of ACC 110
Infratemporal fossa, tumor extension 38
Infratemporal space, tumor recurrence 94
Intracranial symptoms, absence of 39
Intraneural invasion 12
Invasion, perineural 12, 22–23
Invasive tumors 12
Involvement, of brain 59
   of lymph nodes 14
   perineural, ear canal tumor 99
Irradiation, *see also* Radiotherapy
   parotid gland tumor 84, 86
   postoperative, minor salivary gland tumors 24
   response of ACC 100
   tumor management 49

L

Lacrimal gland, tumor site 5, 15–16
   aberrant 15
Lines, of surgical resection 13
Lip(s), tumor, pulmonary metastases 69
   surgical treatment 67
Local recurrence 22, 109–111
   ear canal tumor 99
   incidence 23
   minor salivary gland tumor 109
   parotid gland tumor 86
   sublingual gland tumor 110
   submandibular gland tumor 109–110
Location, of metastasis 23
   of tumor, *see* Tumor, site
Lung, tumor site 5
Lymph node, involvement 14
   metastatic, submandibular gland tumor 93

M

Major salivary glands, site of tumor 21
   surgical treatment of tumor 73–97
Management, of ACC 49–52
   of persistent tumor 109–112
Margins, of tumor 13
   surgical, parotid gland tumor 85–86
Masseter muscle, ear canal tumor 100
   parotid gland tumor 86
Masseter transfer, rehabilitation 114
Maxilla, recurrent ACC 58
Maxillary sinus, tumor site 36
Metastasis(es), incidence 22–23
   location 22–23
   parotid gland tumor 86
   pulmonary 112
      incidence 22
      tumor of lip 69
   regional 112
      incidence 22
   systemic 112
      incidence 22
Metastatic lymph node, submandibular gland tumor 93
Minor salivary gland(s), tumor, distribution 22
   incidence 28
   postoperative irradiation 24
   recurrence 109
   sites 21
   surgical treatment 53–72
   survival rate 24–25
Monomorphic adenoma, pathologic features 6
Morbidity and mutilation 113–114
Mortality rate, 24
MRI (magnetic resonance imaging) 28, 33
Mutilation, and morbidity 113–114
Myocutaneous flap, rehabilitation 114
Myoepithelial cells 13
Myofilaments 15

N

Nasal cavity tumor, distribution 22
   site 21, 36
   surgical treatment 53–59
Nasal sinuses tumor, surgical treatment 53–59
Nasopharynx, tumor site 37
Nerve graft, parotid gland tumor 76
   rehabilitation 114
Nerve involvement 29
Number of operations 23

O

Occult adenoid cystic carcinoma 75
Operations, number of 23
Oral cavity tumor, distribution 22
   prosthetic rehabilitation 61
   site 21
   surgical treatment 60–62
Orbit, tumor extension 55
Outcome at ten years 24
Overall survival rates 25

P

Pain, ACC symptom 27, 29
   ear canal tumor 99
Palate, hard, *see* Hard palate
   soft, *see* Soft palate
   tumor site 60
Paralaryngeal region tumor, surgical treatment 71
Paralysis, facial, *see* facial paralysis
Parotid gland, deep lobe of, tumor site 27
   tumor, facial nerve 84–89
      facial nerve graft 75, 86–88

facial paralysis 75, 84
hair-bearing flap 82
histopathology 86
incidence 28
irradiation 84, 86
local recurrence 86
masseter muscle 86
metastasis 86
nerve graft 76
recurrence 95
site 21, 40
staging 85
surgical margins 85–86
surgical treatment 73–83
survival rate 25
temporal muscle 86
PAS stain 9
Pathology of ACC 5–14
Perineural invasion 12, 22, 23
Perineural involvement, ear canal tumor 99
Persistent tumor, management 109–112
Pharyngotracheal area, tumor site 21
Pharynx tumor, distribution 22
  surgical treatment 70
Philosophy of management 49
Plain film radiography 31, 35
Polytomography 31
Postoperative radiotherapy, ear canal tumor 100
  minor salivary glands 24
Predictables, tumor behavior 41–42
Primary tumor, size of 14
Prognosis, ACC 30
Prostate, tumor site 5, 20
  aberrant 15
Prosthetic rehabilitation, oral cavity tumor 61
Pterygoid area, tumor extension 55
Pulmonary metastases 112
  incidence 22
  tumor of lip 69
Pulmonary resection 46
Punch biopsy 28

R

Radiography, plain film 31, 35
Radiotherapy, see also Irradiation
  lacrimal gland tumor 16
  postoperative, ear canal tumor 100
  tumor management 50–51
Recurrence, local, see Local recurrence
  parotid gland tumor 95
  sublingual gland tumor 110
  submandibular gland tumor 109–110
Recurrent adenoid cystic cancer, maxilla 58
Recurrent tumor 24
  base of skull 40
Regional metastases 112
  incidence 22
Rehabilitation 114–115
  facial paralysis 114
  masseter transfer 114
  myocutaneous flap 114
  nerve graft 114

temporalis transfer 114
Resection, pulmonary 46
Risk factors, ACC 113–115

S

Salivary glands, major, see Major salivary glands
  minor, see Minor salivary glands
Sex distribution, ACC 21, 28
Signs of ACC 27–28
Sinus cavity, tumor site 21
Site of tumor, see Tumor, site
Size of tumor 14
Skin graft, nasal cavity tumor 55
Skin, tumor site 5, 16–17
  aberrant 15
Skull, base of, see Base of skull
Soft palate, tumor extension 38
Solid nests 9
Solid pattern 9
Sphenoid, tumor extension 39
Split-skin graft, buccal area tumor 65
Staging 23
  guidelines 30–31
  parotid gland tumor 85
Statistics and data, ACC 21–26
Subglottic area, extensive cancer 72
Sublingual gland tumor, incidence 28
  recurrence 110
  site 21
  surgical treatment 97
  survival rate 24–25
Submandibular gland tumor, incidence 28
  metastatic lymph node 93
  recurrence 109–110
  site 21
  surgical treatment 90–96
  survival rate 24–25
Supraglottis, undifferentiated cancer 72
Surgical treatment 53–108
  alveolus tumor 67–69
  buccal area tumor 63–65
  ear canal tumor 98–108
  floor of mouth tumor 67–69
  inadequacy 22
  lines of resection 13
  lip tumor 67
  major salivary glands tumor 73–97
  minor salivary glands tumor 53–72
  nasal cavity and sinuses tumor 53–59
  oral cavity tumor 60–62
  paralaryngeal regions tumor 71
  parotid gland tumor 73–83
  pharynx tumor 70
  procedures for tumor management 49
  sublingual gland tumor 97
  submandibular gland tumor 90–96
  tongue tumor 66
  upper trachea tumor 71
Survival rate, minor salivary gland tumor 24–25
  and radiotherapy 25
  parotid gland tumor 25
  sublingual gland tumor 24–25
  submandibular gland tumor 24–25

Symptoms 27–28
  absence of intracranial 39
  pain 27
Systemic metastasis 112
  incidence 22

T

Temporal muscle, parotid gland tumor 86
Temboralis transfer, rehabilitation 114
Therapeutic planning 49–50
Tongue tumor, surgical treatment 66
Tracheobronchial tree, tumor site 17
  aberrant 15
Tubular pattern 9
Tubular type, tumor incidence 22
Tumor, basaloid type 22
  behavior 41–47
    chronicity 46
    predictables 41–42
  distribution, minor salivary glands 22
    nasal cavity 22
    oral cavity 22
    pharynx 22
  extension, base of skull 55, 94
    hard and soft palates 38
    infratemporal fossa 38
    orbit 55
    pterygoid area 55
    sphenoid 39
  histologic classification 113
  histology 23
  incidence, cribriform type 22
    minor salivary glands 28
    parotid gland 28
    submandibular gland 28
    tubular type 22
  location, see Tumor, site
  management 49–52
    chemotherapy 49, 51–52
    irradiation 49–51
    philosophy 49
    radiotherapy 49–51
    surgical procedures 49
    therapeutic planning 49–50
  margins of 13
  persistent, management of 109–112
  recurrent 24
    base of skull 40
    infratemporal space 94
  site 5, 14, 22, 28, 113
    aberrant 15–20
    alveolus, surgical treatment 67–69
    Bartholin's gland 20
    breast 5, 18–19
    buccal area, surgical treatment 63–65
    deep lobe of parotid gland 27
    ear canal 5, 98–108
    esophagus 17–18
    ethmoids 39, 59
    floor of mouth, surgical treatment 67–69
    lacrimal gland 5, 15–16
    lip 67
    lung 5
    major salivary glands 21, 73–97

Tumor, site, maxillary sinus 36
    minor salivary glands 21, 53–72
    nasal cavity 21, 36
    nasal sinuses, surgical treatment 53–59
    nasopharynx 37
    oral cavity 21, 60–62
    palate 60
    paralaryngeal regions, surgical treatment 71
    parotid gland 21, 40, 73–83
    pharyngotracheal area 21
    pharynx, surgical treatment 70
    prostate 5, 20
    sinus cavity 21
    skin 5, 16–17
    sublingual gland 21, 97
    submandibular gland 21, 90–96
    tongue, surgical treatment 66
    tracheobronchial tree 17
    upper trachea, surgical treatment 71
    uterine cervix 5, 19–20
size of primary 14
staging of 23
ulcerated 27
    bleeding 27

U

Ulcerated tumor 27
    bleeding 27
Ultrastructural examination 9
Undifferentiated cancer, supraglottis 72
Unusual cases, of ACC 42–46
Upper trachea tumor, surgical treatment 71
Uterine cervix, tumor site 5, 19–20
    aberrant 15